CEMENTED BEAUTY

A Cancer Story

JACOB JONAS

SpineSun

JACOBJONAS
THECOMPANY

atelier
éditions

BEGINNING

Similar Sufferings

Once you set on the road as an artist, you step into a way of seeing things, a way of doing things. You operate so much of the time on instinct. Almost like a nervous animal, you watch the horizon for some dangers and for opportunity and kindred spirits.

I met Jacob and immediately knew. We met outside a concert in Philadelphia. I knew I was meeting someone with kindness and grace. He told me that he was in the world of dance, and I was drawn to him. Drawn to his spirit, drawn to his energy. I could feel the questions in him as well as see the confidence – and it's a dynamite combination.

For some reason I felt compelled to point him in the direction of my friend Ezra Caldwell. Someone I had befriended, grown to love, and who I can proudly call one of the best friends that I've ever had. I met Ezra in New York, and similarly we bonded. We saw something in each other. There was an immediate connection. And then there was a feverish trading of ideas and thoughts and love. Love of all things forward moving. An energy between us that I can only be grateful for every day.

So, when I told Jacob about Ezra and I told Ezra about Jacob, I thought maybe I'd sent two good spirits into alignment. And it seems that's exactly what did happen.

Jacob has sent me his work through the years and I've always really enjoyed it. Some of the work was actually set to my music, which allowed me to see my own work in a whole new illuminating life. I'm grateful to him.

This life is about walking with kindred spirits. It's about pushing and prodding each other to be better. It's about lifting each other's spirits and souls. And that is really our only job as artists – to somehow elevate the world. To somehow invent the world, or invent a new one. Artists invent cultures, and soldiers defend cultures. And so the whole big dance has a way of meeting in circles.

I read Jacob's book and I was deeply moved by it. Deeply moved by the humanity of it and his willingness to share the journey – every step through the beauty and oftentimes ugliness. Art isn't hygienic. Art is a great big mess. And anyone who makes art realizes just how messy it can get and how chaotic. It's like open heart surgery using screwdrivers and wrenches.

I love the humanity of this book, and I believe that if read in the right light it can be hugely helpful to anyone who is going through similar sufferings.

"We are the music makers and we are the dreamers of dreams" is said by Willy Wonka. Well, we are. I feel blessed every day to live this life. And when I look at people like Jacob, I'm reminded that, yes, I'm on the right path.

If everyone only knew what a

gift it is to be alive.

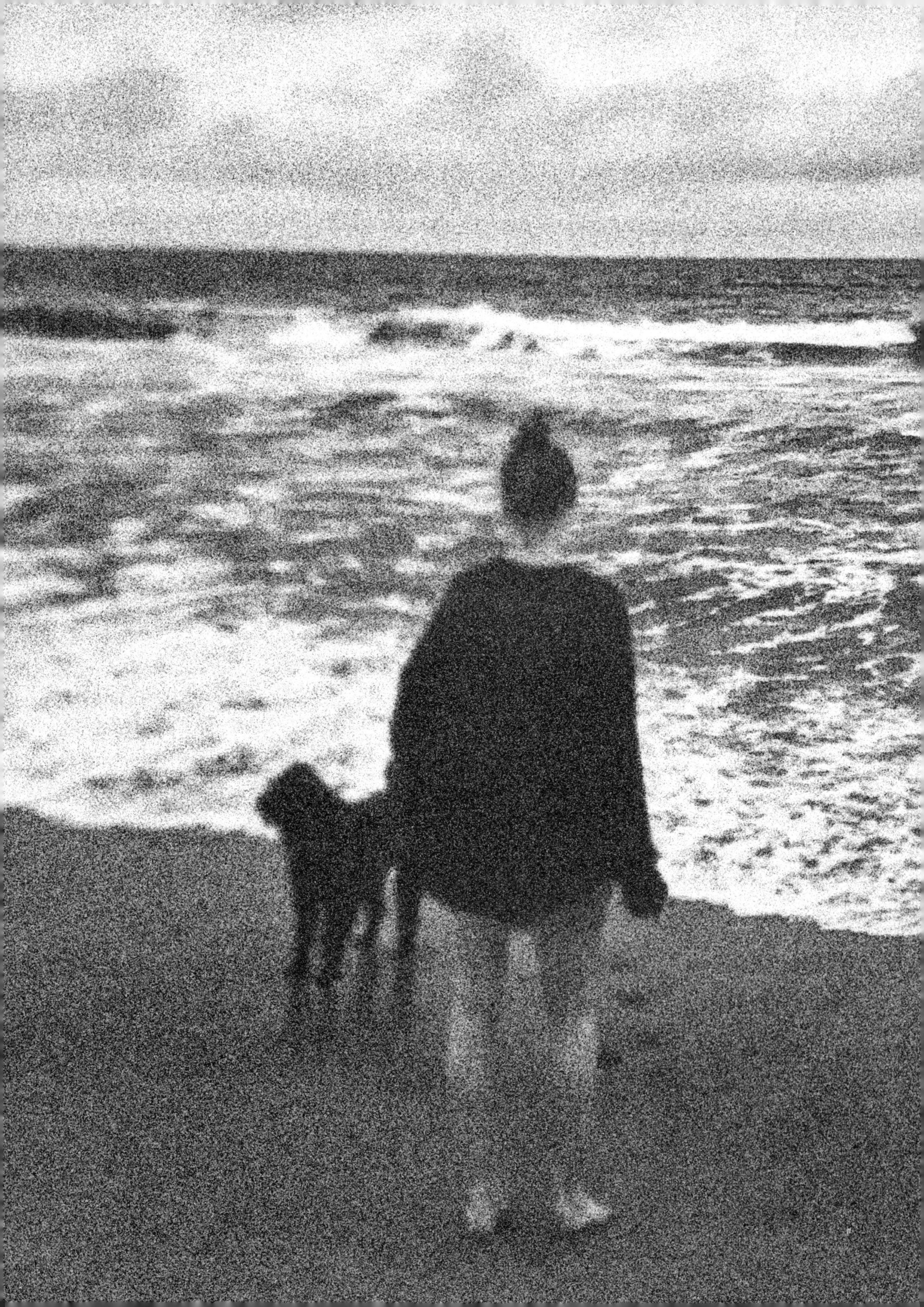

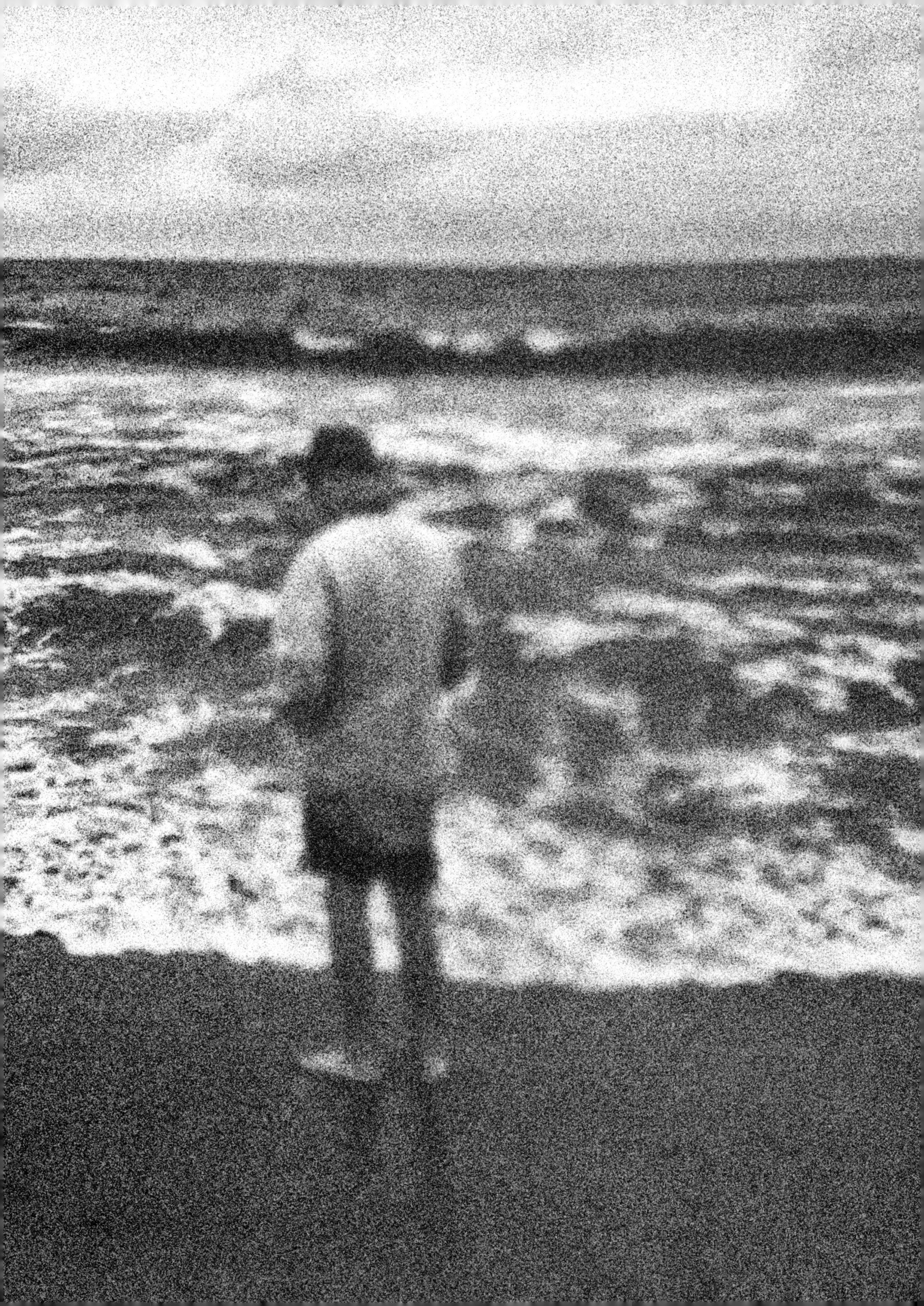

On November 17, 2022, I was diagnosed with stage 4 diffuse large B-cell non-Hodgkin's lymphoma. The cancer developed as a side effect of my Crohn's medication, Remicade, that I was taking intravenously every six weeks for ten years. There was a nine in 10,000 chance that I would get cancer from this medication. I documented my process during this journey.

This book was inspired by two people – Ezra Caldwell and Mallory Smith. When I was a kid, one of my biggest inspirations was Glen Hansard. A self-taught musician from Ireland who made it from being a busker, or a street performer. After falling in love with Markéta Irglová, they formed a group called The Swell Season, sharing emotional ballads about their life and relationship. Soon after, the film *Once* was made about their story, putting them on the map and winning an Oscar for best song. Glen's music always played a special role in my life. His music became the soundtrack to my relationship with Jill, having made multiple duets when I was first starting to choreograph. We had made a duet to his song "Song of Good Hope" and created a short film. When Jill was in college, we went to his concert in Philadelphia. After the show, we waited two hours by the parking lot for him. Finally, his violinist came out for a smoke, and we asked him if we could meet Glen. He took us backstage, and when we met Glen we showed him our film. He was so moved, and this brought so much value and excitement to us. He expressed what fate it was that from all his music we had chosen this song. It was written for his dear friend Ezra Caldwell, who was a dancer and had been recently diagnosed with colon cancer for a second time. Glen expressed the importance for me and Ezra to meet.

The next day, I spontaneously took a bus to New York City and then a train to Harlem to Ezra's home. He asked to go play handball at the park down the street. After a few games, he warmed up to me and shared his story, his love of dance and making cooking videos. When I first heard he made cooking videos, I internally had a judgment and pictured a terrible cooking show. But after I left, he sent me some of the videos. It was the most honest work I've seen. The videos were fast-forwarded films of him cooking. As he left the food to cook, he would spend time in the bath or relaxing with his dog. It was time fast forwarded – it was his healing and story of battling cancer. It left the biggest mark on me and encouraged me to become a filmmaker and tell stories. He also sent me his self-portrait series – a photograph each day of his battle. I was twenty at the time and could never imagine being in the same situation – until I was. My instinct was to document my process the way he did and in his honor. Ezra passed in 2014, a couple of years after our meeting, after six years with cancer.

The second person who inspired me was Mallory Smith. In fourth grade, I switched schools and was a week late from the start of class due to some problems at home. At nine years old, I walked into Ms Lightner's class to a group of strangers. One of them was Mallory Smith. She was tall, beautiful, blonde, athletic, and the most intelligent in the room. It was known that she had some health problems, but no one really understood the complexity of what they were. Mallory was diagnosed with cystic fibrosis at the age of three. Throughout our friendship from elementary to high school, I always admired her and her strength, even though I didn't know the depths of her illness.

Fast forward to when I was 21. I had a serious flare with my Crohn's disease and was hospitalized for six days. Two days into my treatment, Mallory was admitted on the same floor – the fourth floor in the North Tower at UCLA Santa Monica Hospital – and where ten years later I would end up for my cancer battle. It was meant to be. We hadn't talked for a few years since high school. I was overwhelmed with my health, but then I got to learn about the severity of hers. That she'd been dealing with it her whole life. We became so close during this visit. When I was finally discharged, she stayed for weeks after. I would keep coming back to visit her. We would go on walks in the garden, I would take photos of her, she would expose her deepest vulnerabilities and pains in battling her disease. I was shocked that someone could have it so hard. In her struggle there was true heroism and grace. I remember people in society around me talking about their stress and busyness. How clueless one would have to be to express stress from work without gratitude or acknowledgment of their health and well-being – especially in comparison to Mallory's life. Throughout her battle, she journaled. For her own therapy, but also to share her story. When she passed, her mother, Diane, published her story in a memoir, *Salt in My Soul.*

Between Ezra and Mallory, I was inspired to share my story through self-portraits and a journal. My hope is that someone comes across this story the way I did with Ezra's and Mallory's so that we continue to learn from each other's stories. The circle of life. The giving empathy. The mycelium network. There are no coincidences – we are all connected.

Mallory's mom, Diane, shared this with me when I was diagnosed:

J and J, I meet a lot of people going through traumatic circumstances in the work I'm doing now as an advocate. My belief is that for some reason bad things happen to people who have unusual talents and gifts. We know that with Mallory and we know that with you, but I also see it with so many others. You're in for a fight but when you reach the other side, we will celebrate and it will make your heart and art much deeper than you could have imagined. xo

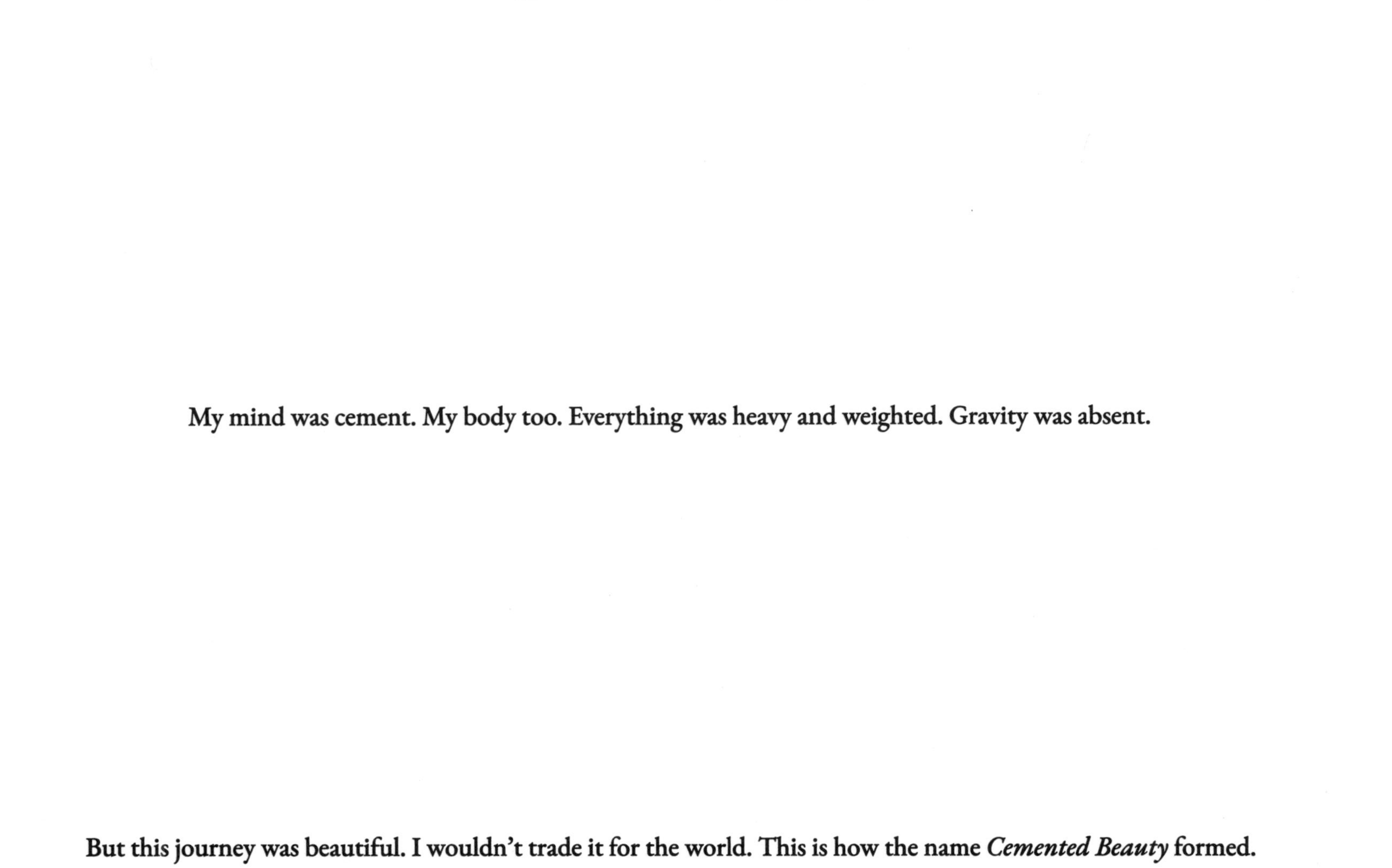

Each time I tried to share what chemotherapy felt like, mentally and physically, all I could think about was concrete.

My mind was cement. My body too. Everything was heavy and weighted. Gravity was absent.

But this journey was beautiful. I wouldn't trade it for the world. This is how the name *Cemented Beauty* formed.

JOURNAL

November 18, 2022

First portrait of knowing.

Yesterday the doctor told me I have cancer. I am destroyed. Broken. Unbalanced. I feel gone. Done. There is support. Pain in sharing, in receiving. I am really broken. I need to take over the world but also come full stop and do absolutely nothing. I see older people and feel mad. I think about death. I no longer care about my impact. I'm at the bottom of the redwood tree, in the forest of many of them. I'm shaking, crying. What's in me? I have cancer. Right before the show. Trying to unplug to watch. See my work through humanity. Through the people healthy in front of me. Diagnosis. It's here. What's the next step? Need to document this whole process. Need to get it out. I want kids. I want a family. I fear I won't have one. Do I have time left? Stomach pain. Knives to the chest. Throwing up. I love you. All of you. Anna Halprin danced through it. Pain pushed down. If I get through, I'll be a survivor. My first reflection. Thanks for listening.

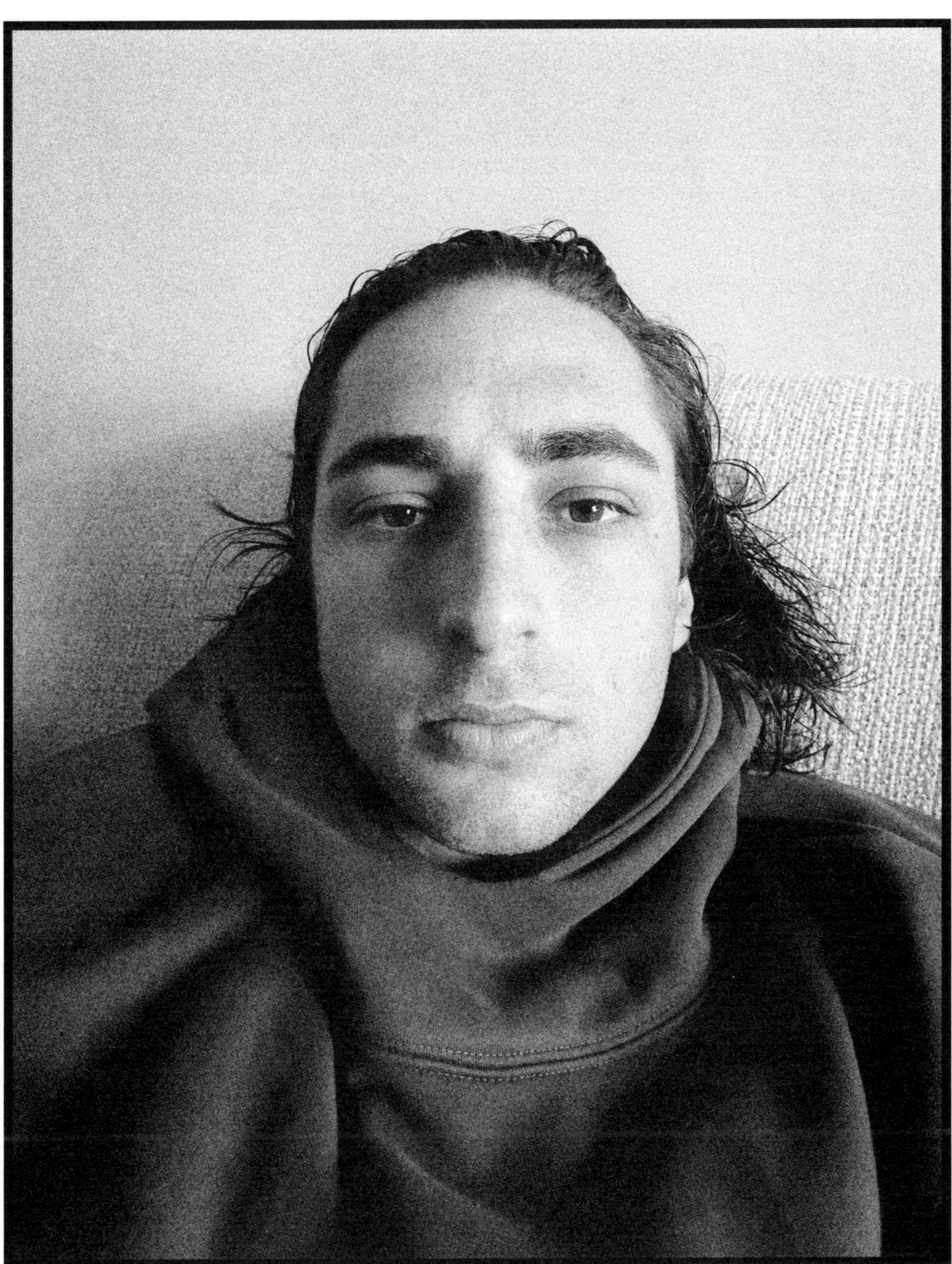

November 20, 2022

Feeling blurry.

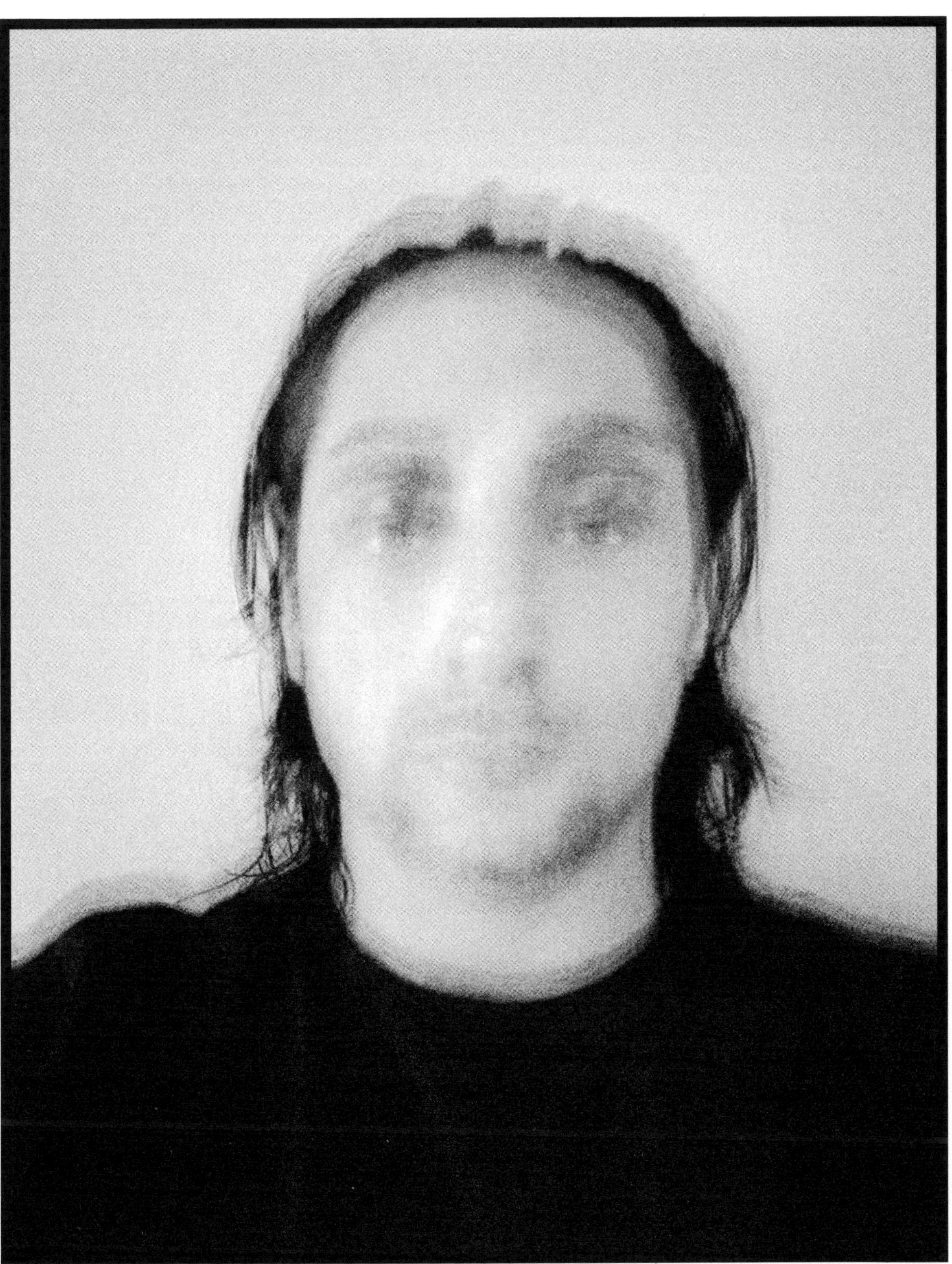

November 21, 2022

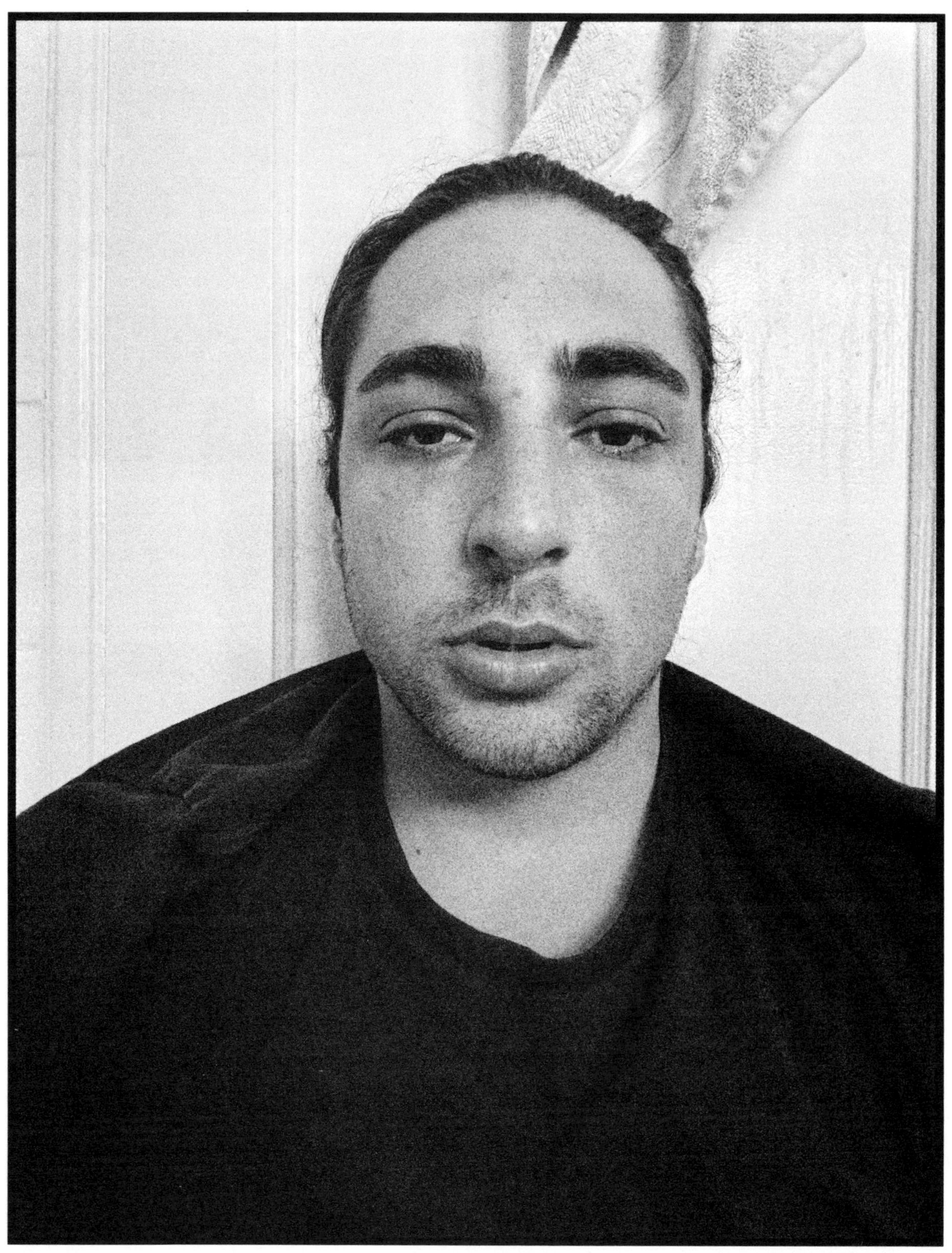

Bathroom floor. Post symptoms. Mind cry.

November 22, 2022

An opportunity for gratitude.

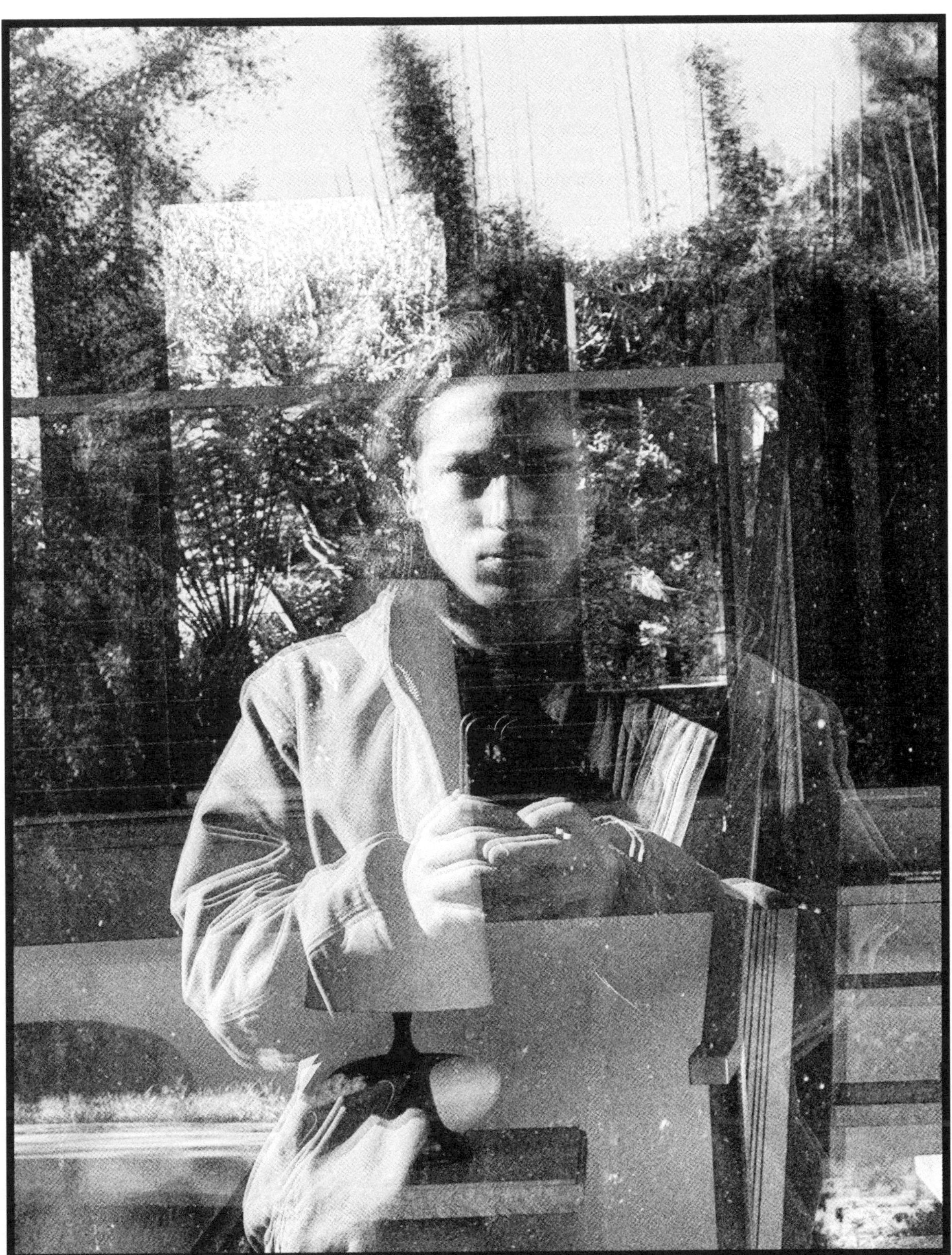

November 23, 2022

Fertility.
Blood work.
PET scan.
CT scan.

First exposure to why they call it a battle.

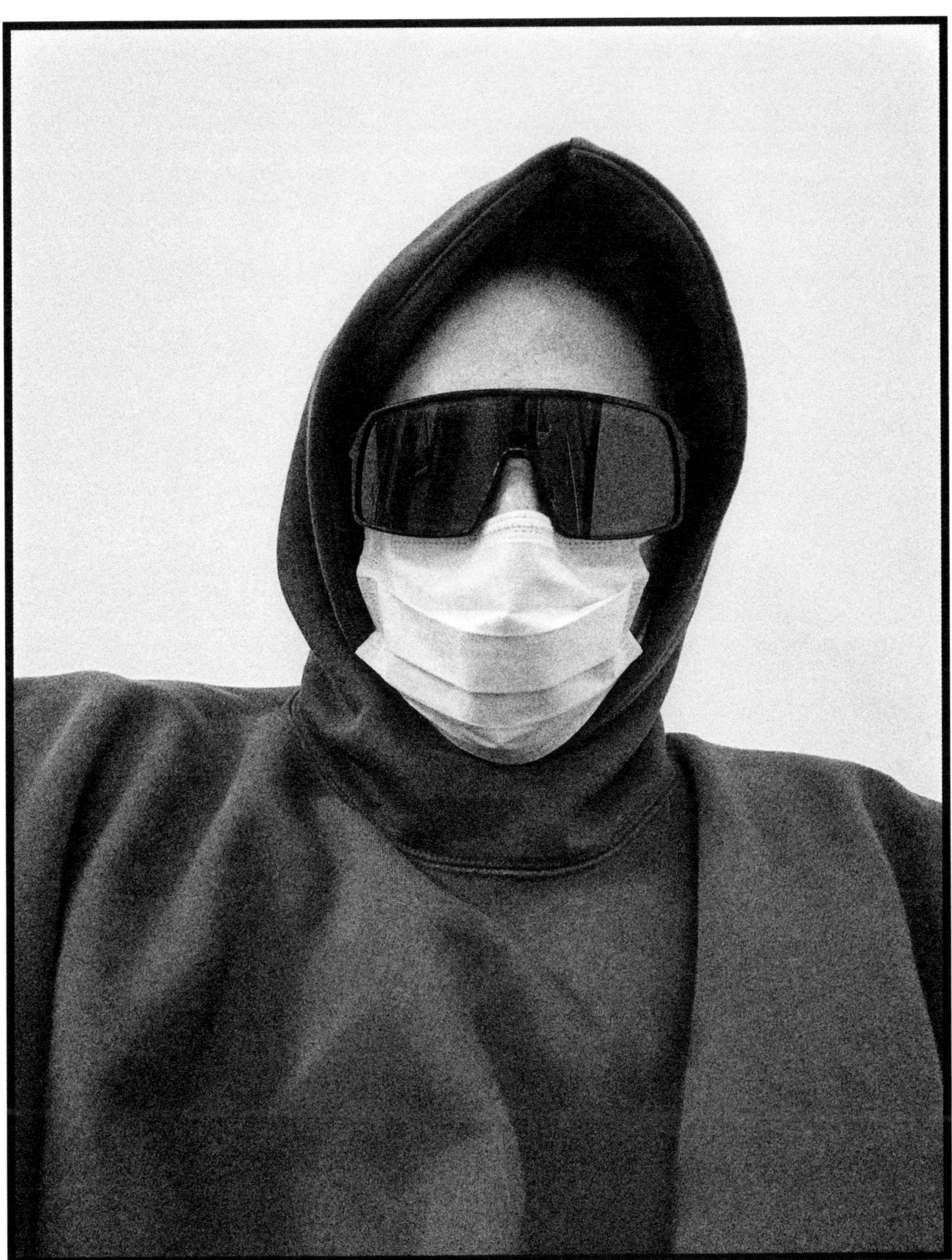

Overwhelmed in thought. Continued bad news – take over of the mind, body, and spirit. An attempt to look at this as an opportunity. Says Maria. I agree. What exactly, not sure yet. I told Alex it's going to be hard. He said, "Hard turns to easy my boy." I still am under the belief everything happens for a reason. I've never thought about suicide before, would never even consider it. Until last night's call with my doctor. The thought has far past but it temporarily existed. Continued thoughts on mortality ... What happens if this does take me out? What impact did I make? What will happen with all my work? Will they continue to work on it? Does everyone's life move on without me? I don't care about the accomplishments anymore. All valid thoughts, but temporary. The doc called to share that the cancer has spread. It's all over. Both hips, three places in my stomach, my liver, and in a bone in my skull. My head has been in so much pain the last month but I had no idea why. There has been pain in my body and now know it's cancer. Still coming to terms I have it. It's stage 4. I'll have to endure a lot going forward. Hair loss, a port, chemo, weakness. Long hospital stays. Everything manageable but difficult to comprehend. After hearing the news I wanted to call Diane. How to deal with bad news? How to navigate this information. She said first by processing shock. Then she got emotional, which made me emotional. Then she connected me to a close friend of hers who survived twice. She brought me great comfort, most of which was saying that the worst part of the process is learning about it. Everything that is happening in my mind is happening visually. Everything is so cinematic. I see the shot overhead, in the bath while my head is submerged and I'm yelling. I see the camera from behind as I walk down the street after hearing the news and crying until my knees hit the floor. Bundled up on the concrete, opening my eyes as my face is against the road, seeing a car out of focus coming toward me. When I am in the PET scanner, left with thoughts. I kept imagining being in the ocean swimming to the pier with Danny. Knowing the only way to finish or get to the shore is by doing it. A terrible day overall. But a forward-thinking mindset.

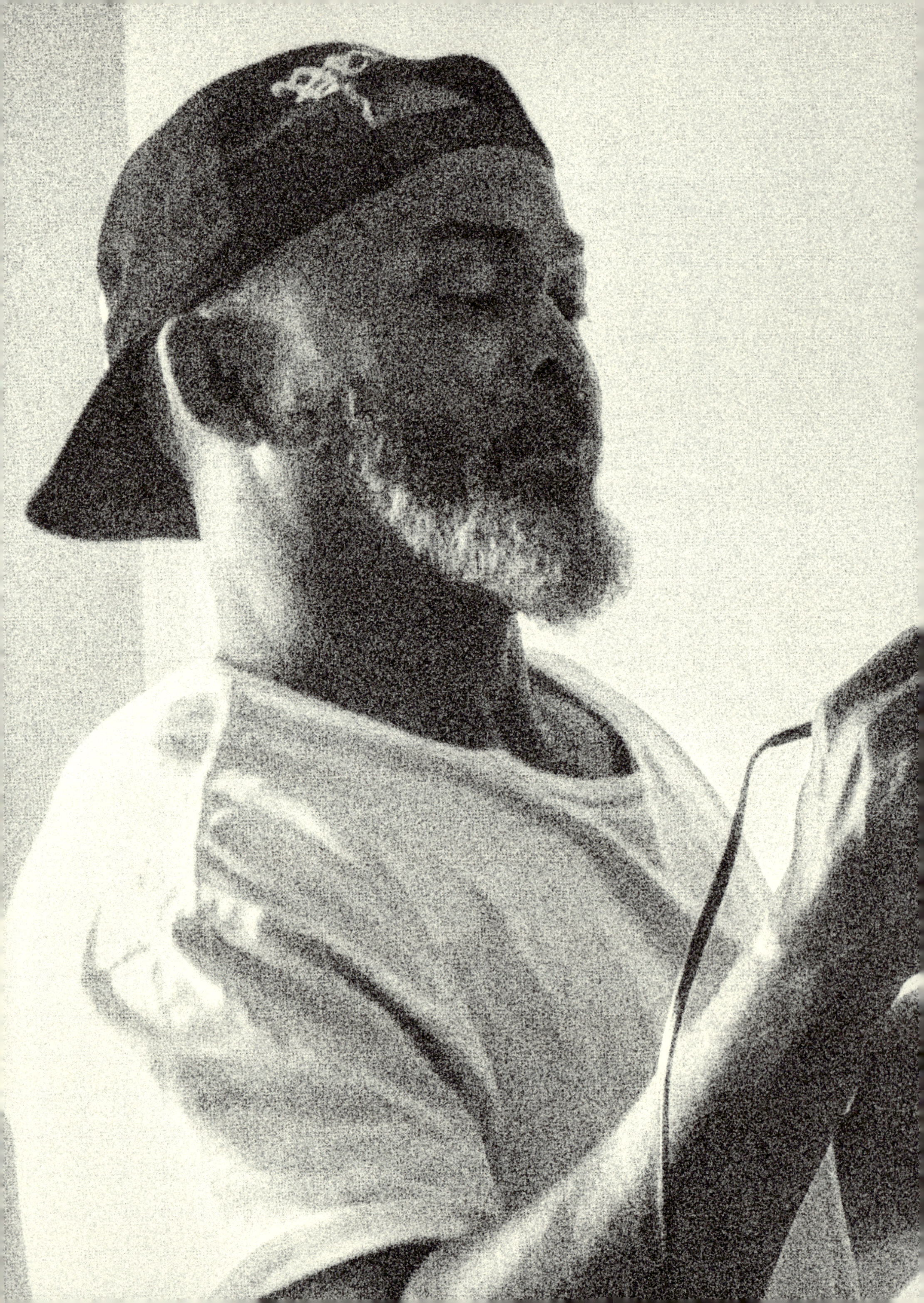

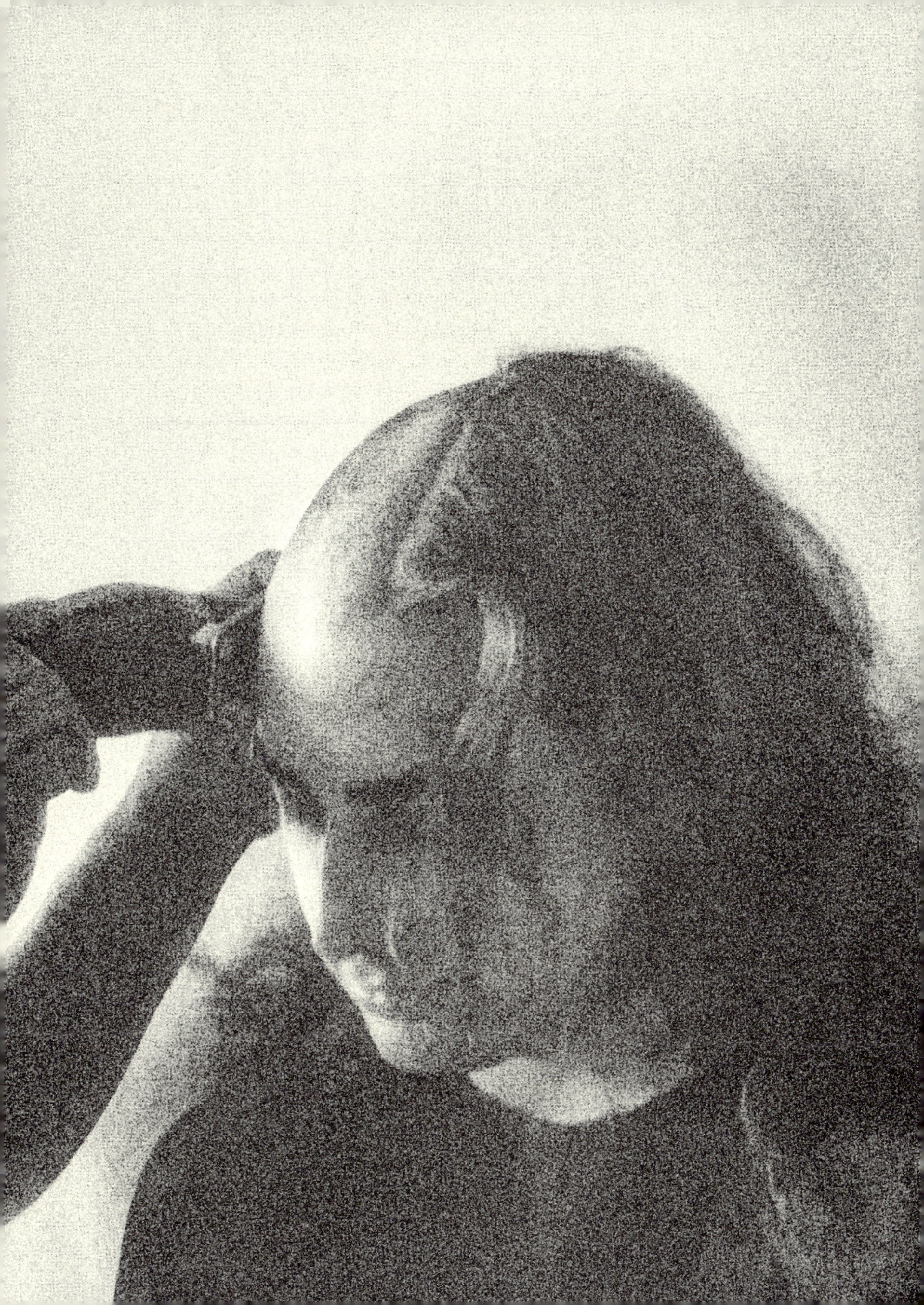

November 24, 2022

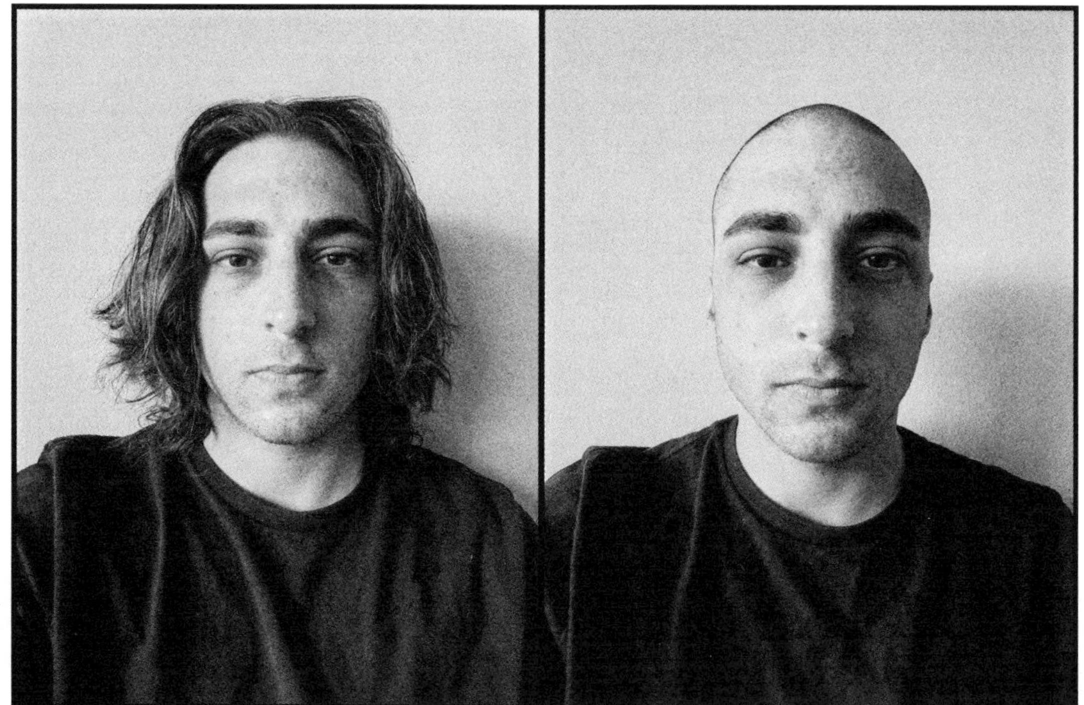

Head shaved, baldness.
A beautiful morning and a last rinse of freedom.

November 25, 2022

Moments before going in for the first round of chemo.

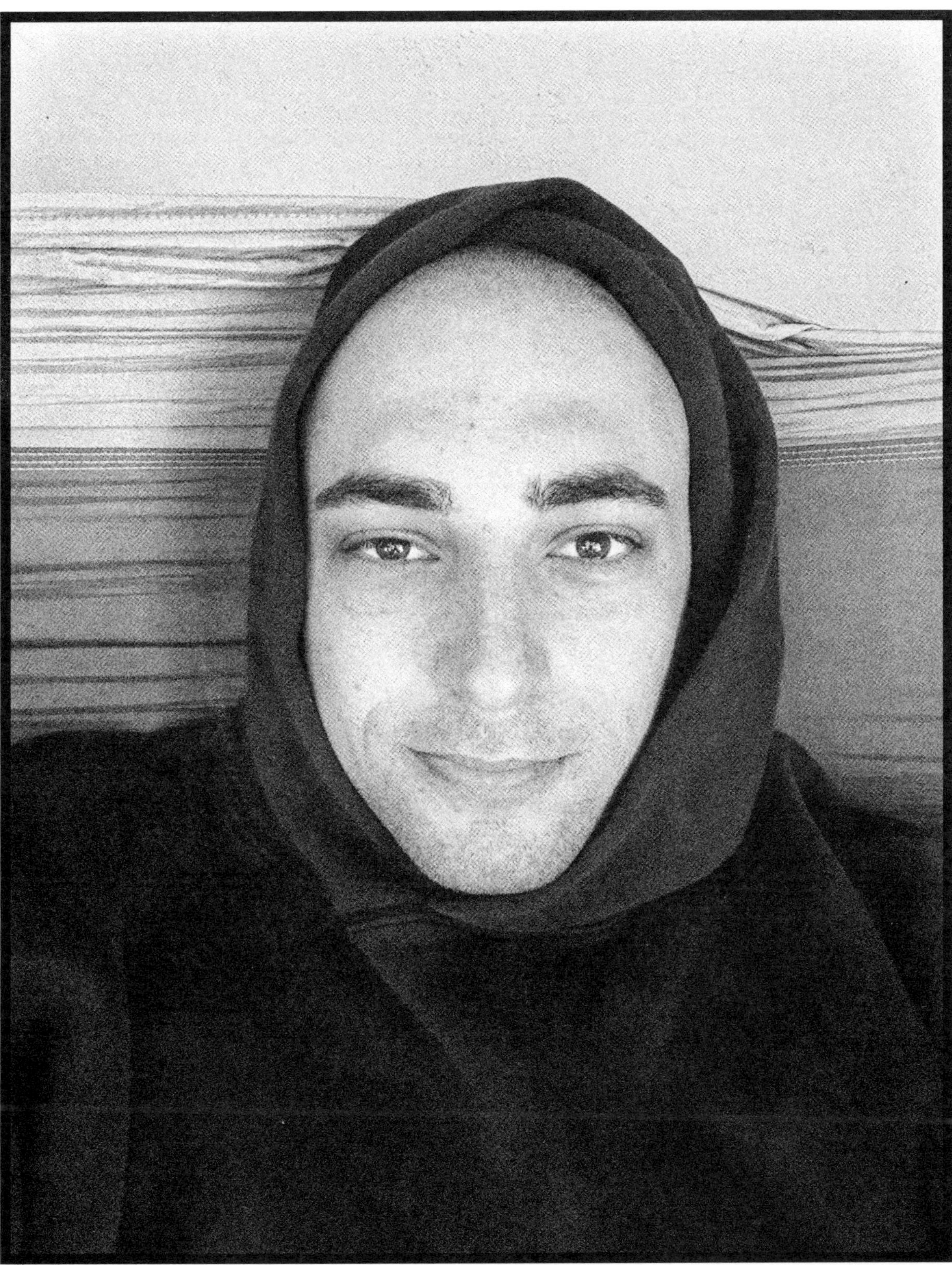

November 26, 2022

Hospital day 2.

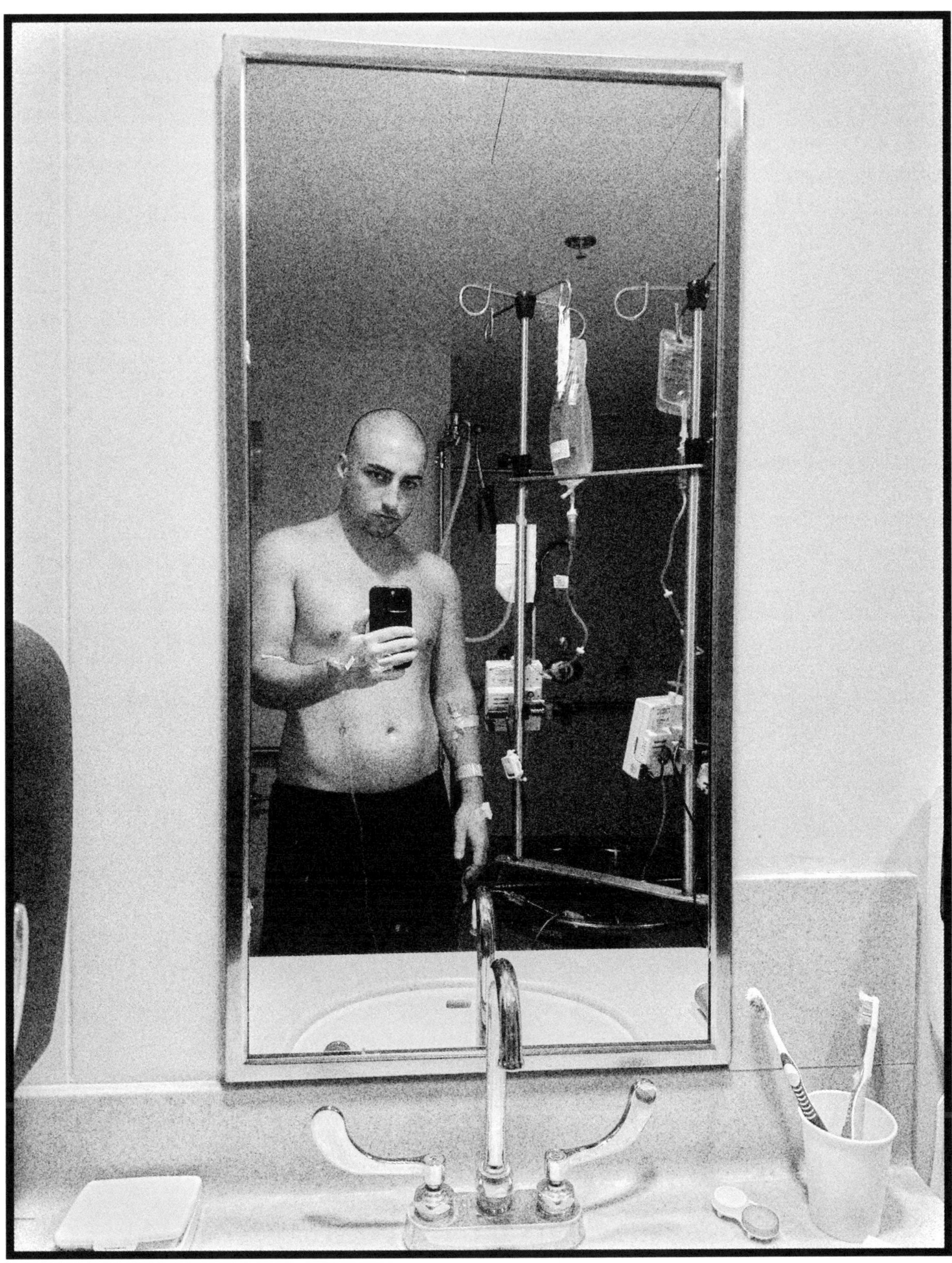

November 27, 2022

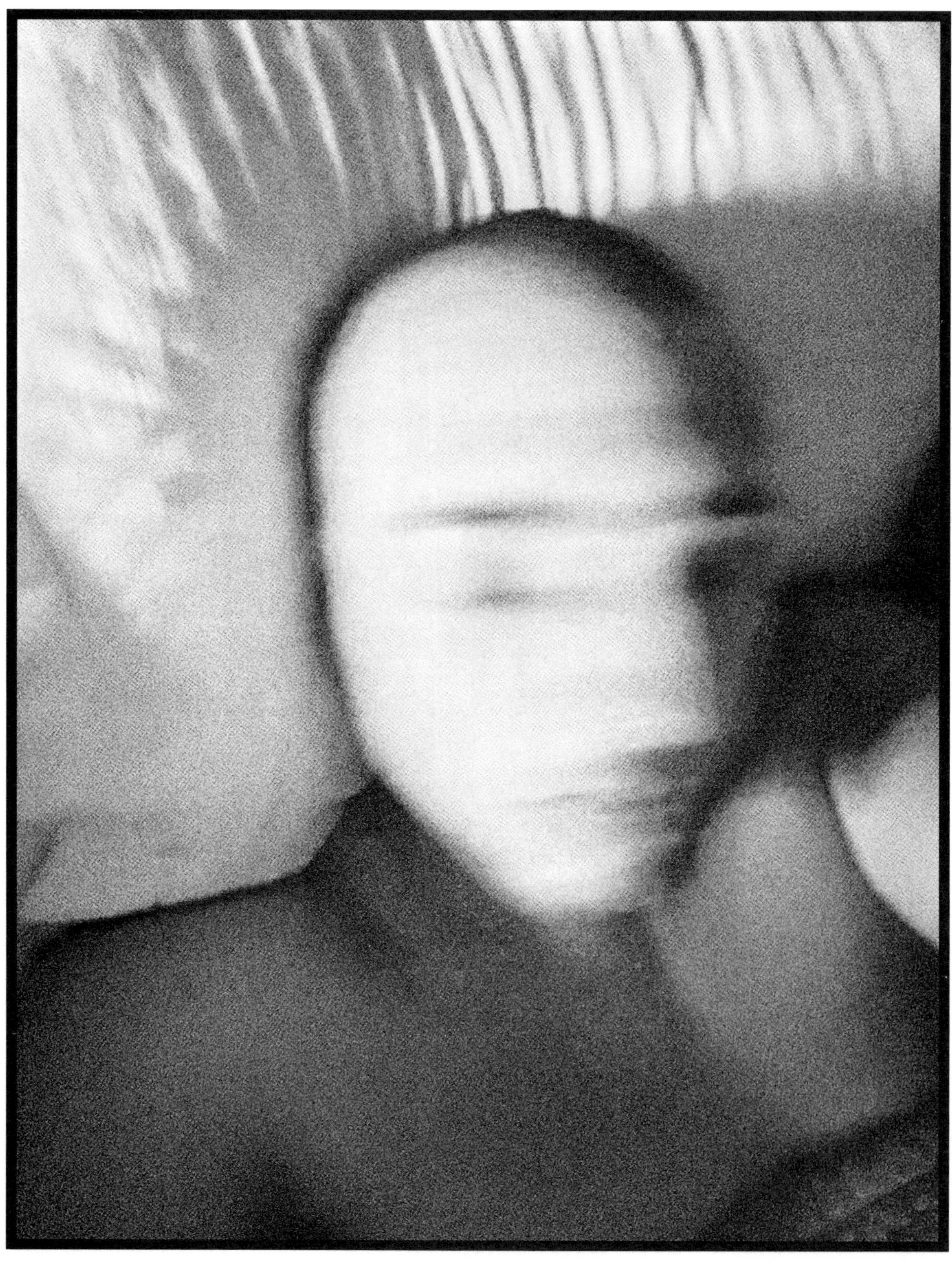

Hospital day 3.

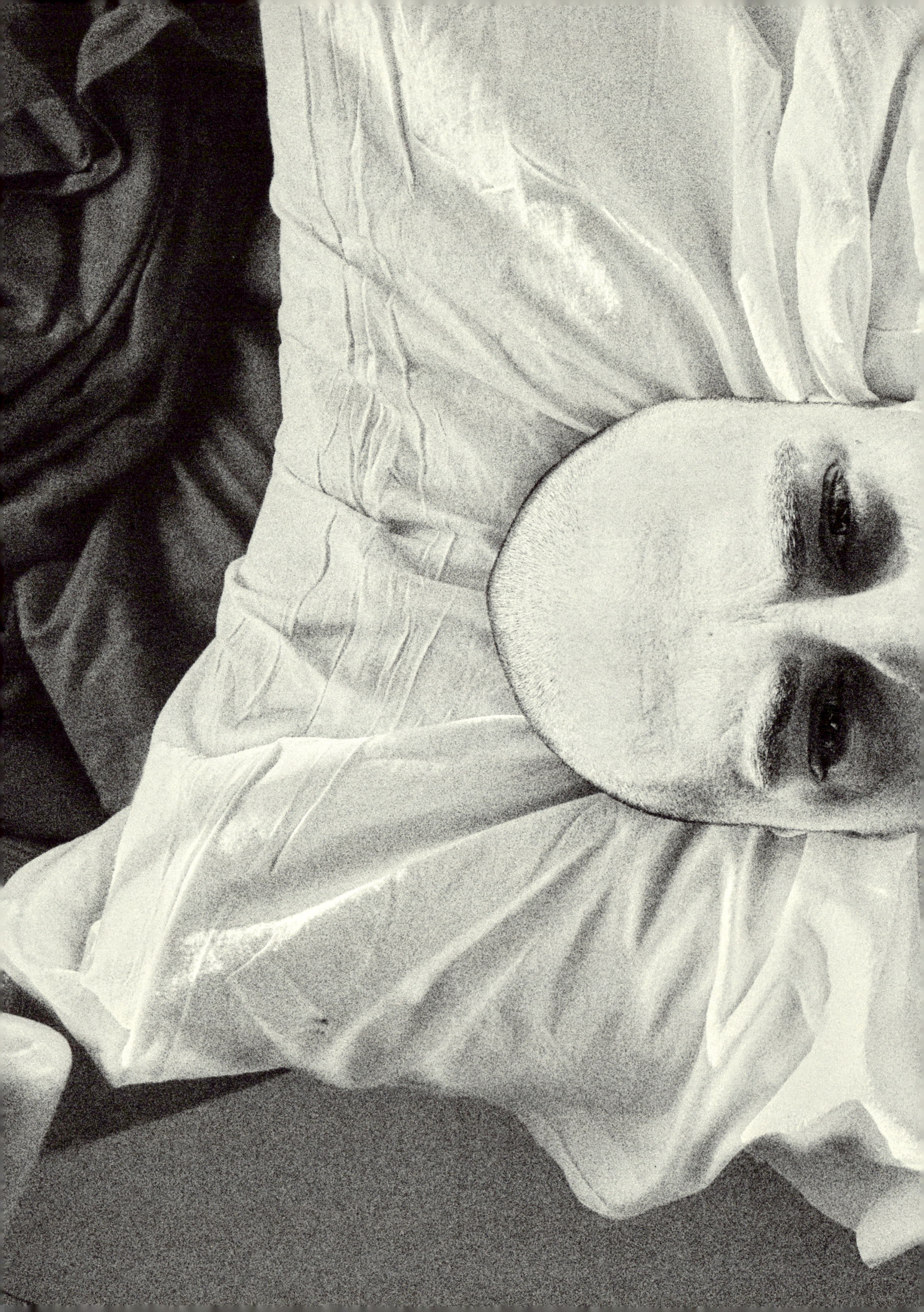

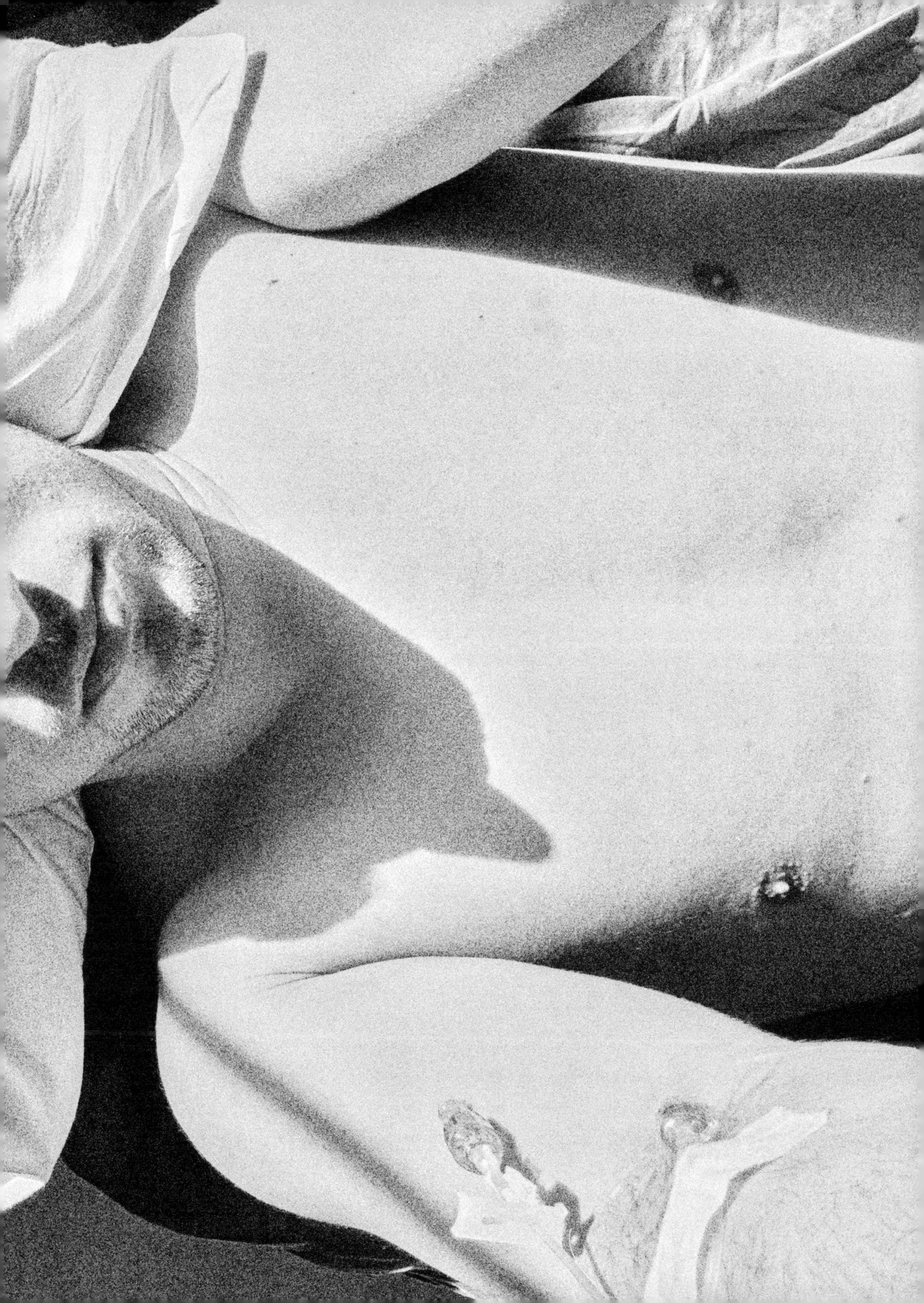

November 28, 2022

Hospital day 4.

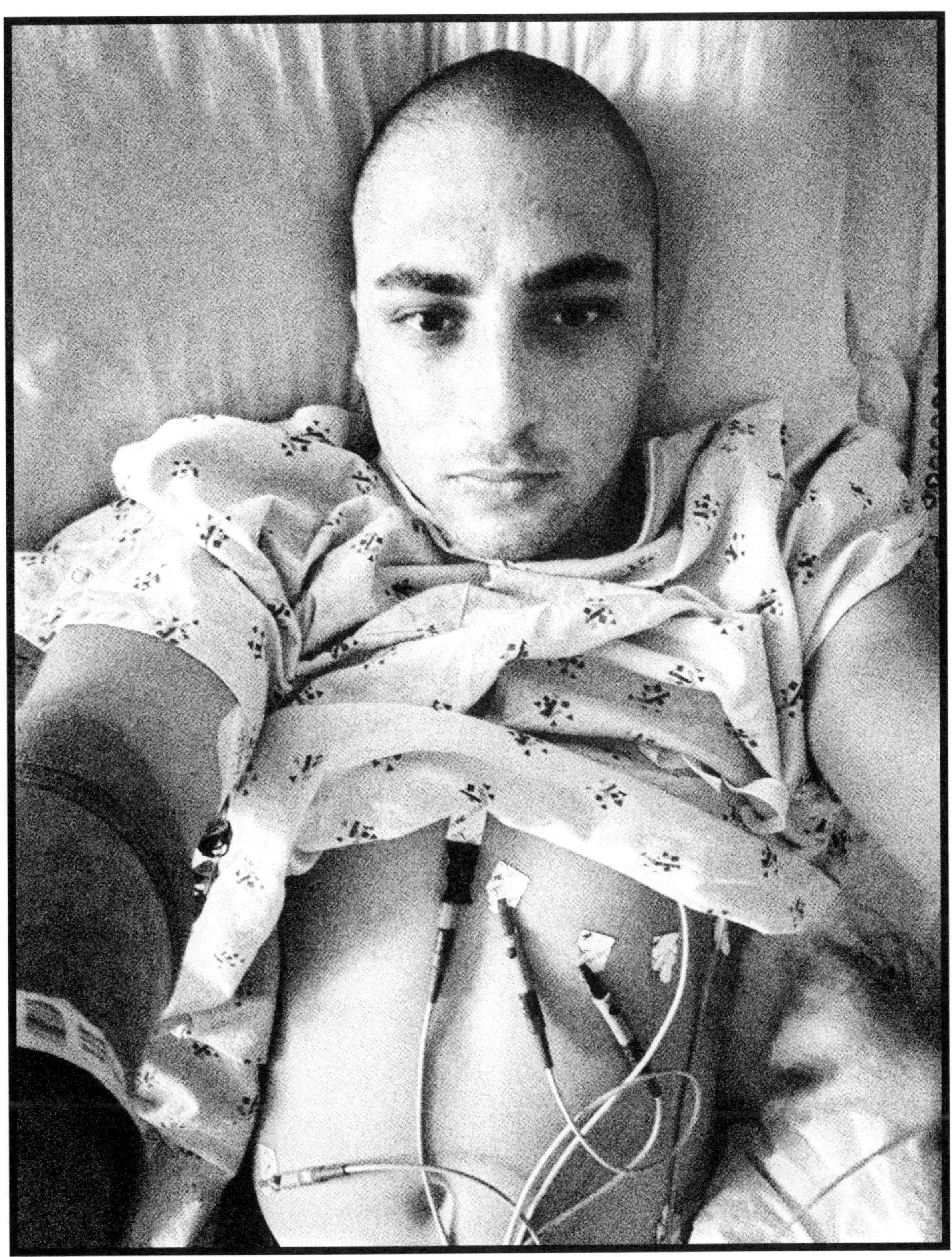

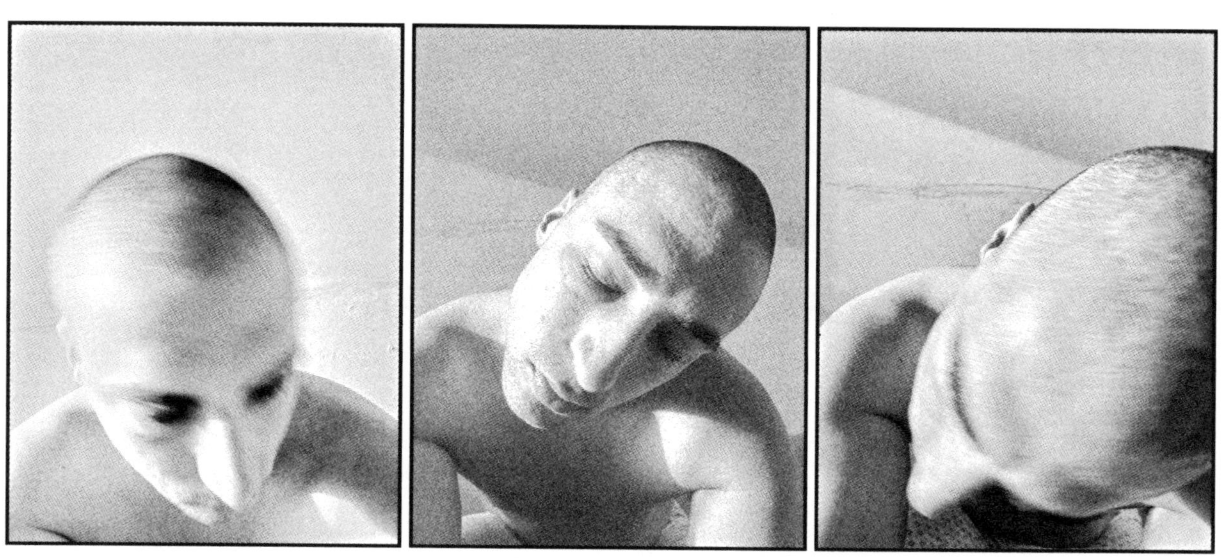

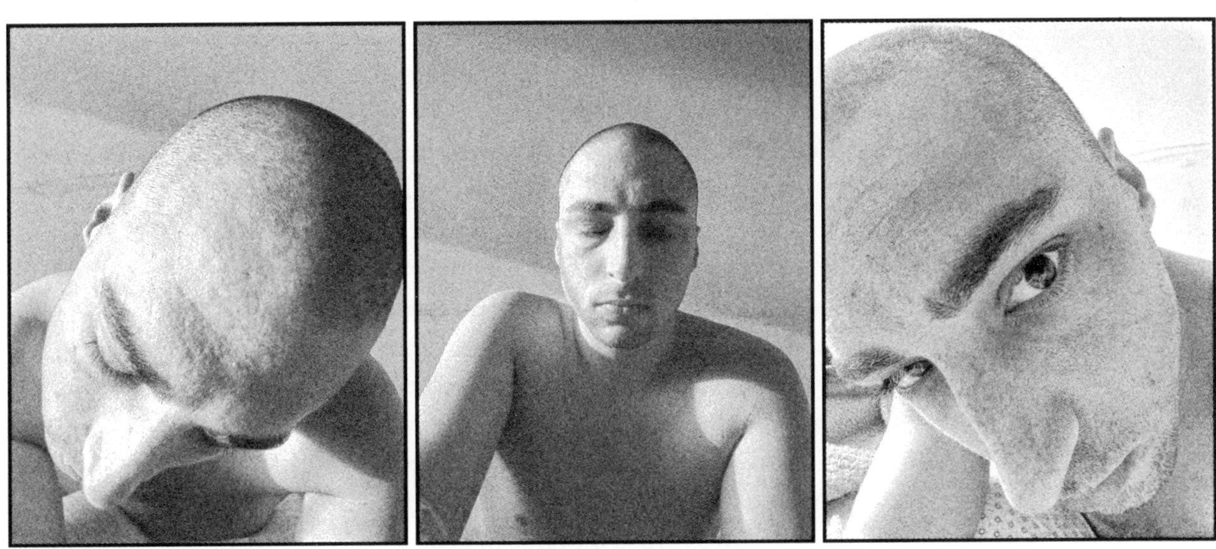

November 29, 2022

Free of thought. Undecided how to feel. Emotions constantly transforming. A predisposed trust but a new learned betrayal. It seems like there is a certainty of how I've gotten here. Side effects from my Crohn's medication. Nine in 10,000. We never want to be robbed or have an accident happen to us, but when really believing in fate, these events can be great shifts in our lives. I'm still trying to comprehend the diagnosis. It still feels so early on for what this all means. But I do feel a sense of gratitude to have this opportunity. In a way, you think about being confined to a bed or trapped in a room as an inhibition of freedom, but in a lot of ways this full stop has liberated my mind. It gave me great peace, like an accident would. I reference a burglary, because with all these cords and IVs going through me I feel there's such a trespassing happening to my body. I know these medicines are good, but the feeling of needing them and being attached to them feels so intrusive. The constant needles poking into my arms of different sizes, the deep inhales, the chin lifts, the hand to the forehead for comfort. Sometimes they get it on the first try. Sometimes a practice of patience. I'm starting to realize this is happening physically to me, but since the diagnosis and especially now I'm really understanding that it's happening to so many people, and in a lot of ways, regardless of how I try not to, I feel responsible.

I communicate with those people to try to offer them a sense of knowing that I'm OK even through the difficulties of this experience. But I see their pain and worry grow. This empathy is so mutual, but whereas most are providing it to me, I feel as though I need to be providing it to them. Too often in my life I'm the rock. I'm the leader. I'm the powerful one. Weakness unexposed. In this circumstance I feel as if my weakness is under a magnifying glass. Like a caged animal at a zoo. Everyone watches from afar and stares at me, in awe of my beauty and rarity. But cry inside because they know where I should be. Free. In a wilderness somewhere else. I'm curious how this will all turn out tomorrow or the next week, month, or year and how this time will change me and change those around me. When this started I could have chosen to meet it with anger or with an opportunity. And I really do feel grateful for what is happening. I feel these drugs entering my system. There's a deep war going on inside. But on the outside I'm comforted by my love. She's with me every step. And it's happening to her as well. And we are going through it together. This morning was special. A cuddle in the bed and time to reflect. Thanks for writing this, my love. I love you.

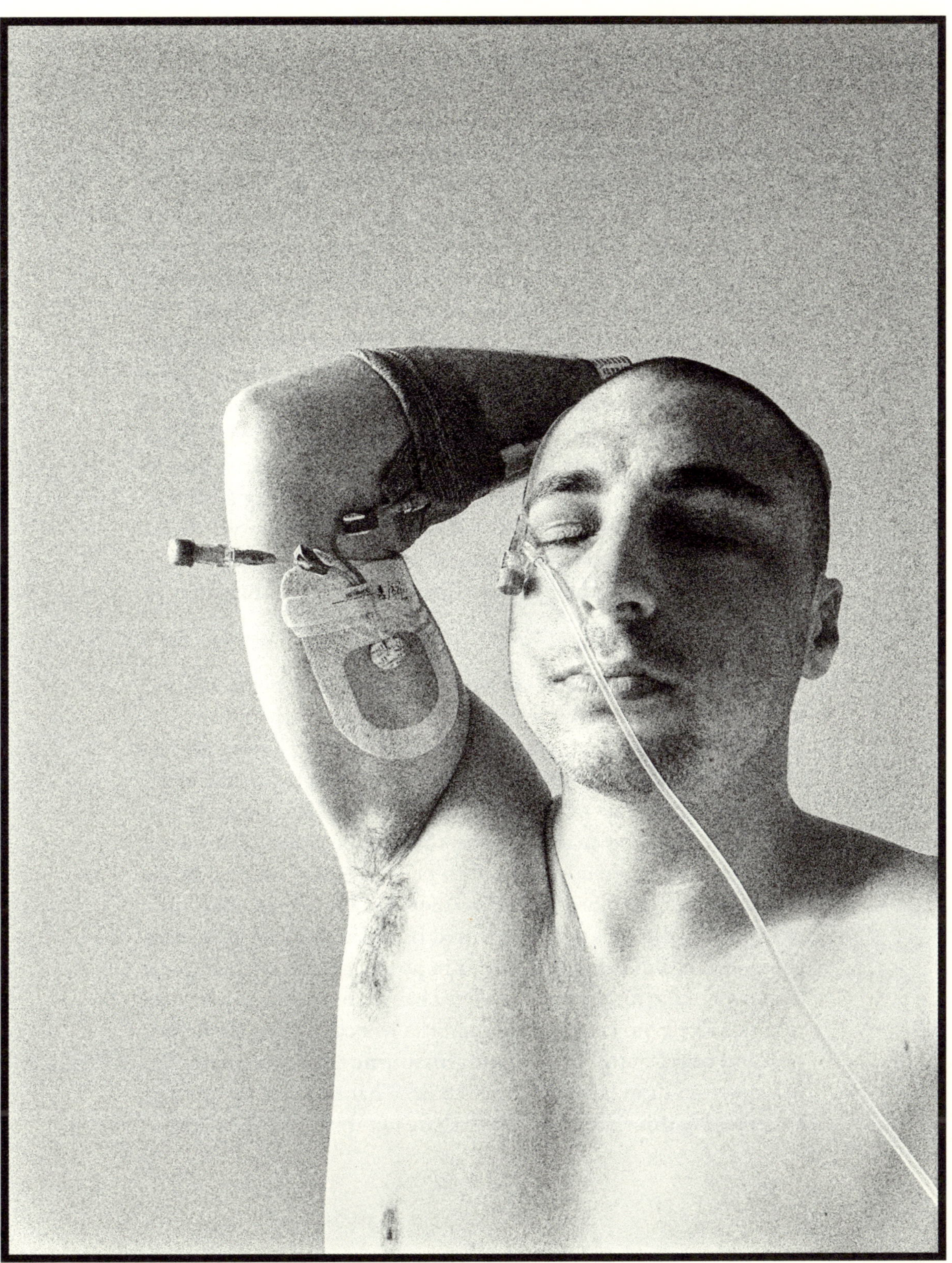

November 30, 2022

An effort of interrogation to find peace of mind. In this process I need to find myself as the dancer again, not as the director. I need instruction and perspective to facilitate someone else's vision here. I'm not the one in charge. The highs and lows are starting to become more extreme. I'm feeling pretty low right now. But I enjoy it. I've never been one to think about challenge or anger or pain as an emotional pursuit in the bigger picture. It's been more expressed through my physical health. Last night was very rough. I woke up and got to spend time talking to Donald Byrd. He's a real gift and a real friend. He offered me so much peace this morning. I'm continuously confronted by the depths of humanity in these circumstances. The things we take for granted most outside of these hospital rooms and diagnoses are viewed under the biggest microscope lenses in here. The care and sensibilities your friends and family share and their deep sensitivities and reflections offer so much meaning. It's been so gratifying as well to connect with these nurses and staff who sometimes outwardly express their motivation to be economic as a means of fitting in with society, but in truth their care and passion for what they do is so rich and meaningful.

This chemotherapy is bringing me down. I feel weak physically and emotionally, but I still find gratitude with every drip that goes through my IV. Since my diagnosis I've been craving having my feet buried in the sand at the beach. My body connected to the earth. The cold temperature of the water against my ankles. I've more and more been noticing seagulls flying toward the ocean. They are a reminder for the direction I need to be going. My love and Maria have expressed the word "dense" to me – I really love it. The fabric of my being also feels very punctured from the amount of needles going into it. I'm being threaded. I'm just a hamster with all these doctors looking for my results. They change the numbers and sizes to make sure I can keep spinning on the wheel. Within my depression and pain I'm still in love with this journey. It's time to put the pen down so I can have another cuddle. Thanks again for writing. I'm enjoying this time with you to share my thoughts in no rush.

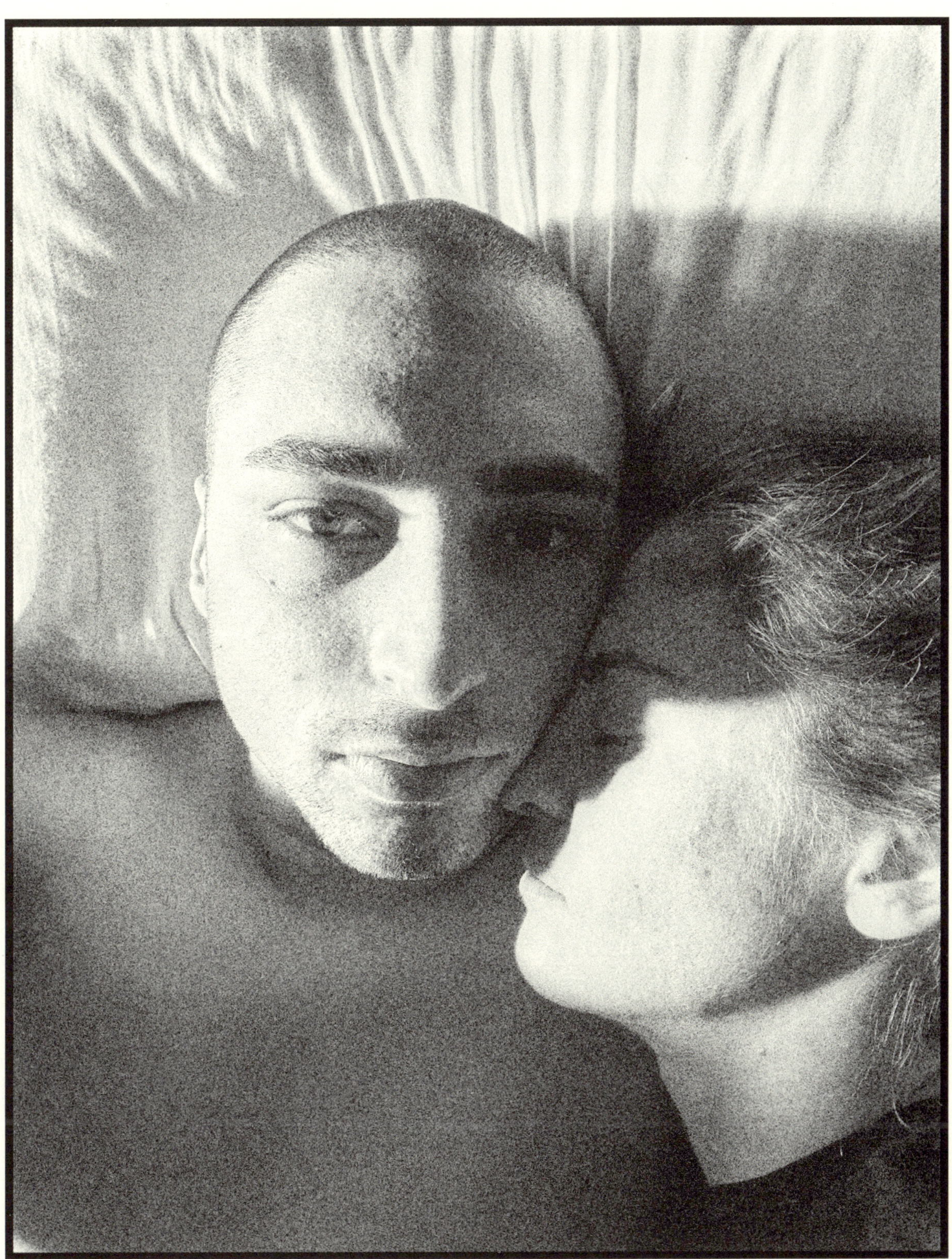

December 1, 2022

An examination of youth.

I woke up in the middle of the night in a panic.

I was 30 with cancer lying in a hospital bed.

The internal experience has been surreal, but visually seeing it from the outside through my brother's video pregnancy announcement made it feel so dull. The conversation about the baby, the new life, the adolescence. You're confronted by the possibility of play. Two great events happened yesterday. I spoke with Anibal, and he shared Pilar's frustrations with him about how Lucas isn't good on the monkey bars and it's Anibal's fault. Although a joke, it struck a nerve in Anibal because he saw himself in the little Lucas and wanted to make him better. Then Danny came over and had me imagine myself being held by my mom and dad – really being held where I don't have control over my head. Walking down the street holding their hands, learning how to crawl and walk, thinking of myself free and adventurous with the little diaper on my butt. I think about that visual with Lucas, and I remember a photo taken of me as a kid holding two rings on a playground. When I woke up in this panic and reality struck, I felt an end much closer than a beginning. We all know I will be OK. But the comprehension in the news over the past month has made me acutely aware of the end rather than the beginning, even if just temporary.

When you think of the Redwoods or the Grand Canyon or the great Pacific Ocean, there's a realization this is all just bullshit. There are these complex battles that happen in an instant through inner dialogue, through conversations with others, through daily or annual conversations of professional ambitions, but in truth these moments pass by so quickly.

I lay here from

7 to 7

During the same amount of time as the shift of my nurse. Thinking how aware and productive my thoughts have been in my inactivity than their thoughts in their activity. What if I had a rehearsal where we internally just lay there the whole time and the manifestation of thought and being resulted in the real work? The work of the growth of the trees or the waves crashing or the kid's curious mind.

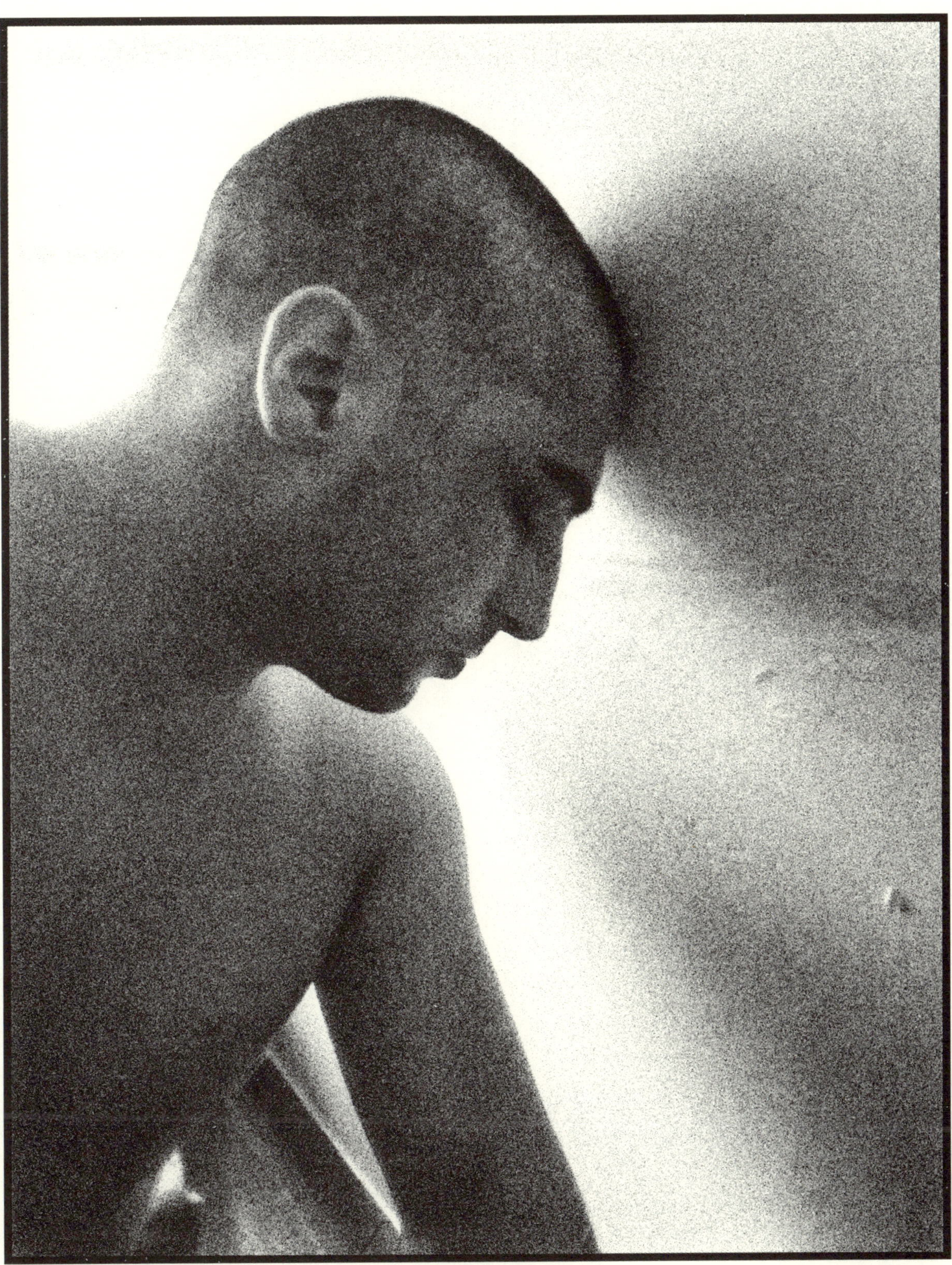

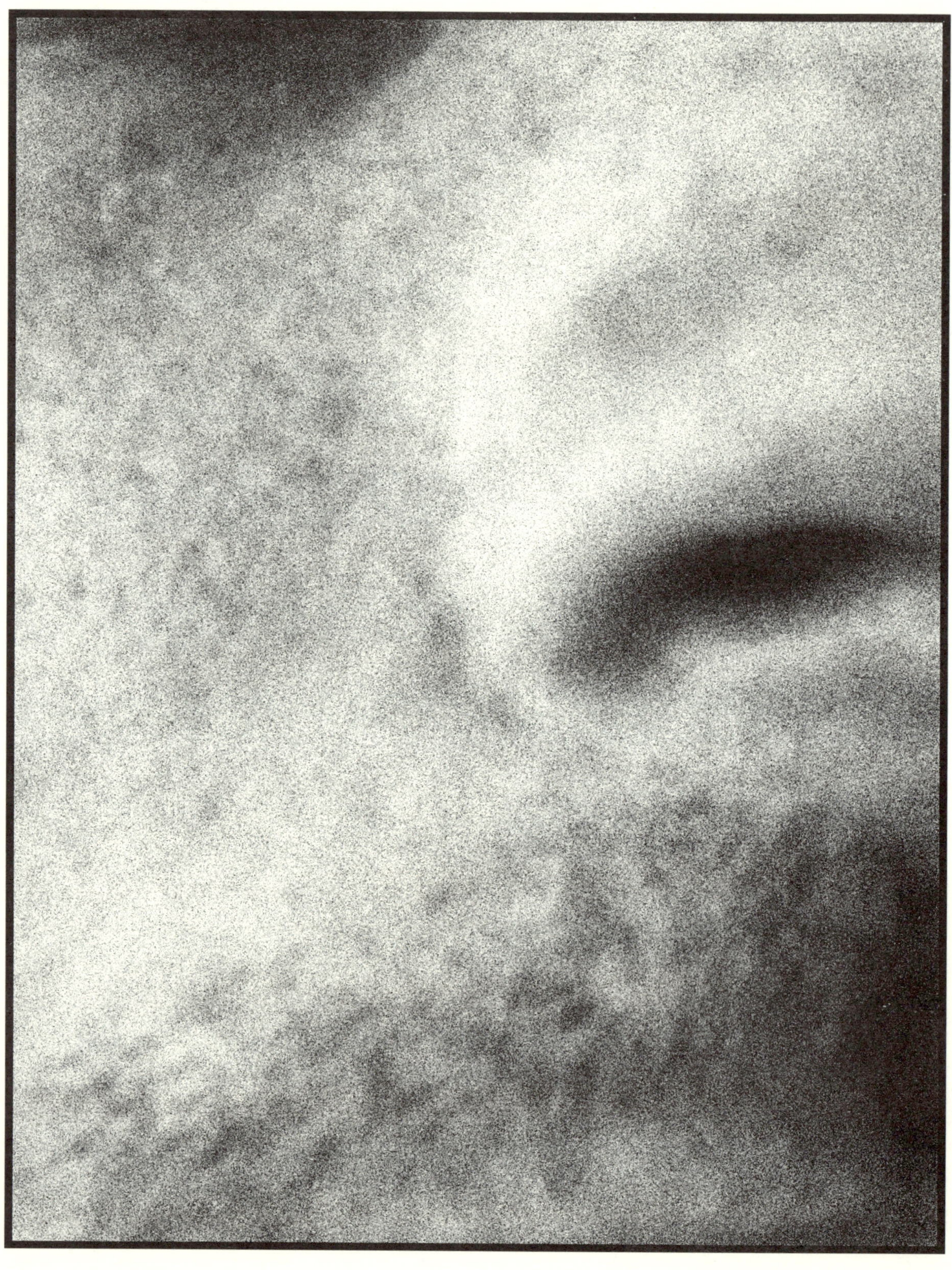

Let's not take for granted walking outside any more. I want to feel the butterflies landing on my arms and the snail crawling up my leg. I want to tilt my chin down and feel the cold water on my spine as my back leans against the rocks. I want to feel your nose circled against mine. Thanks for another beautiful morning sharing my thoughts, my love.

December 2, 2022

Acceptance through opportunity and gratitude versus anger and fear. Throughout this process so far, people keep acknowledging my resilience. They have great knowing that I'll be OK. I have that feeling too. There can be the temporary lows and doubts, the collisions of fate, but they pass effortlessly. They often say "opportunity meeting readiness." This is just another opportunity all along. As the last bag of chemotherapy goes in, knowing I'll get discharged soon,

I find these eight days in this hospital room so peaceful.

It was a challenge but one where I gained so much more than I lost. I haven't really stopped like this since I was 21, when I was here last. In the real world I fear stopping, taking time off, having intimate time with my love. It feels somewhat unproductive, but how are we really measuring productivity these days? The only way for our roots to grow is through sunlight and water, through oxygen and photosynthesis. Being physically here in this box has formed my identity in some ways – and how people perceive me. I will leave here soon without my association to it, but still have this invisible illness. I'm early steps down this road. Ready to manifest my authenticity of what this little eight-day experience has been so far and the diagnosis leading up to it. I've also reflected on the need for physical warmth. There should never be a circumstance where someone wants to touch you and you stop out of the assumption that it provides another person discomfort. Cuddle people. Hug them. Hold hands for hours. It's the real connection of our cells moving through connection. It's the only way to feel if someone else is alive through their heart and breath. Never find embarrassment through touch and never allow someone else to feel envious by touching you. My love, these mornings have meant so much to me. From waking up with your hand in mine, to opening the window and letting the light in, to sharing these thoughts with you. You've been craving this time with me for so long and I've been so blind to the value of why we needed it. Although this hospital visit was no Big Sur, I've enjoyed this time with you so much. I love you.

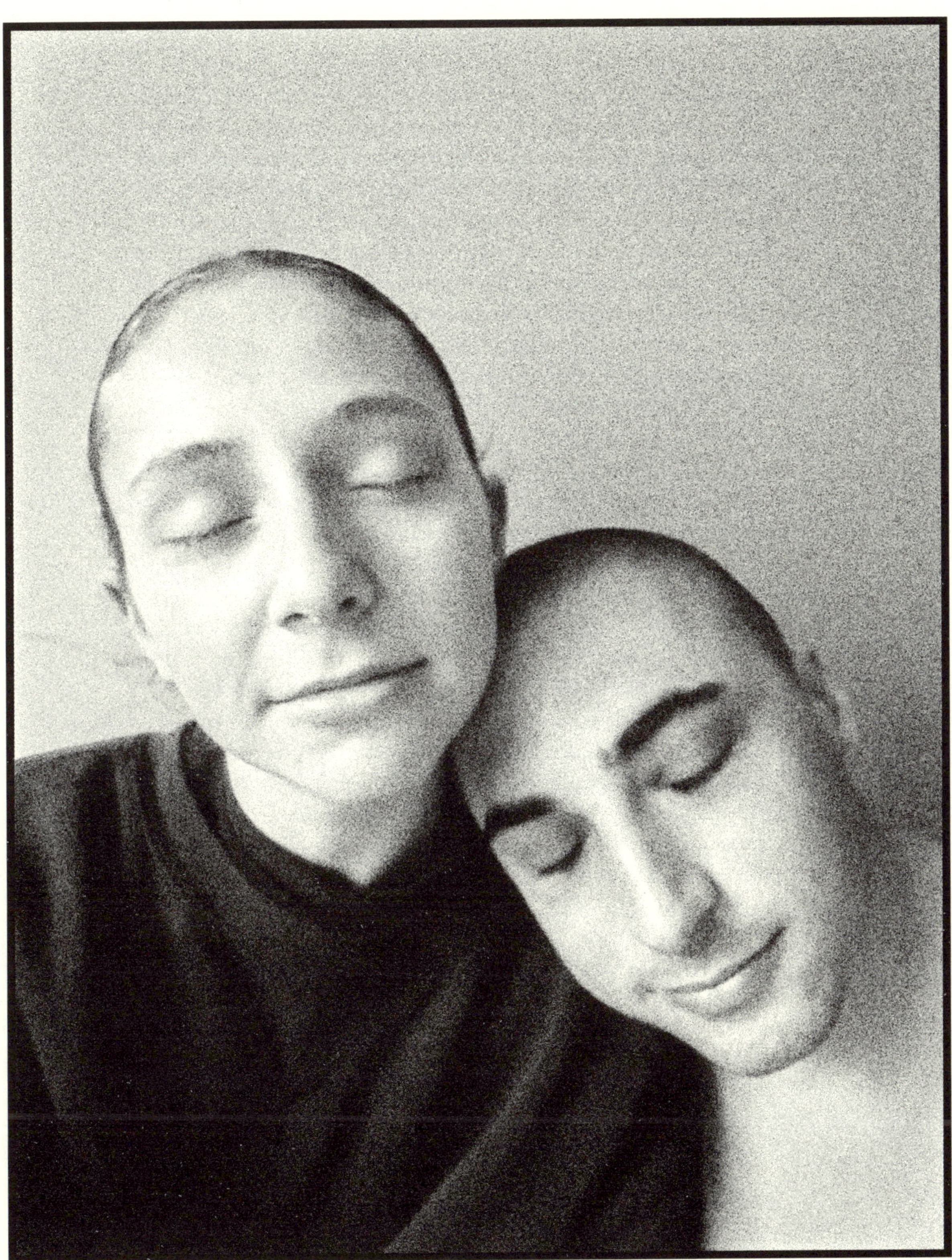

December 3, 2022

Discharged after 9 days. One down.

A deep breath. An introduction of the light. My arms pulse. I feel my cells doing the work. The work is the nothingness, just the being. I'm still on an incline to healing, to understanding how to naturally grow instead of forcefully grow. It comes with great pause of thought. I don't want to lose this poetic mind or leave him behind. I don't want to shelve the importance of connection with others to prioritize professional ambitions. With this discharge, my mind explores old habits of things to do, jobs to get, emails to respond to, and dance compositions to create. These are all things I'll knowingly return to, but for now I'm not ready yet. Since the diagnosis and more recently, I've been thinking deeply about marriage and kids. I think the true agreement of asking someone to marry you though is rather not to agree to a partnership between the two, but to have the expectations that the marriage would always keep your partner feeling whole as an individual and that the wholeness of that individual is what would benefit the partnership. In speaking to Maria yesterday and going through this experience with my love, there's been a deep comprehension, especially when briefly met with mortality or the possibilities of it, that we really belong to our cells. That the empathy, the love, the worry, and the healing are shared by so many and are mutual, but the real process is an individual experience. We can never really truly be exclusive to someone else but only to the moment or circumstances that we're in, but what you can do is commit to loving someone so deeply that you support their journey of wholeness, and they support yours. Thanks for writing in my journal.

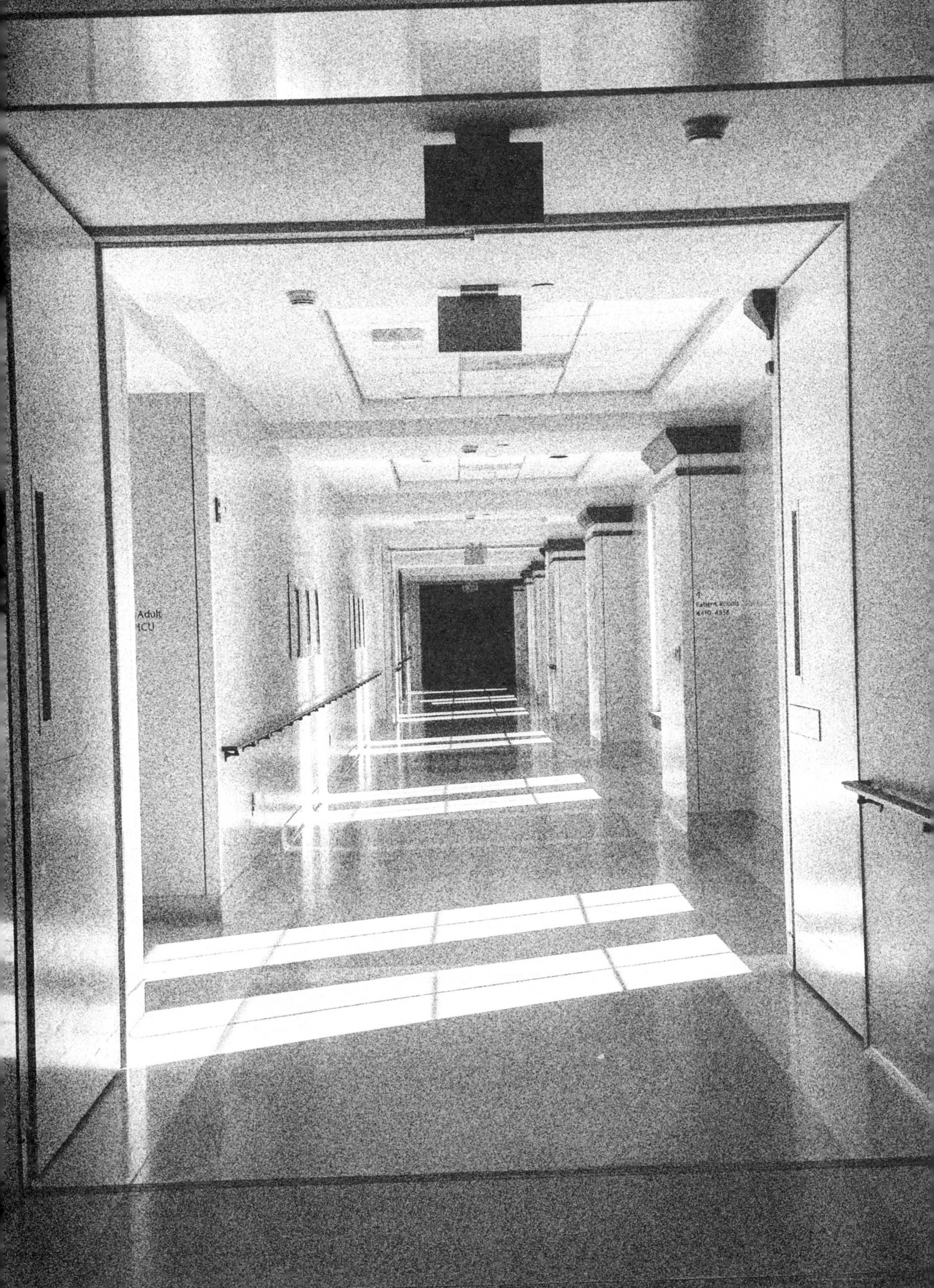
Adult
ICU
Patient Rooms

December 4, 2022

There's new sounds this morning.
The light's entering the room from a different place.

I'm in my home now but it feels different. Everything feels different. The walk to the bathroom, the routine, and the expectations of self. The future is still so unknown. There's this temptation to jump back into the way it was. I'm having small glimpses of fear, but also trying to start my day right. As I looked out the window, I saw a singular seagull flying west. That will be my big activity today. Last night I had all these visualizations – feeling the rubber from the bed, feeling like I was plugged into an IV, seeing that green bag staring at me, the nurse knocking and coming in, the monitor illuminated from the meds I need to take. Yesterday, leaving that space was so overwhelming but also so peaceful. Nine days to now explore my new physical form. Having two visitors at a time felt so intimate and the dialogue was so whole. Last night was the first time I was a part of a group but not the focus of the conversation. There was a lot of stimulation. I have this instinct now that I'm home to appear and to communicate to everyone that I'm OK, but I was reminded by my love that the more I suppress these thoughts the more they will overcome me. My professional life has always had something to look forward to. And right now I really need to focus on being in remission and celebrate being treated because there's a minimal fear that I may not be. There's still a minimal fear. Thanks for writing. I love you.

December 5, 2022

beginning

effects

of

chemotherapy.

*D*iscomfort.

Labs.

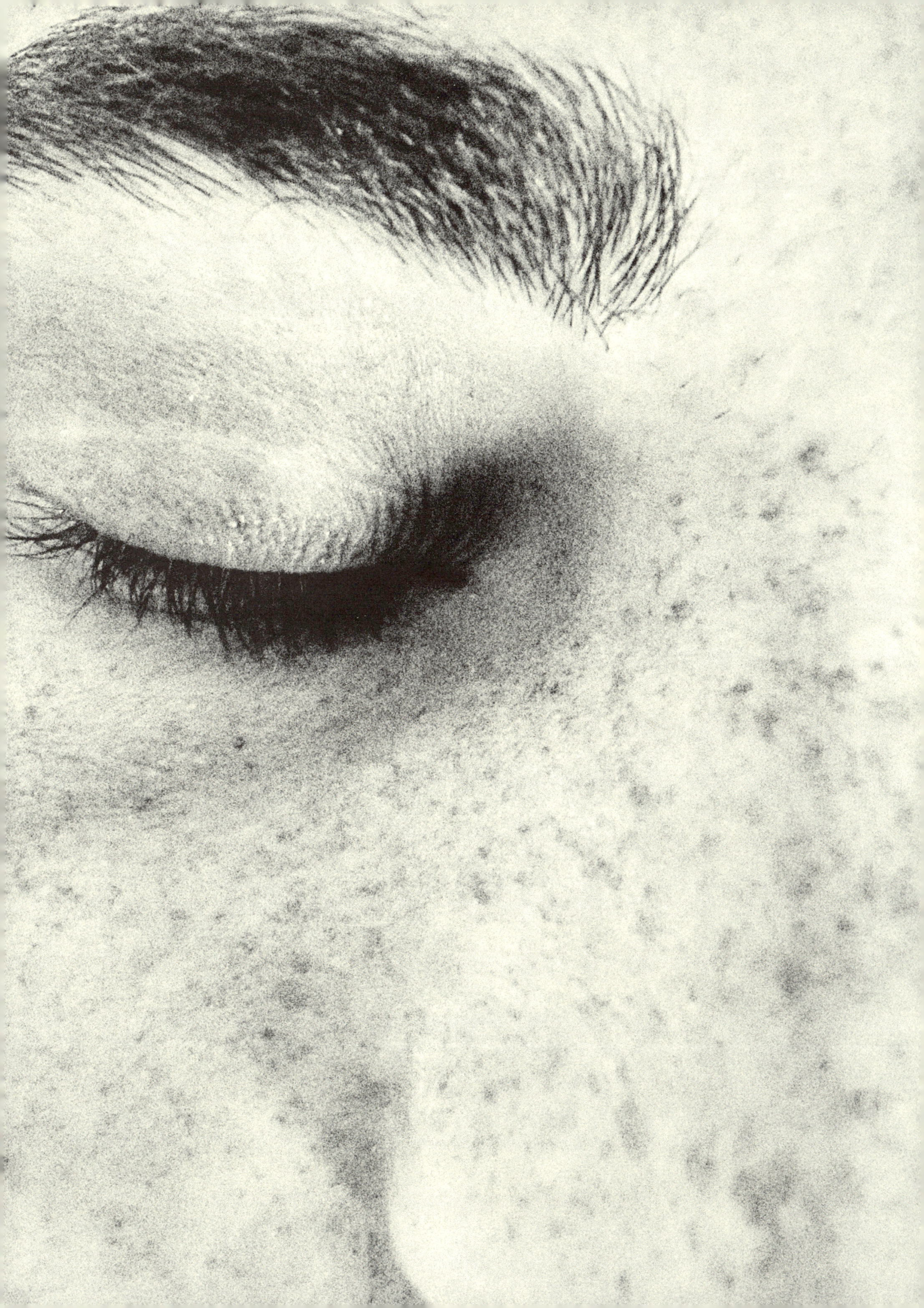

December 6, 2022

Have never felt this uncomfortable.
Height of chemotherapy symptoms.

Haven't slelpt in three days. There's no
one position that feels good.

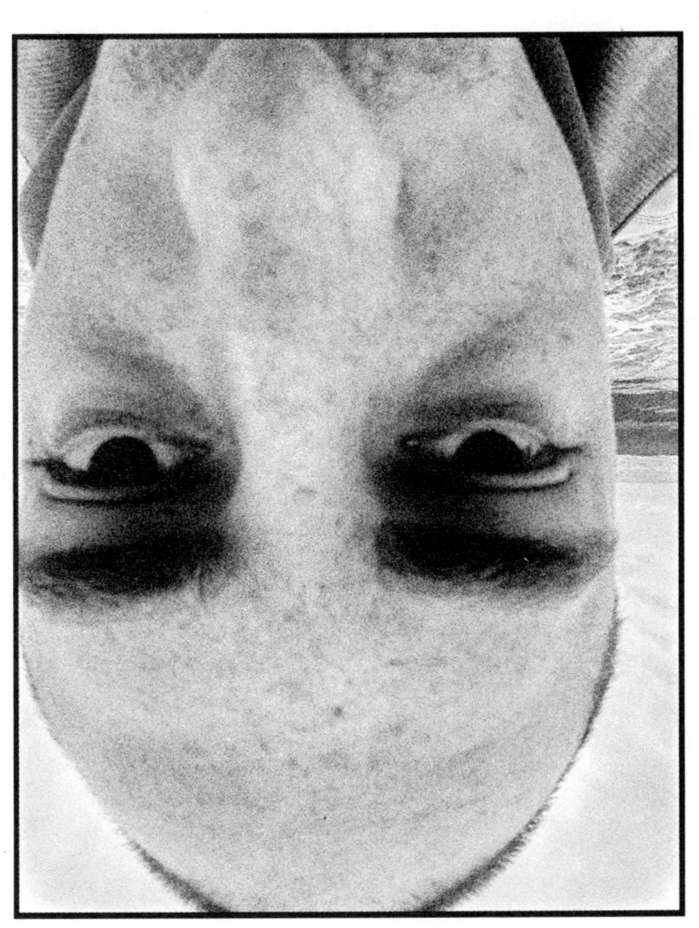

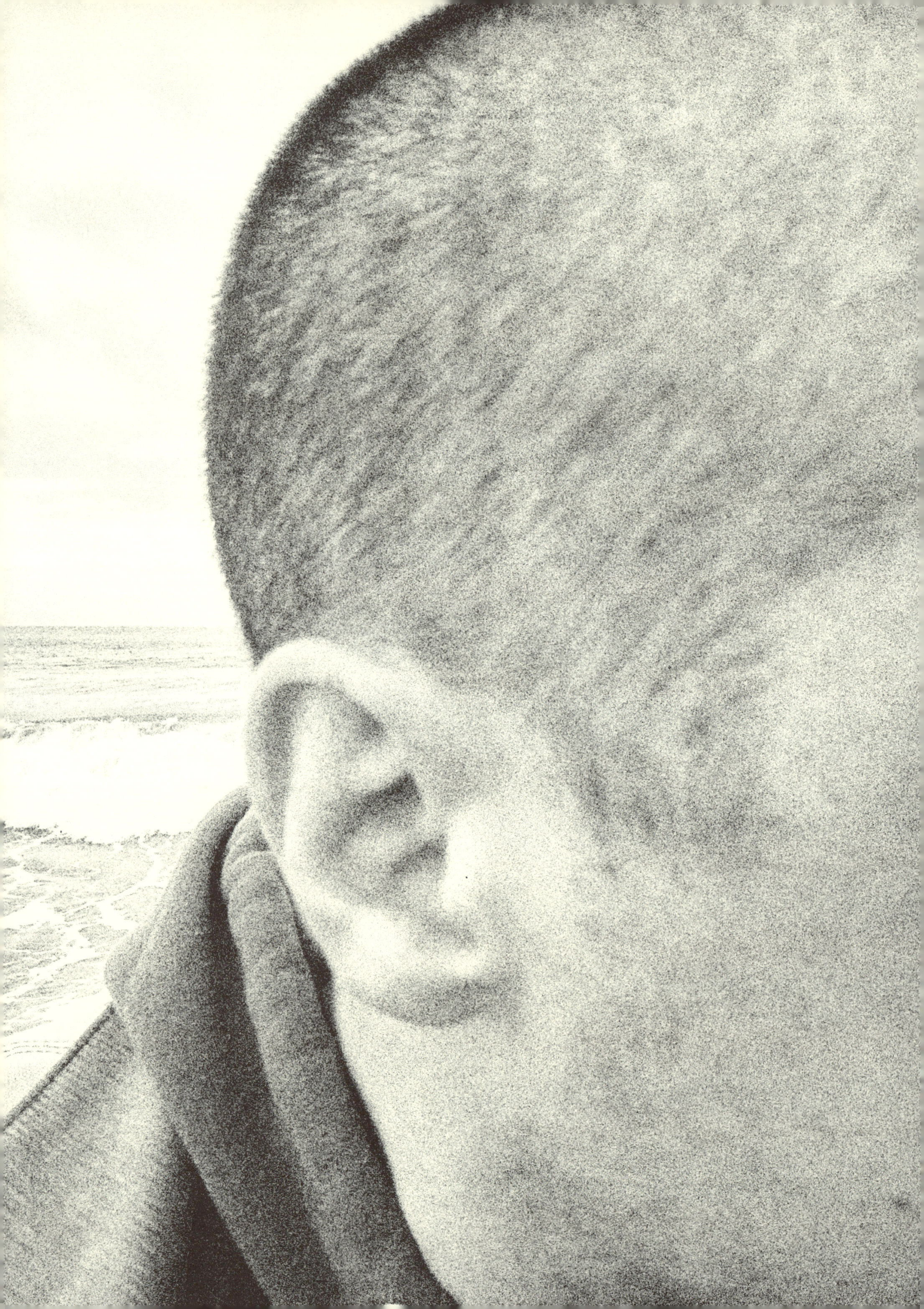

The hair is so long. There's hundreds around like bushes tangled around me.
Their eyes like waterfalls of tears.

I feel billowed in.

Like in a cave of fear.
The visuals are so loud.

My lips tingle since the bone marrow shot.

There's specks all over my chest like stars.
My nervous system is shutting down.

I can't feel the strength of the touch being given to me.

My body and mind try to rest but the uncomfort battles against itself.
I just want to sleep.

The gas leaves my system like a hurricane.

It may sound funny,
but the compression of my abs and ribcage forces such abruption

of weakness.

I can't feel my flesh.
But this too shall pass.

My lips still tingle.

The time goes by so slow, with fear to make it to the next hour.
I still follow the seagulls.

The sun peeks through the clouds.
I stare at the morning swimmer with great envy.

Through each stroke the dolphins appear.
Pelicans in fives fly north.

The frustrated sea lion and the salt water against my feet.

A small circle in the neck.
It's as though I'm dancing again, but did anyone tell me to stop?

I need to find my dance.
I'm in discomfort you see, but this too shall pass.

Until the next dose of chemotherapy.

December 8, 2022

Park time. Finally a smile. Nice to be outside.

The true lowest lows and highest highs. A rocket ship of bipolarity. My body couldn't get comfortable. I couldn't ease my mind. It was crying. Continued symptoms, thinking the worst thoughts. Feeling like time won't move. There's a realization that I can't fight this poison with natural remedies. I need to put this shit to sleep and to come to bat with the hard stuff. After a new cocktail of big pharma, I finally got some rest. Waking up I finally felt normalcy again. I had the energy to move around the house, to walk down the block and to lay down within my own body. Since talking to Govindha, I feel so inspired to look at the nutrients I take as part of my medicine and healing. Walking into the studio yesterday was the best moment I've had post the chemo trespass. Working with the dancers, bringing their best to life, brought my best to life. This morning, I got overwhelmed by the perception of nothing I had in front of me, but my mind all night kept spinning with the many things I want to accomplish. When faced with a cancer diagnosis, being the producer doesn't fucking matter any more. I'm an artist. I have such a deep and complex body of work that I need to communicate. Last night, watching *Mind Cry* and *In a Rush to Do Nothing* were two of my favorite moments as a choreographer. I really love what I do. I was so honored that they danced them. I'm also incredibly proud of Emma. The saint who held down the fort. Her growth as a leader in such a short period of time is mind blowing. I'm not sure if my poetry is dissolving, but that's all I have for now. Thanks for writing, my love.

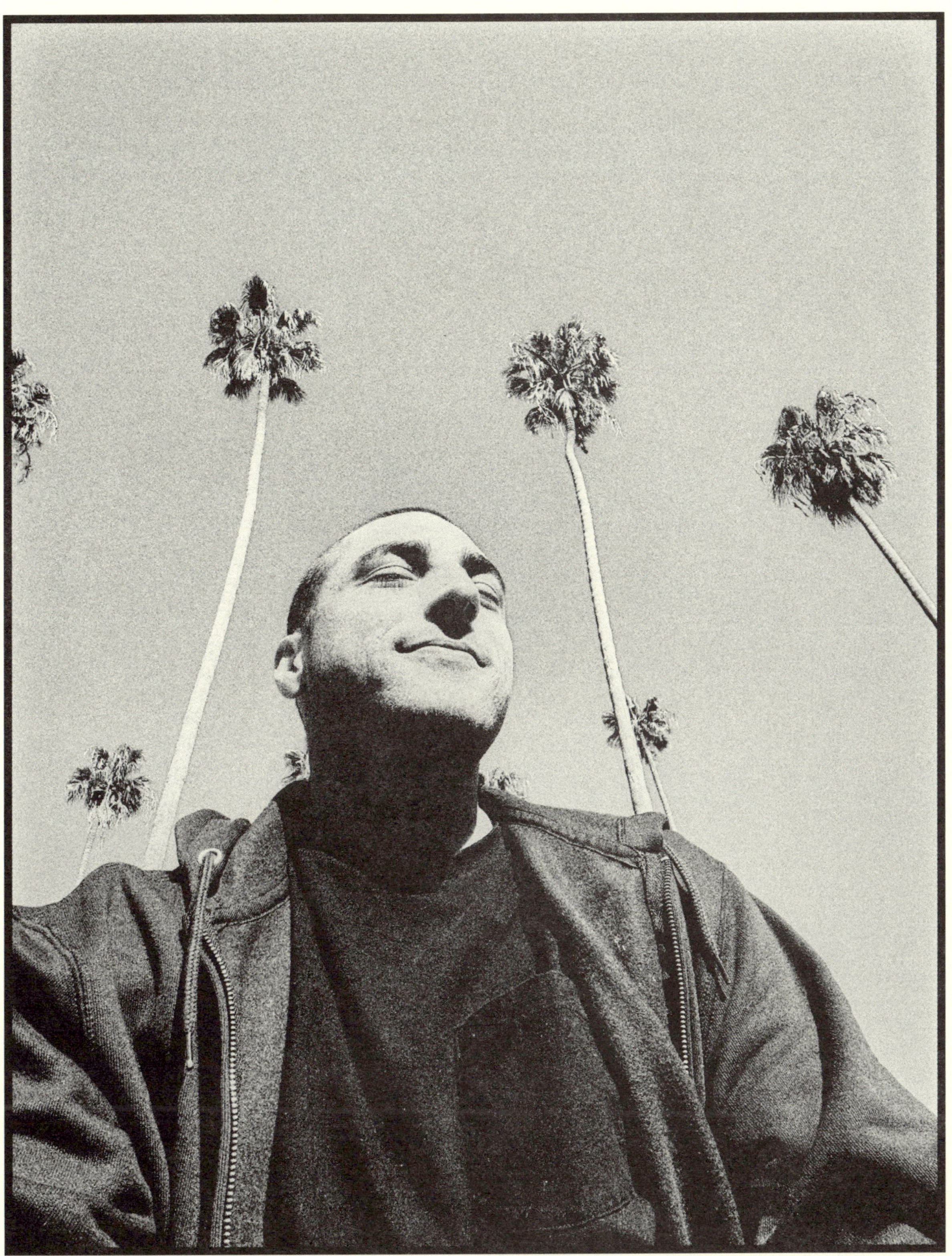

December 9, 2022

Show time.

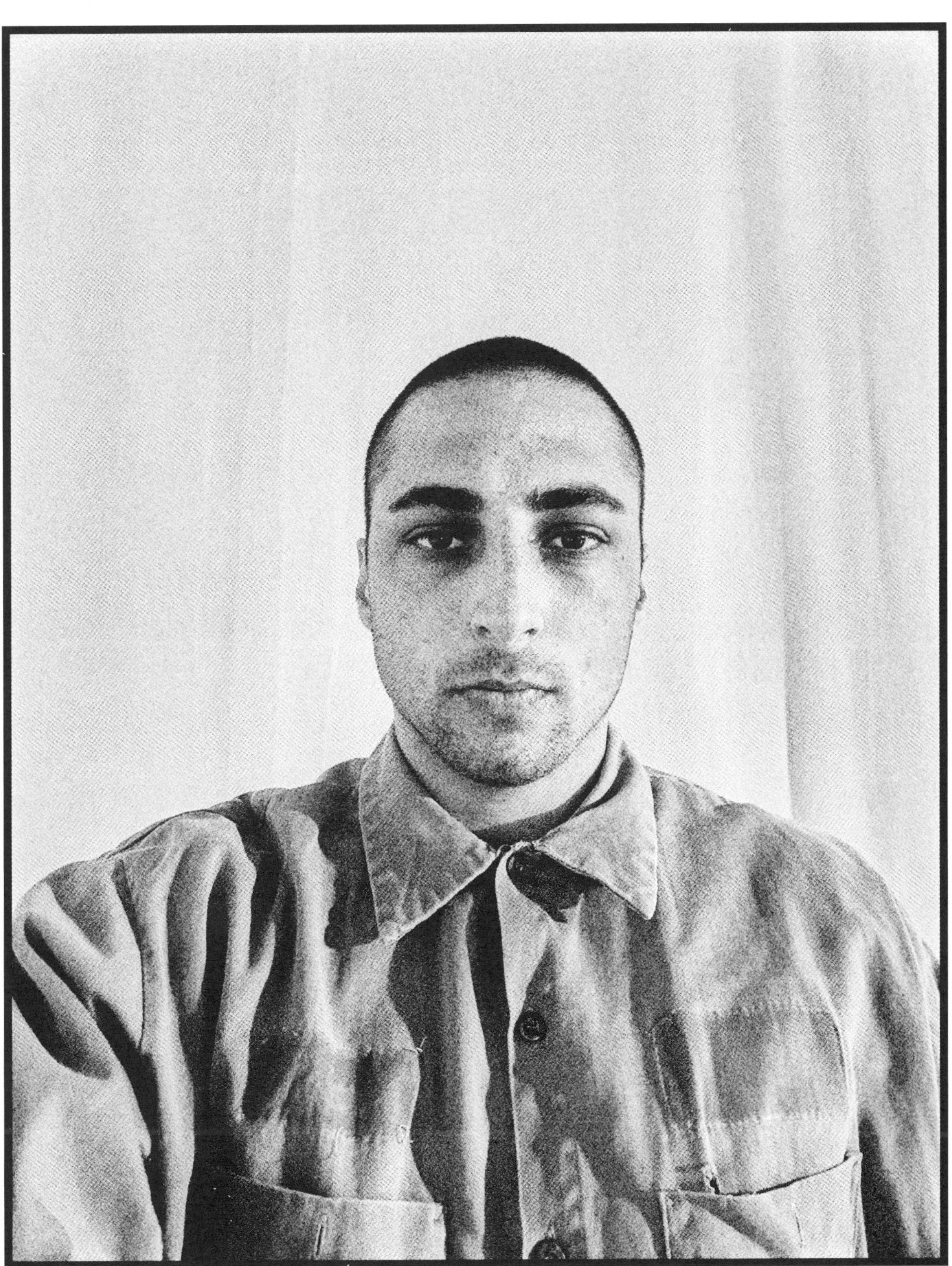

December 12, 2022

Capturing freedom.
Head against Point Mugu.

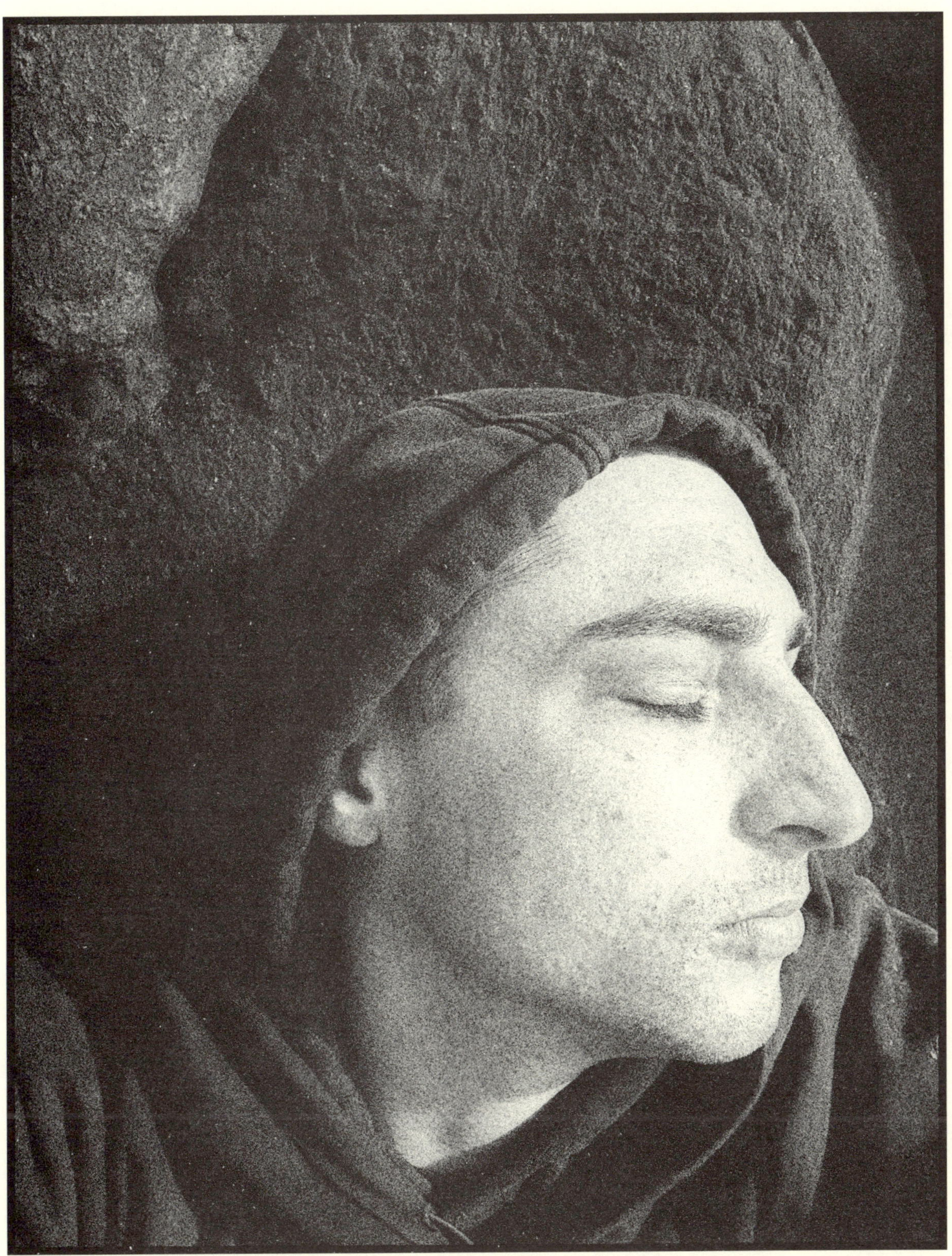

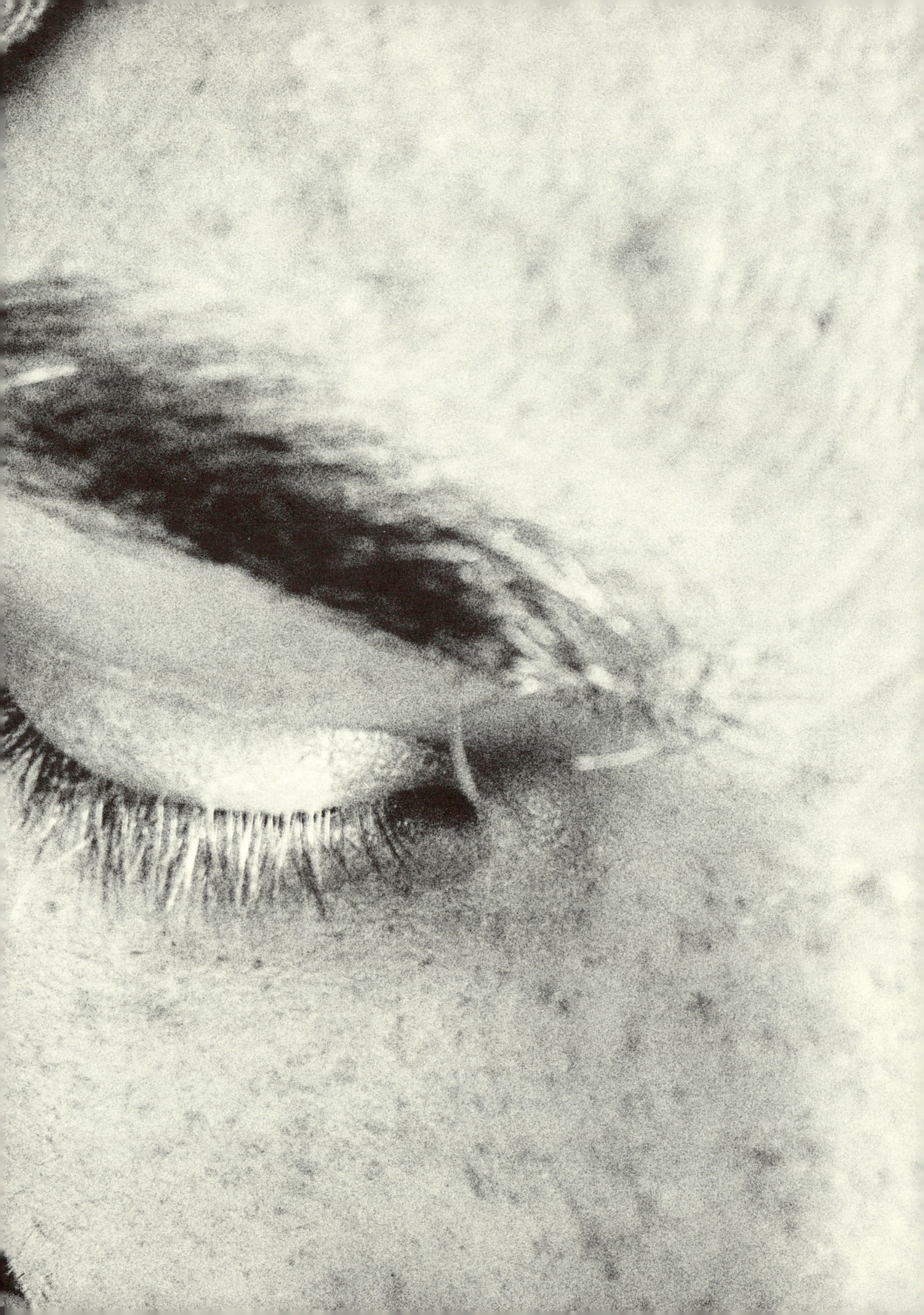

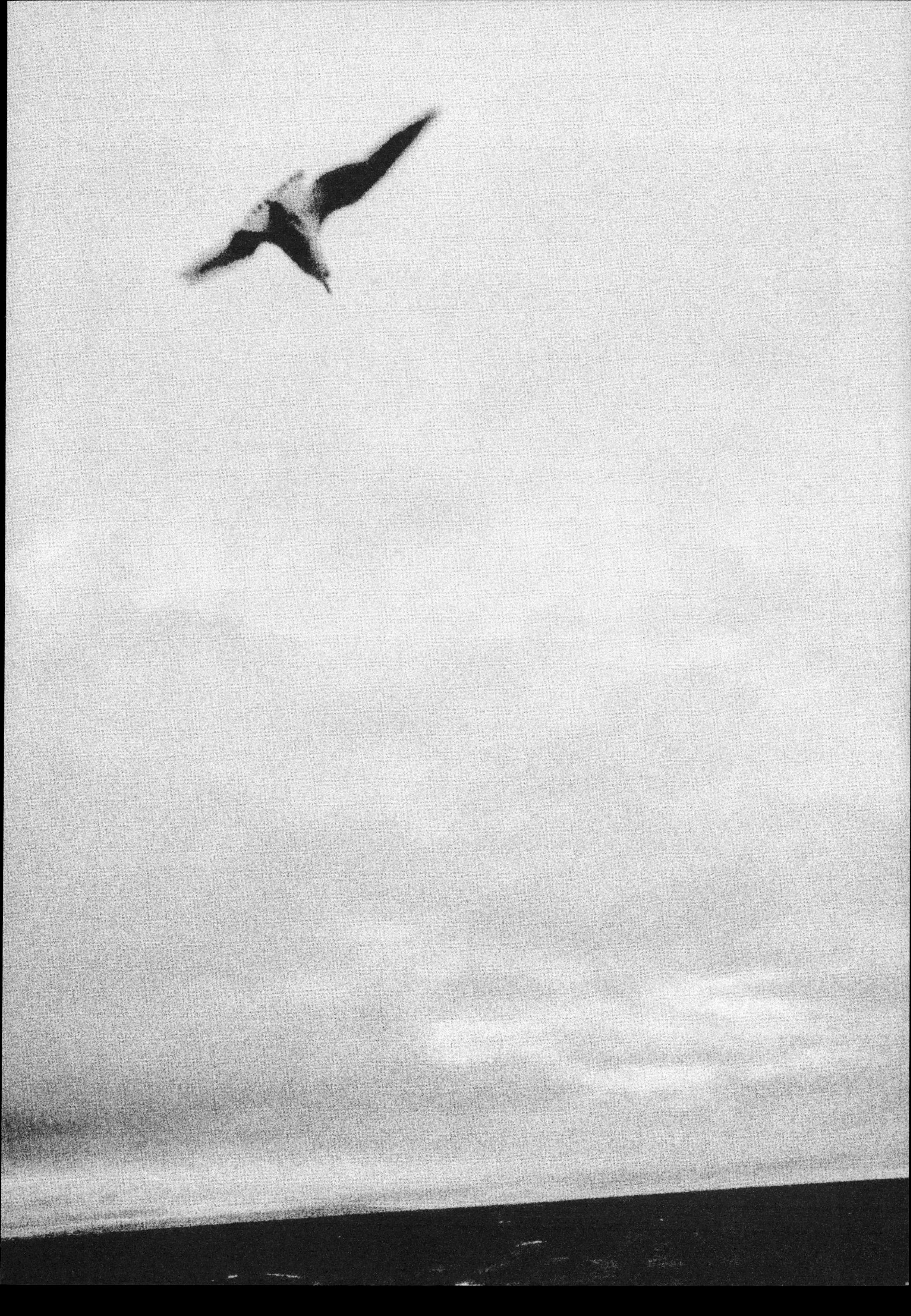

December 13, 2022

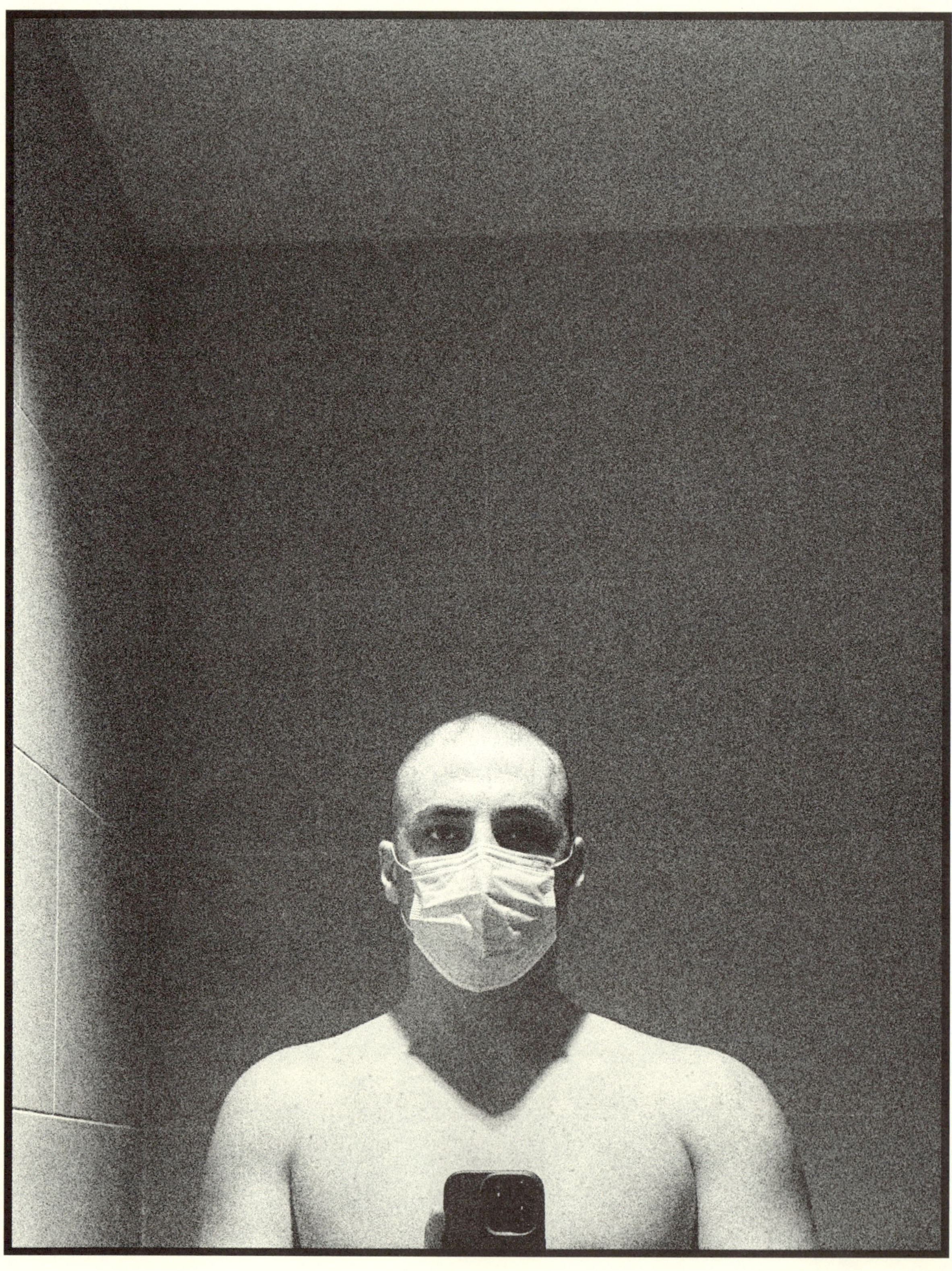

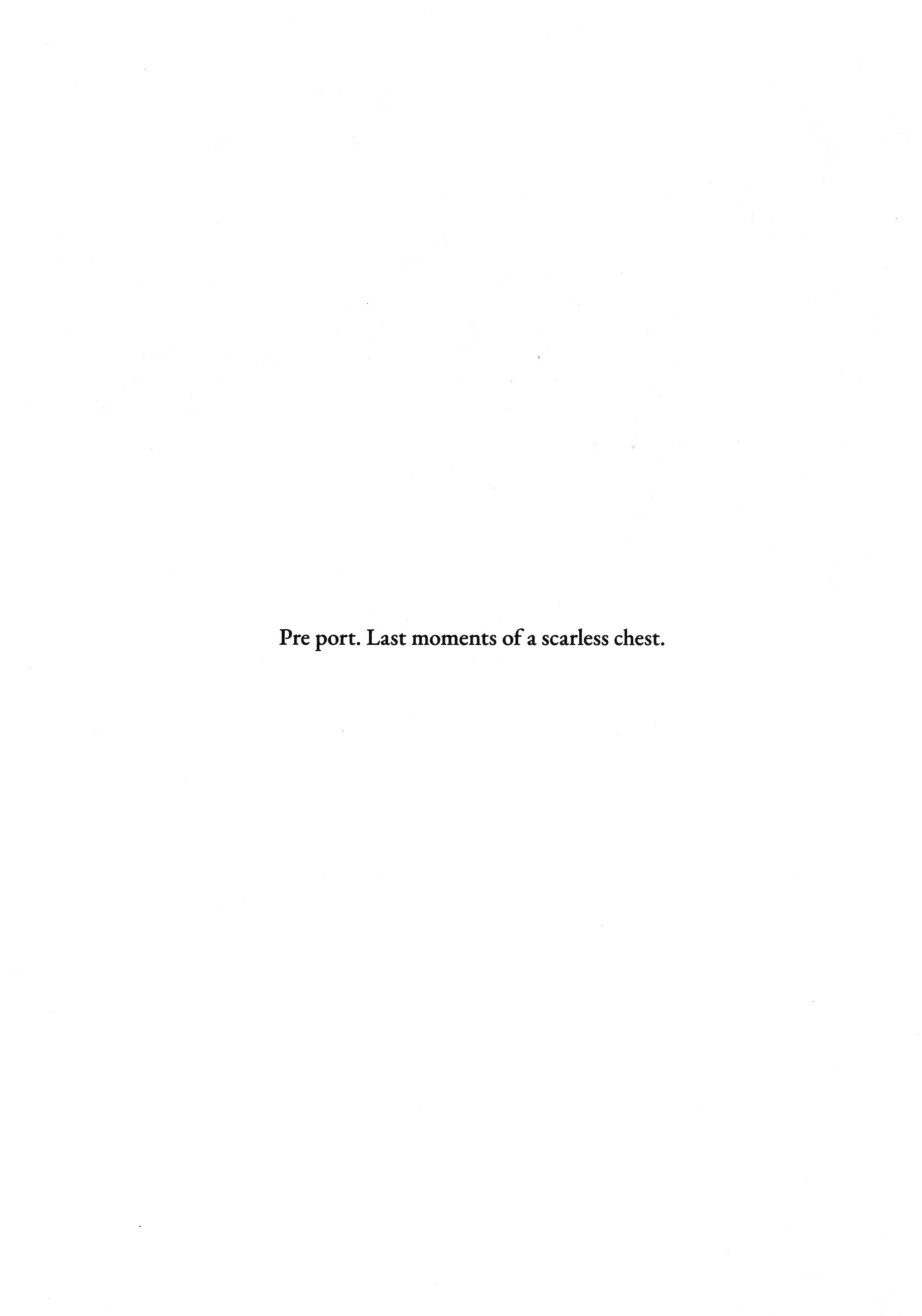

Pre port. Last moments of a scarless chest.

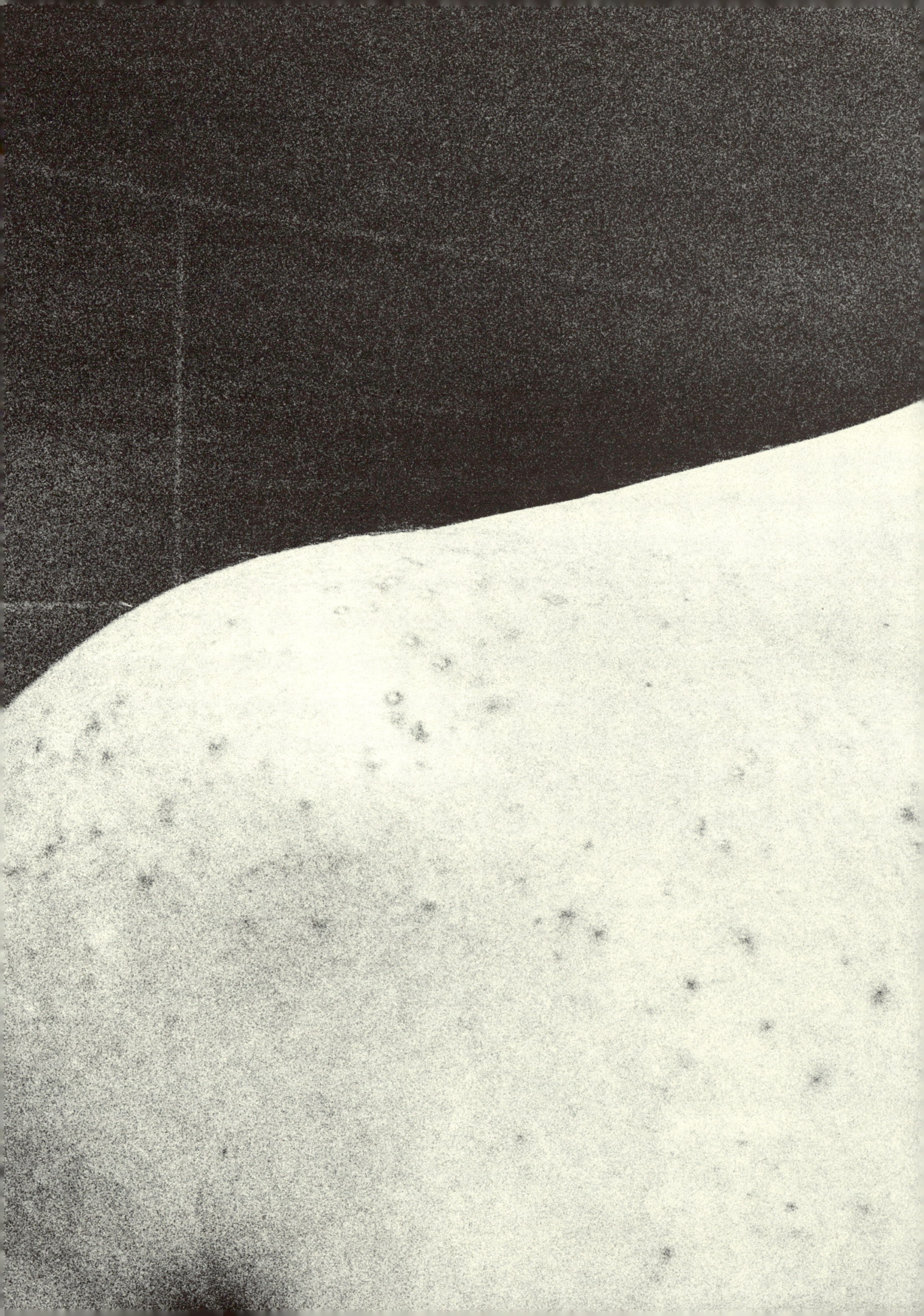

December 14, 2022

When people feed you grapes
just open your mouth
and eat them.

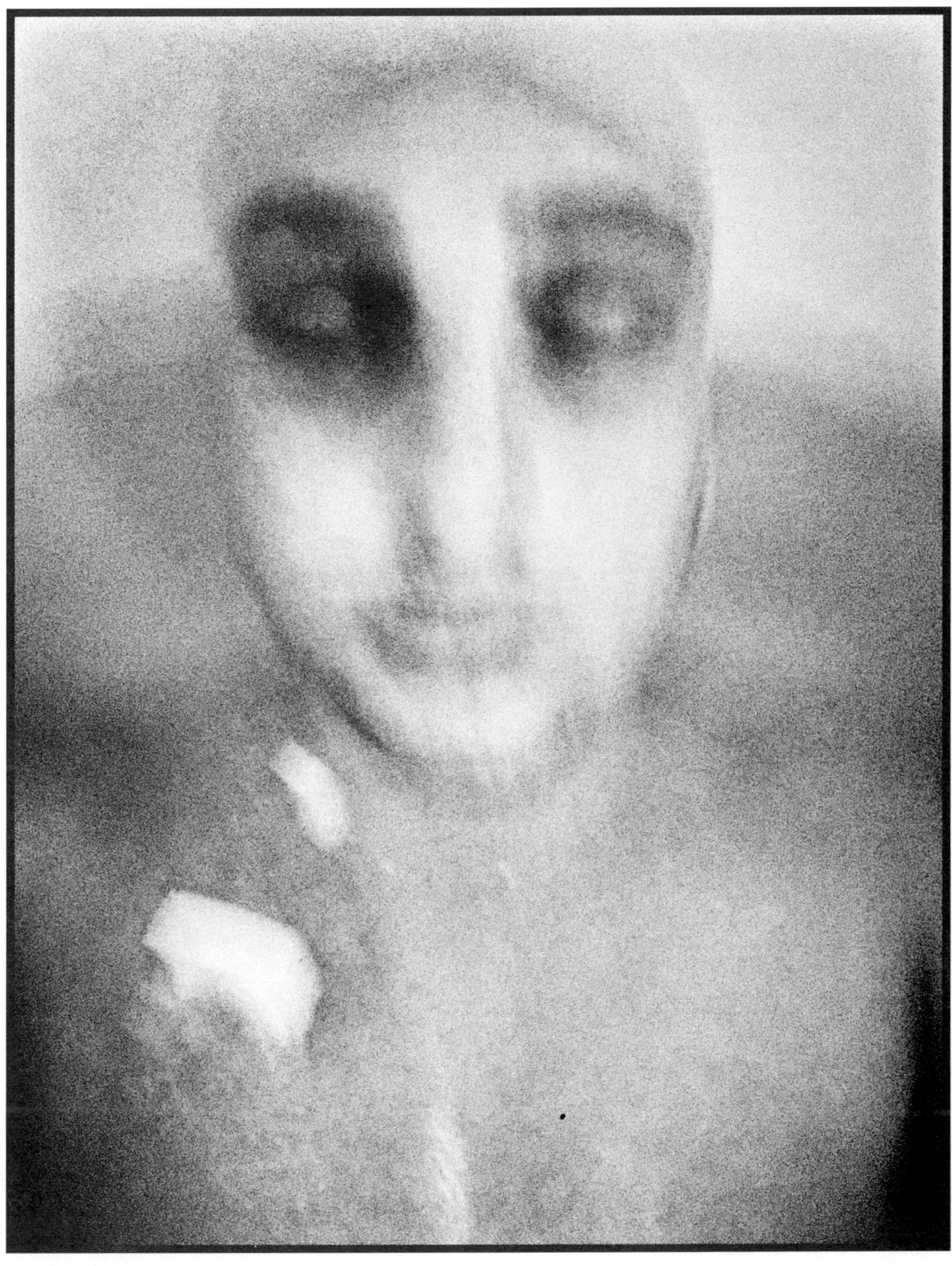

December 15, 2022

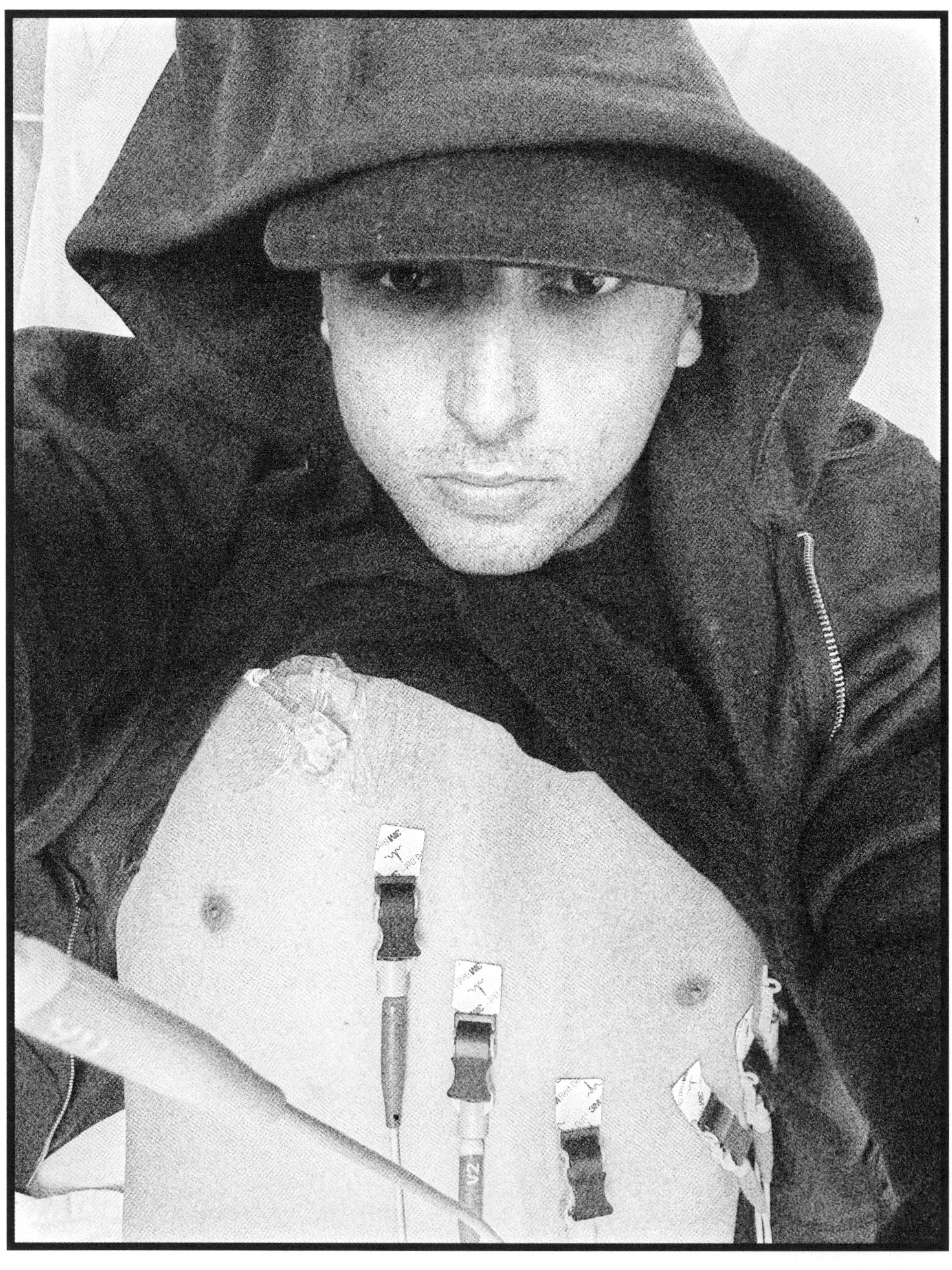

Embarrassed weaknesses.
Fainted with
wet pants.

December 16, 2022

Stopped by cancer. Overwhelmed by normalcy. Desiring productivity. This past week has been one of the greatest of my life. Mainly because of my new perspective. I've learned how to disconnect two things – art and business. Too often they were intertwined, and my desire to be productive was led by an insecurity to run my business, answering emails, talking about budgets, strategizing over and over and over again. Competing with my ambition and constantly losing to it. Prior to my diagnosis, my motivation was in the wrong place. I had my most successful year yet and worked on the largest projects and made the most money, and yet I was the most unhappy. My motivation was to chase money, to desire the inbound commercial job, to care about how many audiences were in the venue, to be in the biggest venue, and to care so much about the outer perspective – the likes, the engagement, the visibility. This past week I got to watch *In a Rush to Do Nothing* and *Mind Cry* come to life. I got to see the power and success of my team and their ability to perform at the highest level, especially in my absence. I've never felt so happy and proud seeing my work before. Night after night I cried so deeply. It felt like a visual and sonic medicine healing me in real time. The audiences came, they were really there. The dancers poured their hearts into the work. Their bodies were given – from the calluses on their feet to the sore back, the bruised shoulder, the tight neck, and the fragile wrists. They gave everything and they were going to not care who was in the audience. The shows concluded, and I was filled with so much inspiration and energy. I went to the Water Garden the next morning at 6 a.m., when Liam and Robert met me and helped to redesign the physical space and the spiritual energy. One moved table, a few moved chairs, a swept floor, and a deep consideration of how a space is designed completely shifted my attitude and love for the Water Garden.

My motivation now, especially having the stillness, this questioned mortality, and this poetry injected into me – I now know my motivation is fully my art and not my business. I've set up all the space boards to identify each project. I'm more inspired than I've ever been to only focus on my work. Each night my mind is powerfully shared ideas from the universe, and I fortunately write them all down and am making them come to life. Prompts of ideas, projects, directions, people, and things to stay passionate about. I feel like prior to my diagnosis I would start each day blindly driving on a road in front of me. Whereas now I feel I have a map for a road trip across the whole country for exactly what to do and what direction to go in. And who to go with me. I've had so many deep conversations recently. Many of which have had so much purpose, and have felt like I'm speaking to a mirror in a lot of ways, advising people with the lessons and realizations I've learned. One powerful conversation was talking to my love about the official passing of my baton of caring about the business side of things and focusing fully on being the practitioner while she fully dives into running our business. I've talked to Ryan and Jordyn so deeply about life and sharing with them my new love and appreciation for family. And how before I felt family was something I belonged to and wasn't necessarily something I wanted to take part in. Whereas now I feel it as something that's mine that I lead and design, and choose to bring the best out of each person individually. It's something my family belongs to as opposed to the reverse. I had a great conversation with Ray, who shared his experience of cancer from 40 years ago in great detail – and it was exactly reflective of mine. From ceremonially shaving my head to comprehending that the most difficult part of having cancer is how those around you react and worry about you. We talked about how much this disease is a positive thing in our lives and how we equally share this deep acceptance and beauty with our mortality if it happened. I talked with Ivan, and so powerfully shared the importance of gratitude and stillness. The more we do what we do, things get harder rather than easier. That our most valuable investments are those around us. Our saved wealth gives us the flexibility to explore what we want and our own mind to purposefully explore and pursue what we love. I talked to Jonathan and Tal individually, and shared my excitement and interest in diet, nutrition, and exercise.

That health is the most important thing in our lives and that I was motivated to explore it further. I've prompted many people in my life recently with the question, "What would you do if you had one year left to live?" Now that I've reframed my motivation with this new gift of having cancer, I've questioned everyone's motivation around me, to bring out the best in them. I've talked to my love more about marriage, as there is such a readiness and deeper understanding for it now. I'm not necessarily ready this second but deeply understand the commitment so much more. The need to commit to somebody else's wholeness, to their growth and love of themselves. That this is not a piece of real estate. A marriage doesn't allow you to have someone else belong to you, but rather agree to share their whole being. What I believe from this pursuit is that it's not a commitment, but rather an agreement to share love. There's nothing exclusively binding about it. As we will never belong to each other. We will just share indefinitely. I also expressed my need for physical expression and the ability and interest to always be able to explore that need. And that it's a two-way street. It's not a singular desire. We discovered if this marriage ever didn't work at any point that it would be a mere transition for growth for the individual with a commitment to the friendship and relationship – as opposed to using the word "divorce," which exudes so much negativity and destruction. My love tirelessly writes in my journal today a collection of thoughts from the past week. We stopped writing daily for a while because of my exposure to normality and my distance to pain. Yesterday I was reminded of my cancer, the symptoms came to haunt me again – throwing up all night, pain in my liver, soreness in the back of my skull, fainting on the hospital floor while urinating in my pants – an embarrassing and physical takeover exporting illness and fluids from my body. It's in this moment of weakness I'm reminded to journal again. The pain and trauma humble me and remind me to record my thoughts. This past week I escaped into a normalcy, but I've returned to my relationship with my cancer, and in great coincidence I completed the choreographic score for *Mind Cry,* a piece exploring these deep symptoms. There have been so many newfound realizations recently. I'm grateful to my love for continuing to write them down.

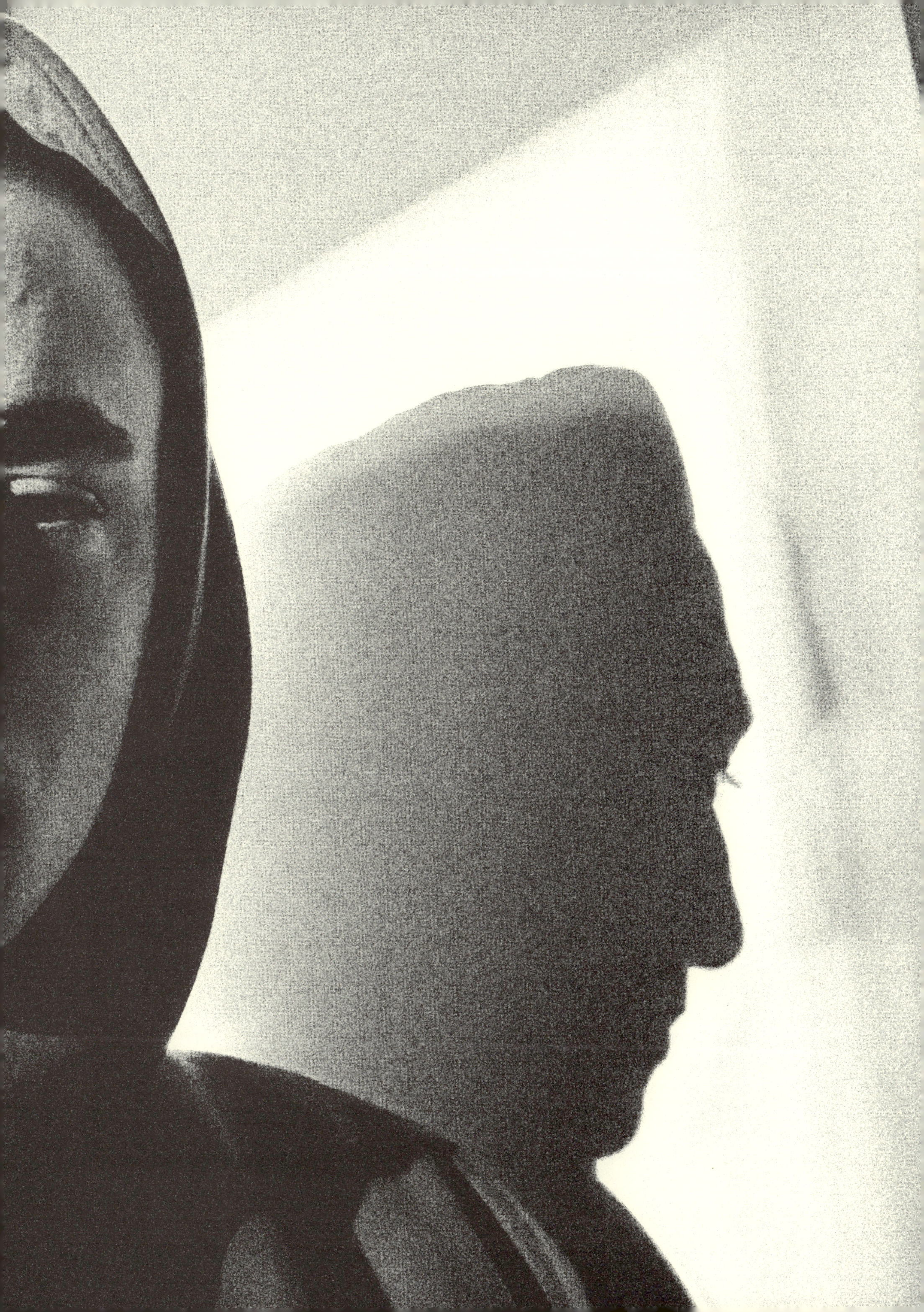

December 17, 2022

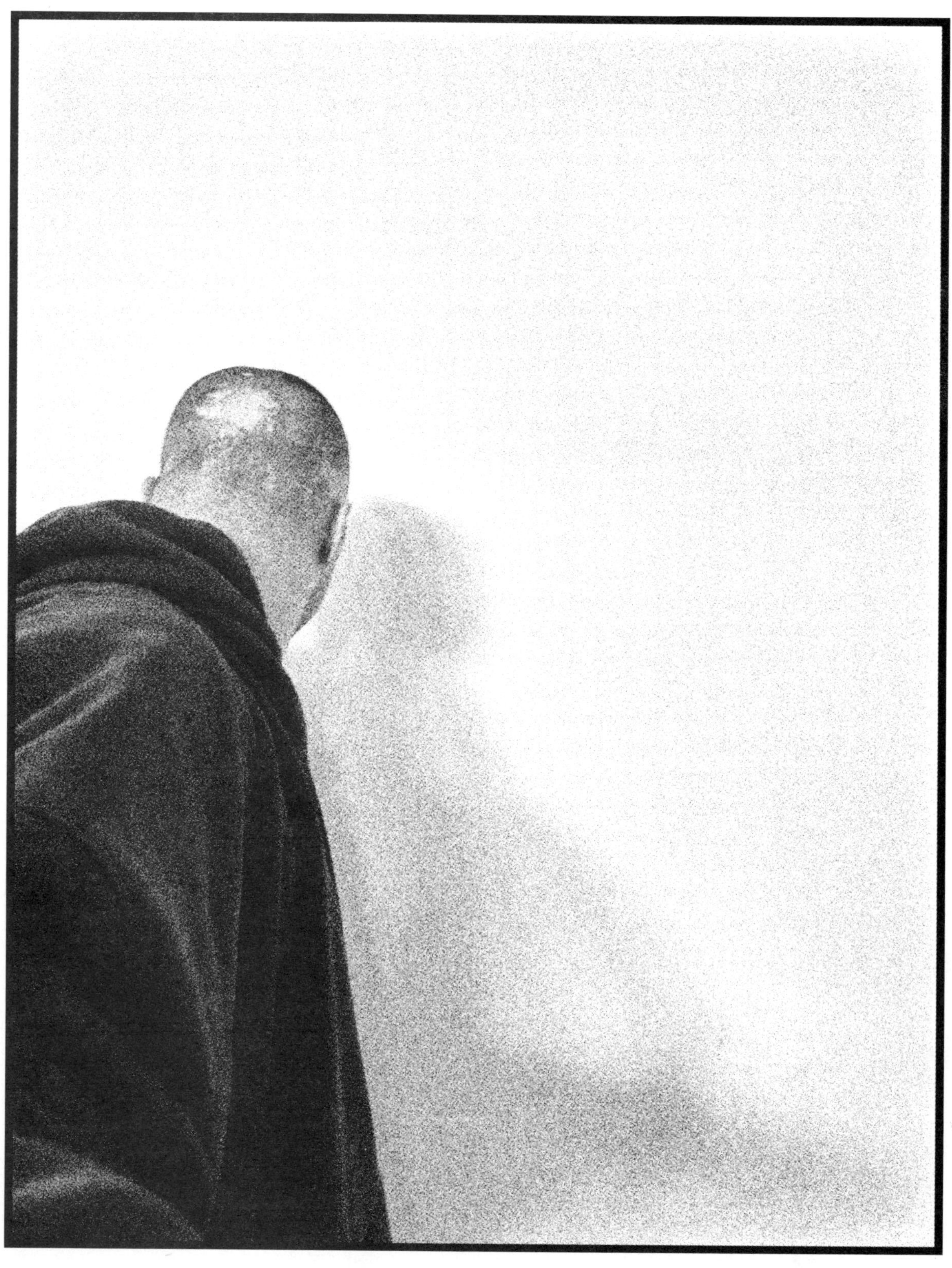

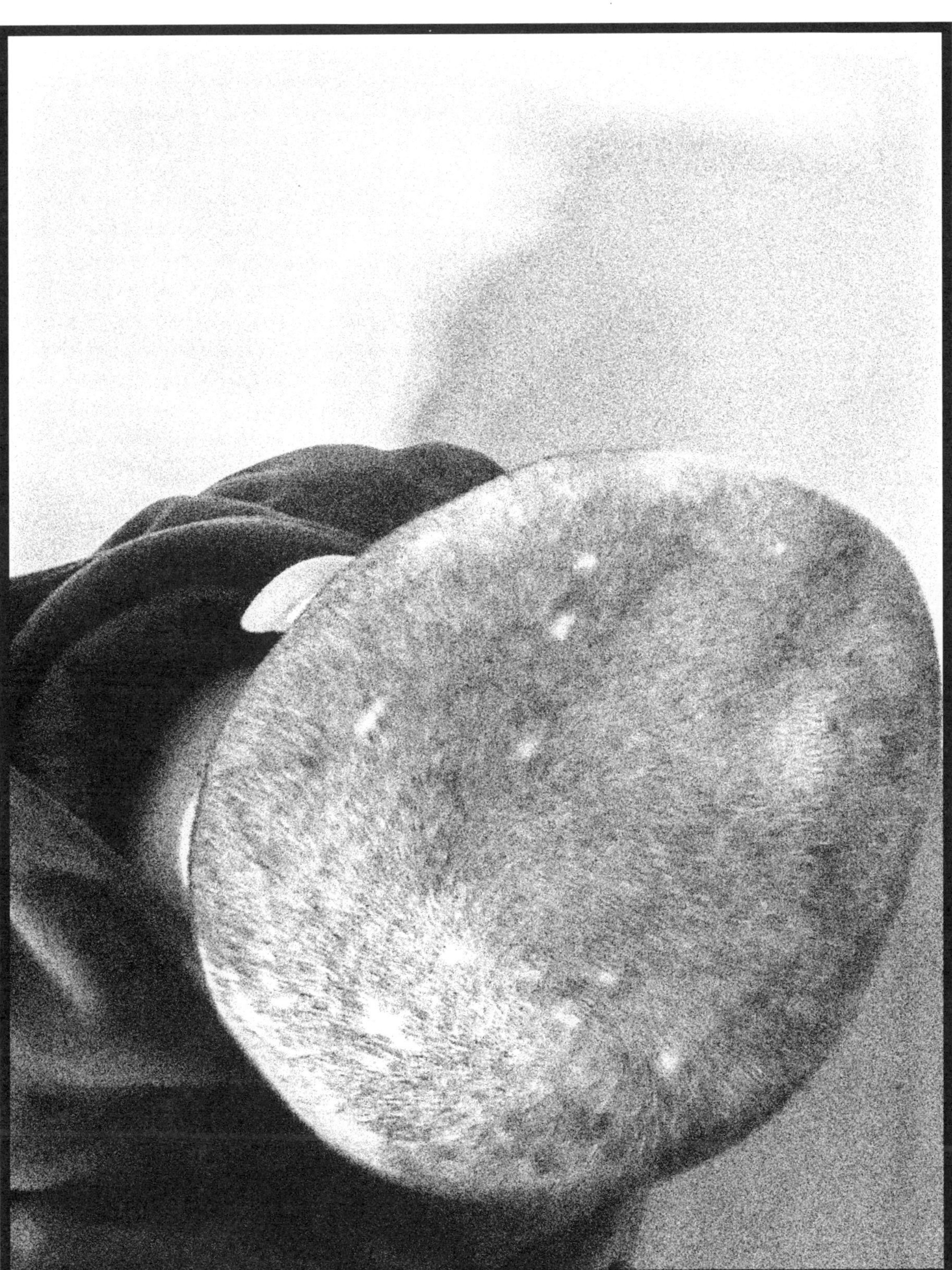

December 19, 2022

Hair fell out.
A soak of sadness.

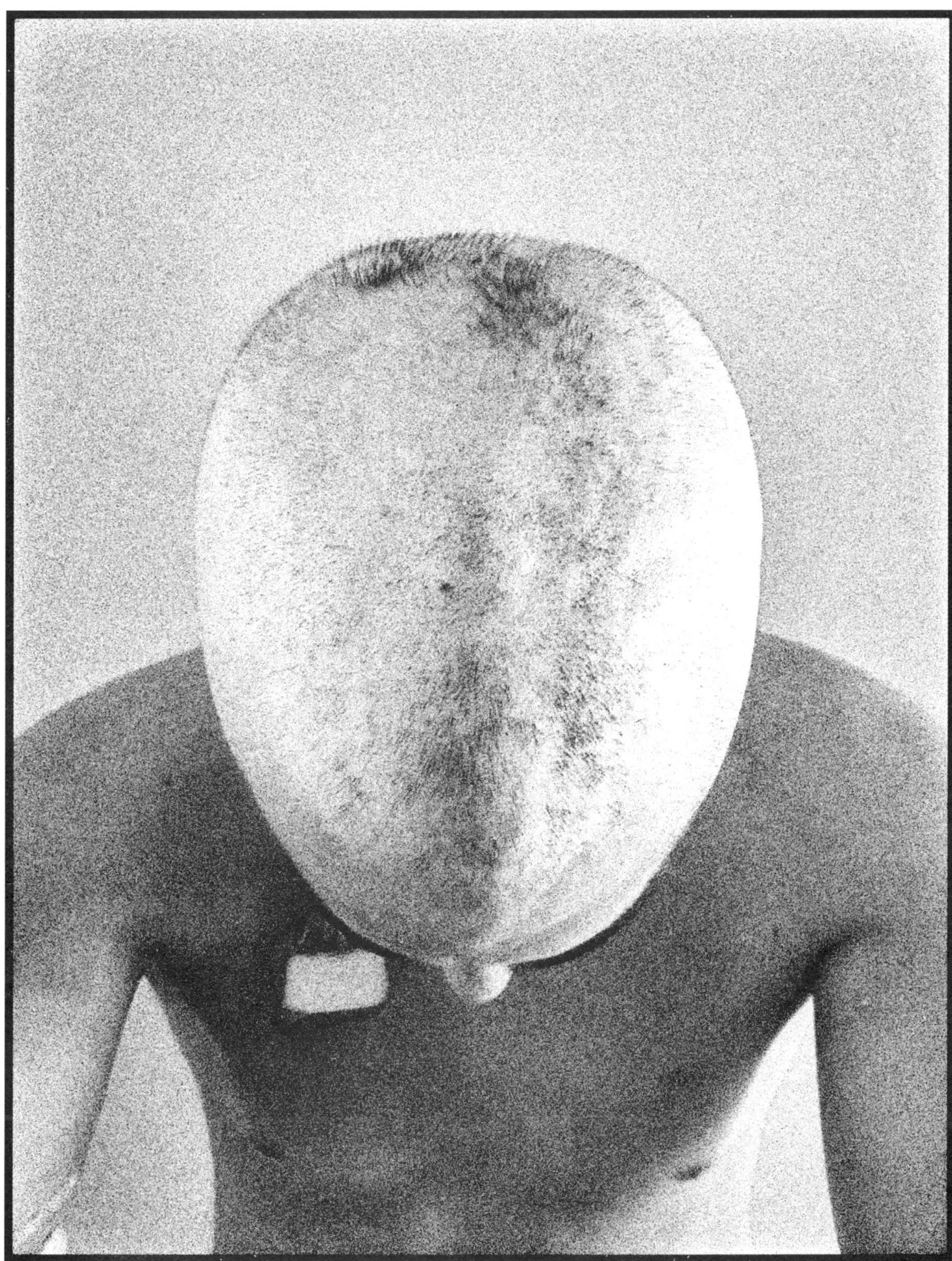

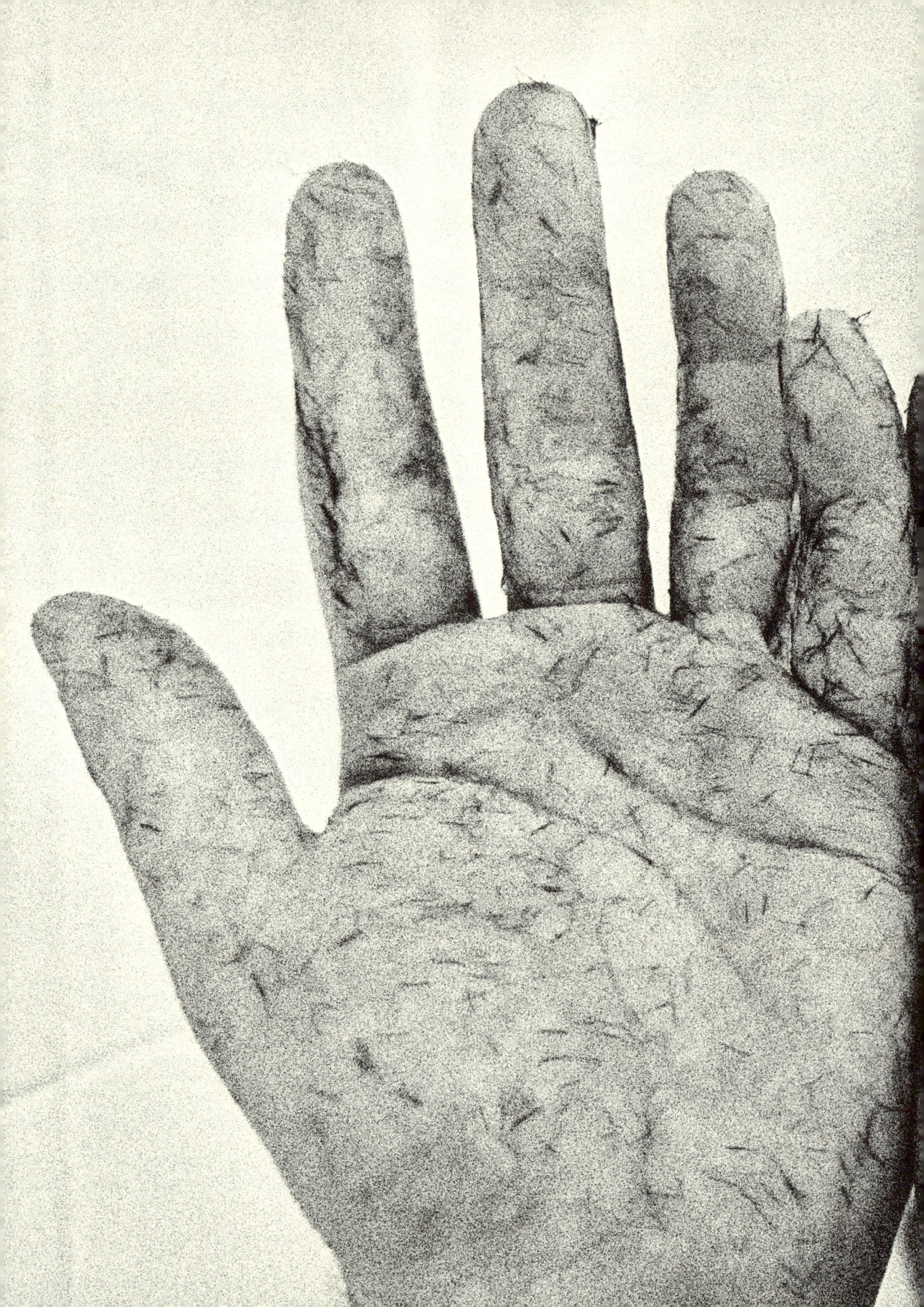

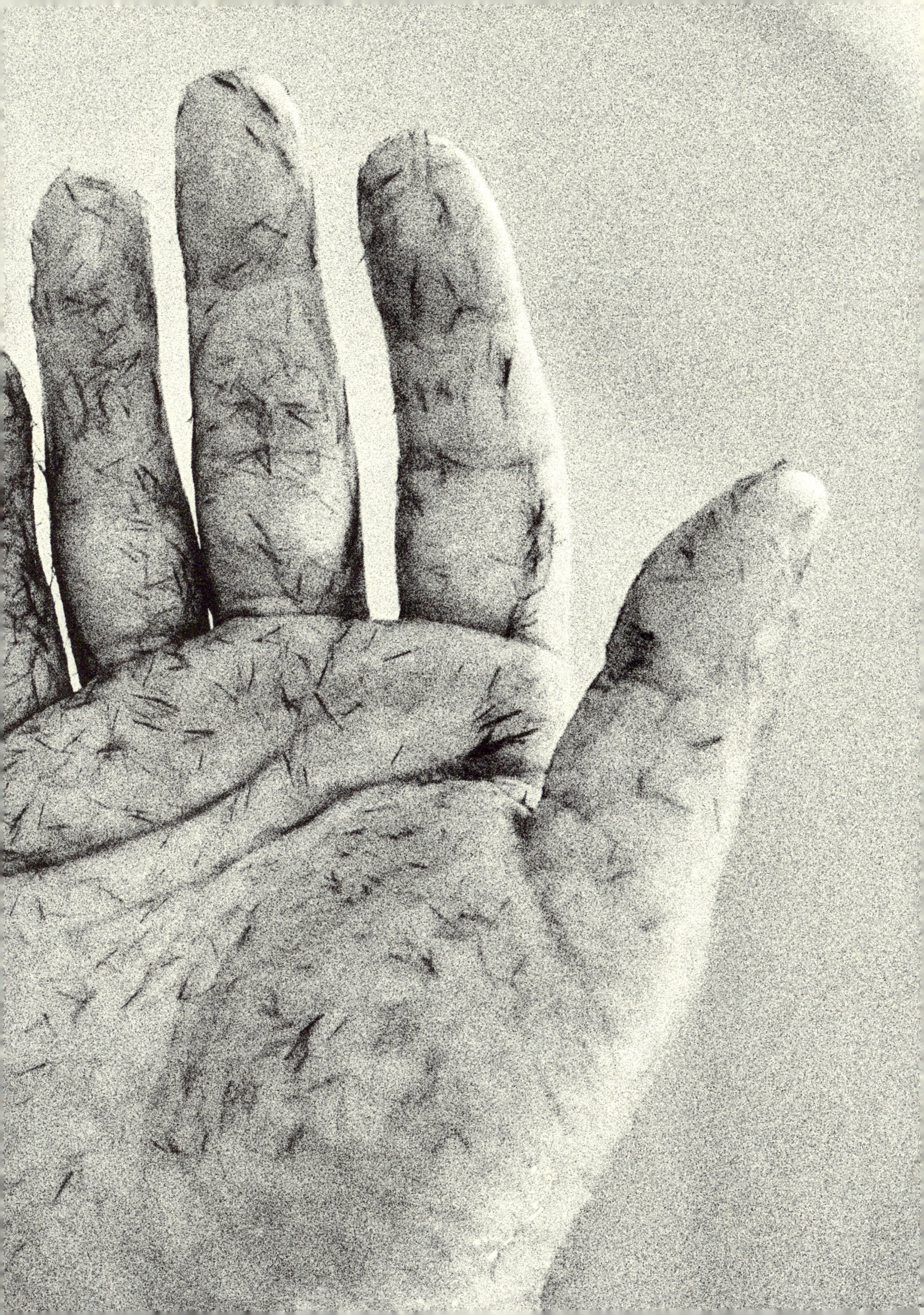

December 20, 2022

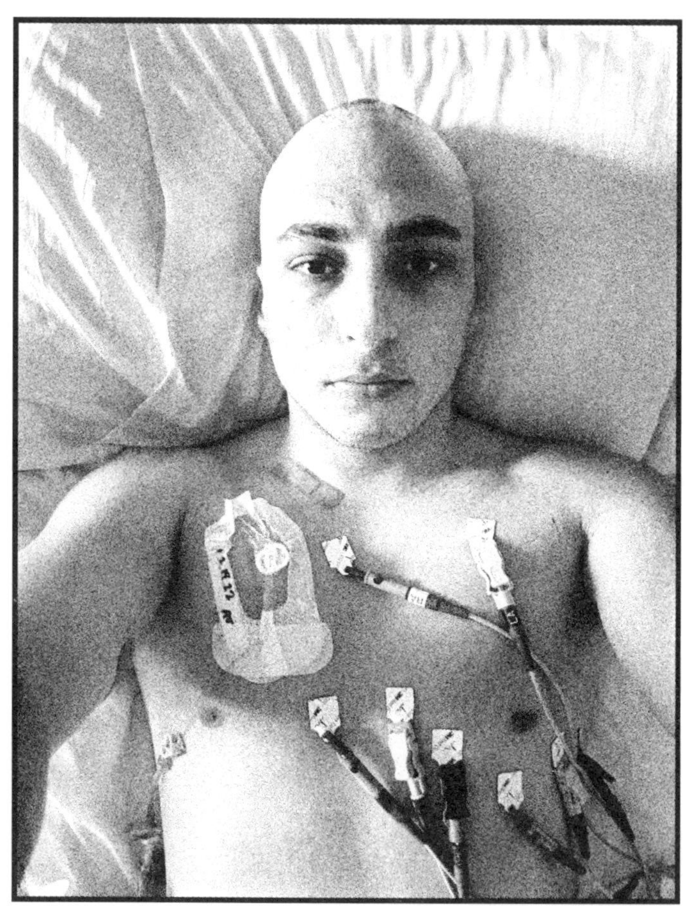

Day by day. Future fears expressed. Tomorrow is undetermined. Our wholeness is ours. Societal belongings are false. We're not exclusive to anyone or anything. We share, commit, support, and love, but we're all really on a selfish journey. Most hear the word "selfish" with a negative connotation, but in truth being selfish is a protection of wholeness. We can never stop our own curiosities from being explored. We're all on a timeline whether we like it or not. Be it for a project or a lifetime. We try to design our future paths, but there's an unpredictability of experience and events. You'll never really know what will happen to your health. Exhibit A. You can't know what's going to happen in the next day, week, or year and how it will affect you or those around you. Something may happen close to someone you know that will in turn affect how you behave or how your relationship with them is. We compare day by day to the artistic process. We go into the artistic process with false confidence, making everyone around us believe we know what the result will be. But in truth all we have is our instincts, experiences, ideas, tools, and belief in ourselves and those around us.

And with our shared experiences and some leadership, we journey to the finish line together with the circumstances that are available. Life is simply a creative process. The night of December 18: on my grandmother's balcony. With traces of the sunset as the night sky appeared. A winter chill in the air. The hot soup against my throat. The high temperature forces a slow swallow when we move too quickly. We don't enjoy the digestion of food. I had a little pause and became deeply present, realizing this was my last moment of normalcy before heading to the hospital. A wave of depression hit. A celebration with family all around. Echoes of their life whisper through my ear from the periphery.

The minimal stresses of work and relationships and the daily issues that they interface with toyed with me. I was quickly reminded of the severity of my diagnosis. The next day before going back into the hospital I spent time working at the Water Garden. I like the word "selfish." I've realized "working" oftentimes has a negative connotation in society too, but in truth I deeply love working. I deeply see my responsibility, or at least one, is to acknowledge the creative potential and ability of those closest to me. And share my ambition and drive by giving them tasks to see their work through and make sure it's shared. I'm simply giving more people homework assignments so that their work is more visible.

After a beautiful walk in the sun, I entered the glass sliding doors to my new home this week. I took a moment to pause under the tree in the courtyard at the hospital. After entering my room, I lay down. Accepted stillness. New nurses. New room. New perspectives of the same experience. One mission: to get this chemo into my body.

Drip.

An immediate humble reminder that I'm not here for it, but rather it's here for me. I surrender to it with gratitude. The sun slowly comes up. The light peeks through the window shade. My love patiently writes my thoughts down. I'm not sure who will ever read these again, whether my future self or someone else, but but these moments of expression are therapy to me. A selfish act of expression. Thank you, my love.

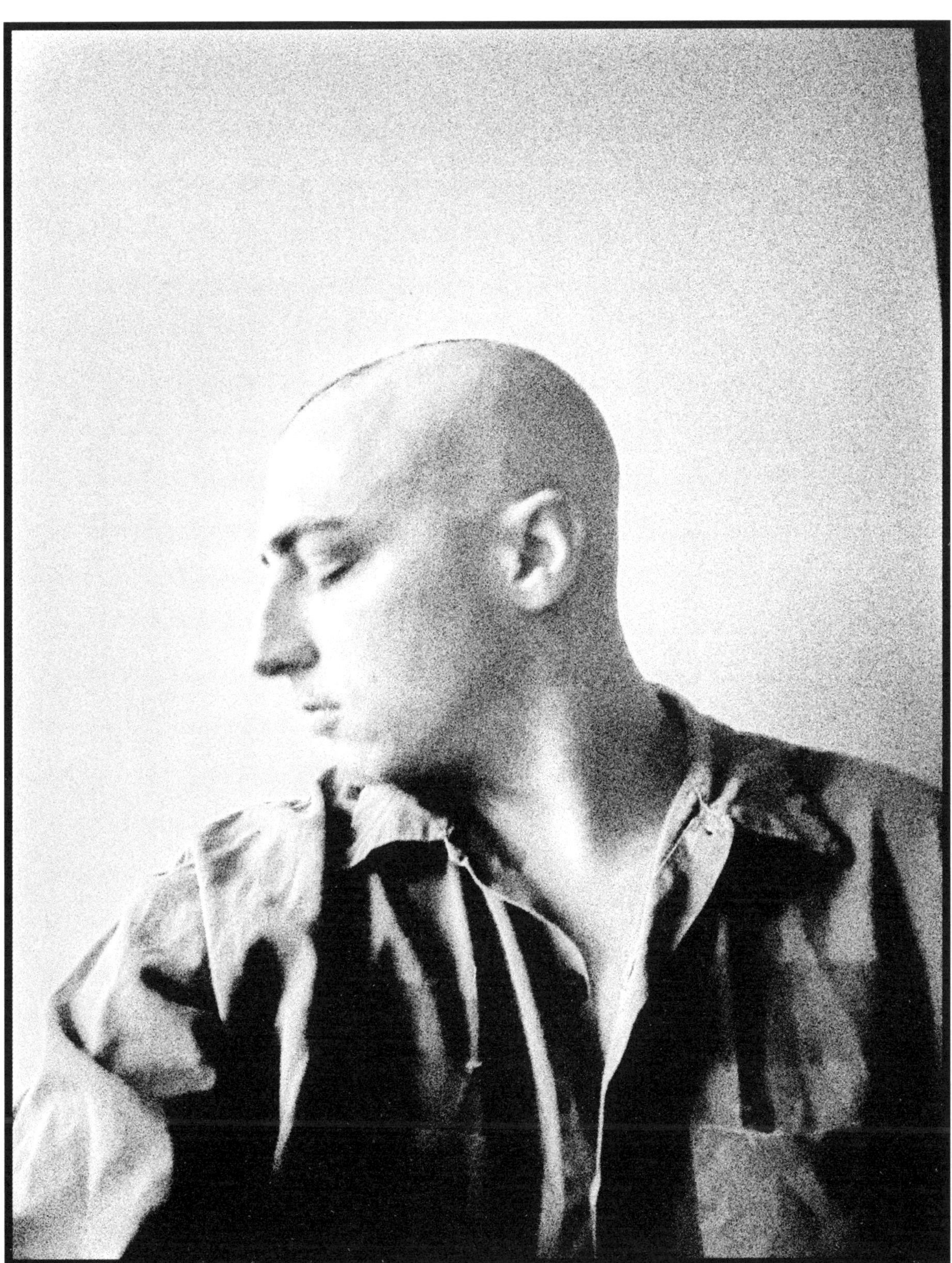

December 21, 2022

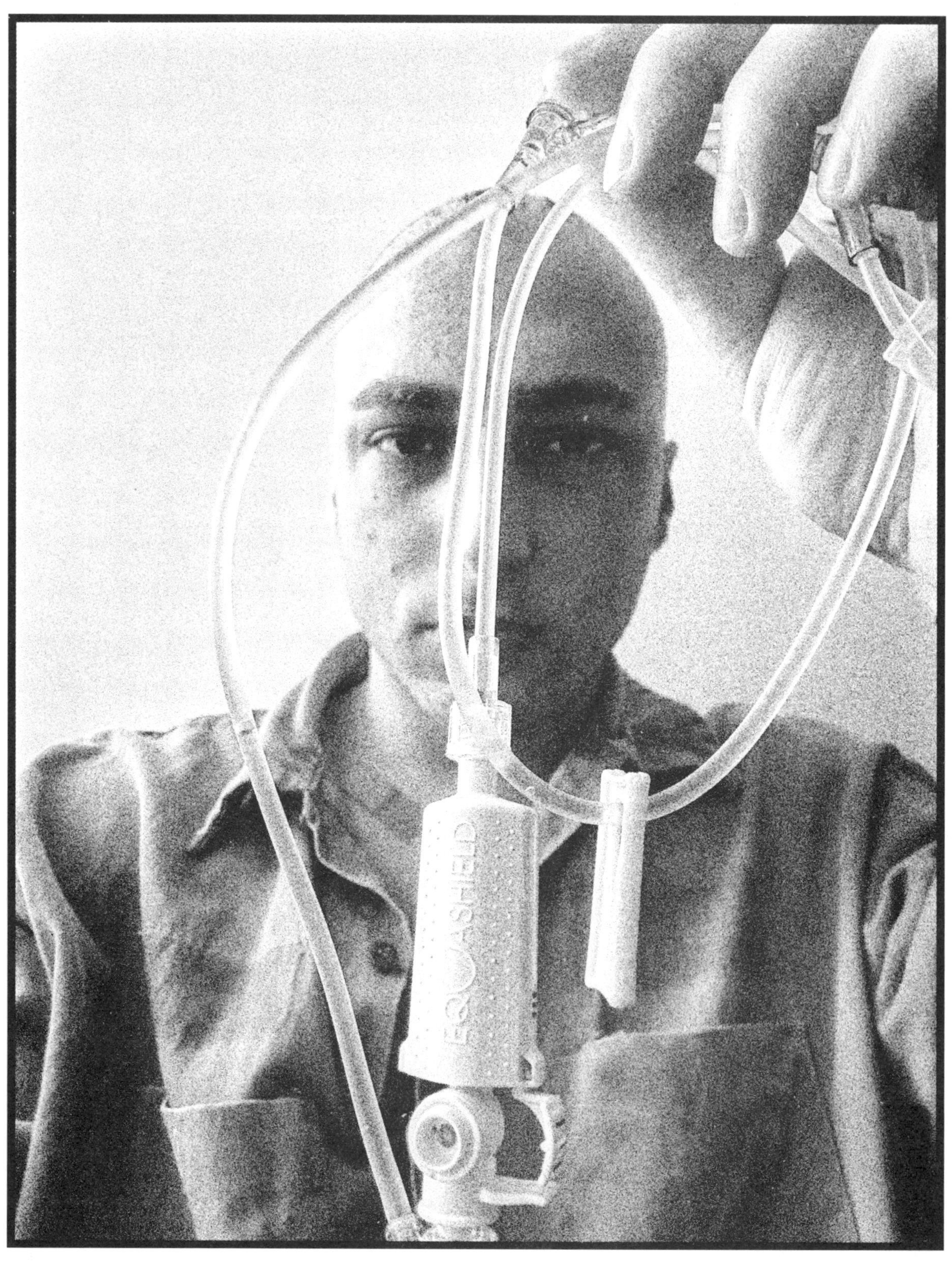

Finding peace in forgiveness. Sometimes holding space in past relationships or traumas can cause you more pain than the person you're in disagreement with. Letting go of that pain is a selfish act. Strength sometimes comes in the little things. There's a deep effort in vulnerability. There's no need to fight between right and wrong. The strength comes in moving on. We've been taught all our lives that exterior strength, appearing to others to be strong, is most important, but after learning about Twitch's death and the need to hold grudges, you realize that internal strength and understanding supersede all else. I lay here watching the continuous bronze drip. I watch the chemotherapy enter my system. My inner being becomes weak and depleted again, while my mind strengthens with sensitivity and poetry. I had a wave of depression coming back in here. Until I was humbly reminded that I'm not here for it, but rather it's here for me. Yesterday I shared a moment with my love, starting a new creative process for a new work called *Drip*. A series of solos verbally communicated from afar. All made while being infused with the chemotherapy. Yesterday's rehearsal felt so healing and purposeful. As artists we continue to pretend we know what we are doing, but we're all really just following a need to solve a problem in real time. As the momentum continues to slow down, the clarity and purpose tend to speed up. Thanks again for writing, my love.

December 22, 2022

Pain so deep and so unfamiliar. I've never experienced this before and it won't go away. I see my mortality again. The internal dialog is toxic, like the chemo entering my system. I try to use visualizations to breathe, but nothing seems to help. What's the opportunity here? Where's the gratitude? I just feel fear and anger. I'm really scared right now. The worst part is there's nothing immediate. It goes too good and then it stops. The slow pain is too deep.

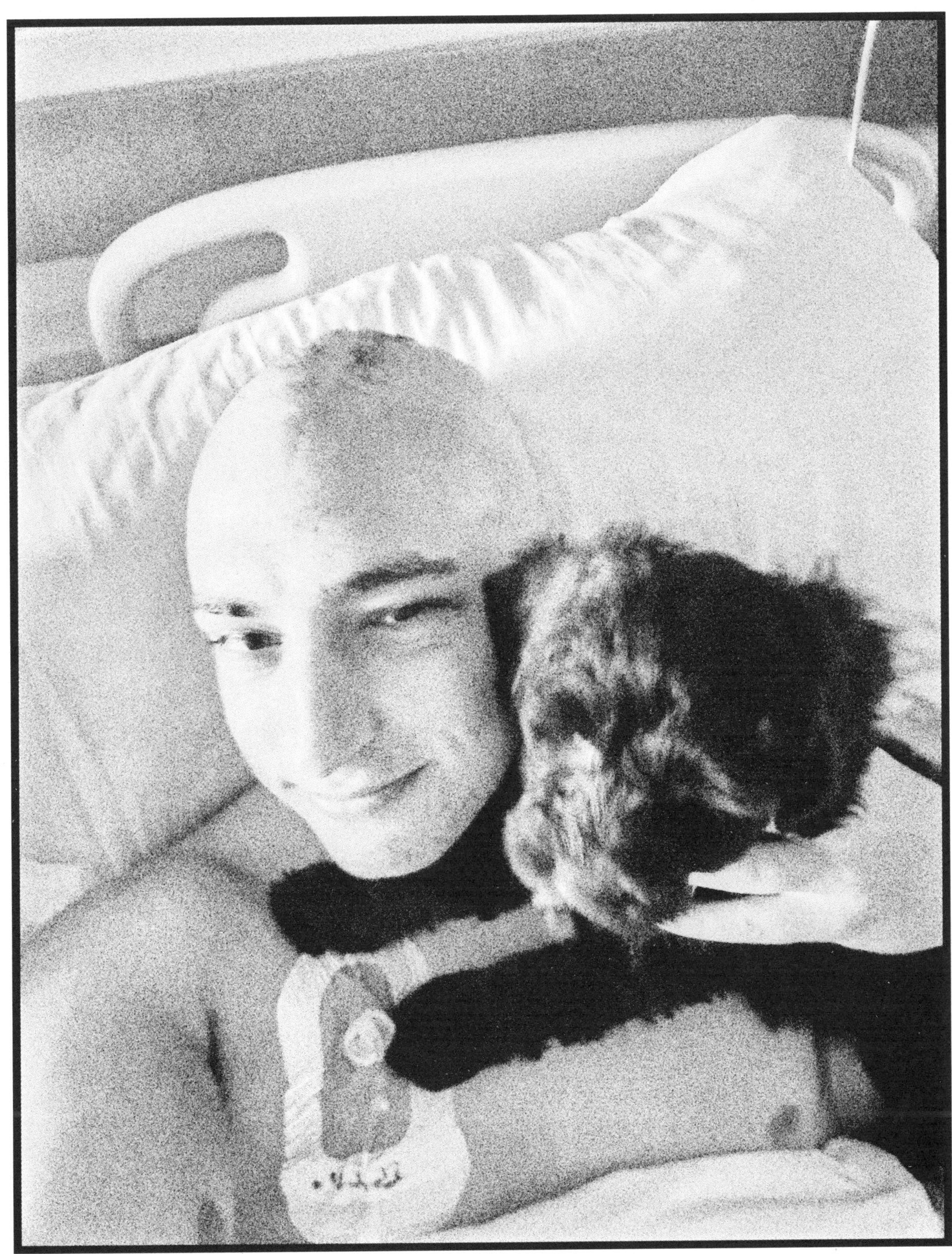

[illegible]in

part

December 23, 2022

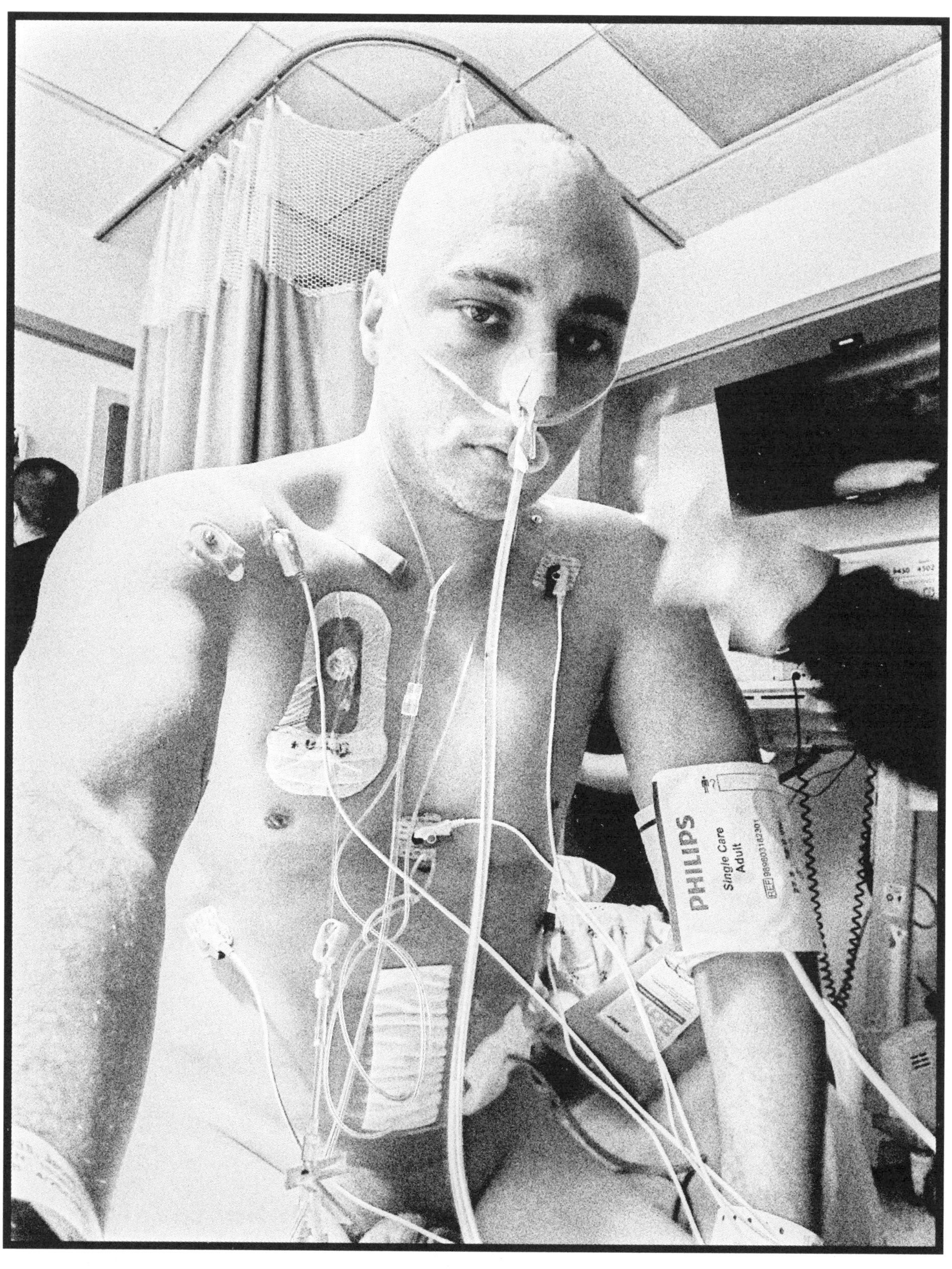

A comprehension of oxygen. A trust in their experience. I've been good at leading with optimism until today. The fear crumbled all down. It's not so much about what I have to do, but rather the scars that last. It's only up to me to communicate I'm not another hamster. I forcefully remind them that I'm a human of great value. There's an accessibility of gravity on a day-to-day basis.

This time though I felt the solar system.

Felt like I got diagnosed all over again. There's a crash course of what could go wrong. The possibilities of "what if." The pain deepens. I just need a solution. You can never really measure somebody's ego versus helpfulness. The overexertion of communication is sometimes not necessary, and with all my fear I'm still conscious and trying to insert my good character. In moments like today I've been recently feeling like my only relationship has been with my lymphoma, but I was slapped by my Crohn's and this existing threesome of self, stomach, and cancer. I'm sure a lot of things could have gone wrong and might still go wrong, but you can only lead with optimism and fate. I'm not leaving here any time soon, but some of these conversations exacerbate the possibility in my mind. I seek so hard to find peace in myself and in others. I reached out for forgiveness and relationships that ended poorly not because they were my fault but because they were occupying space in my mind. Anesthesia. Perforation. Emergency colorectal surgery. Waking up not knowing what happened with acceptance. Upstream. Air in the line. You can't go outside. Privileges.Hydrogen wash cloth. Group therapy. Normalcy. Rarity. Till death do me part. Blindfolded soaks in the sun. Watch out, a bump. The pain was never that deep before. Came to. It's over. I'm fine. The universe did its part. A few small discomforts. Inner tubing through my holes. A desire for a deep breath. I'll be good soon. But will I remember these great details? The ocean's calling my name. The salt water along my face. My feet buried in the earth. The waves crash just to my ankles. Thanks for writing, my love.

December 24, 2022
Morning

Searching so deeply to find the lesson here. The value of a nurse and care partner is indescribable. I thought the vulnerabilities of shitting myself in the middle of the night and fainting and urinating was as worse as it could get. I learned I had to get surgery to my stomach yesterday, and it was very clear I couldn't hear the details. I learned about the possibility of having a colostomy bag attached and I absolutely lost it. Again, I'm open to the lesson, but that's not it. Adaptive versus submissive. I can't submit to the bullshit. I'm not a fucking hamster. As I rolled through the hallway and finally met with the anesthesiologist, he wanted to go into great detail about what the surgery was going to be. I told him to just stop and do it. Put me to sleep and get it done. As I came to and I didn't have the bag connected to my body, it felt like the biggest win, but yet I was still deeply uncomfortable and aware of all the new attachments to my body. A tube down my nose, a new IV in my left arm pumping new fluids, oxygen in my nose and also measuring my carbon dioxide. A little red ball coming out of my left hip connected to my digestive system, but I can't get the courage to ask what it is although they say it will be temporary. Last, amongst other things, are constant vitals. When I finally get some shut eye, my blood pressure wakes me. Or this little green trigger that communicates when I need pain medication.

I don't care whatever happens to me in my life, one of the things I'll always most value is my hygiene. I woke up in the middle of the night smelling like absolute shit. I haven't showered and I've been so desperately trying to pee lying down. Each time I urinate it burns so badly, and just recently learned they stuck a catheter through my penis for the surgery. After a thoughtful and patient cleanse and a brushing of the teeth, I felt ready to return back to bed.

It's unacceptable now that we have hoodies that anyone visits me without being in uniform. I've never been in this much pain in my life. Or endured this physical vulnerability, but I'm still investigating what's to learn here. I've always had this inner drive deeper than anyone else when it came to my life's approach. I don't know if it stemmed from family trauma, being bullied, not succeeding academically or what. I do remember, when I was hospitalized here nine years ago for Crohn's, there was a great threat to my life physically that gave me a motivation like no other. This experience since being diagnosed, I've authentically questioned my mortality on a weekly basis. I really don't feel confident in my future health right now. That's a statement I feel and I'm worried. Although it's a temporary worry. Maybe I'll be fine. This too shall pass. But it is also becoming the biggest infrastructure for drive and motivation to take over the world when I'm good and able to. There's not enough time in the world. There's not enough time in the day. There's not enough time to tell those that you love them. I'm dealing with forced maturity here. I'm ready for it to be natural again.

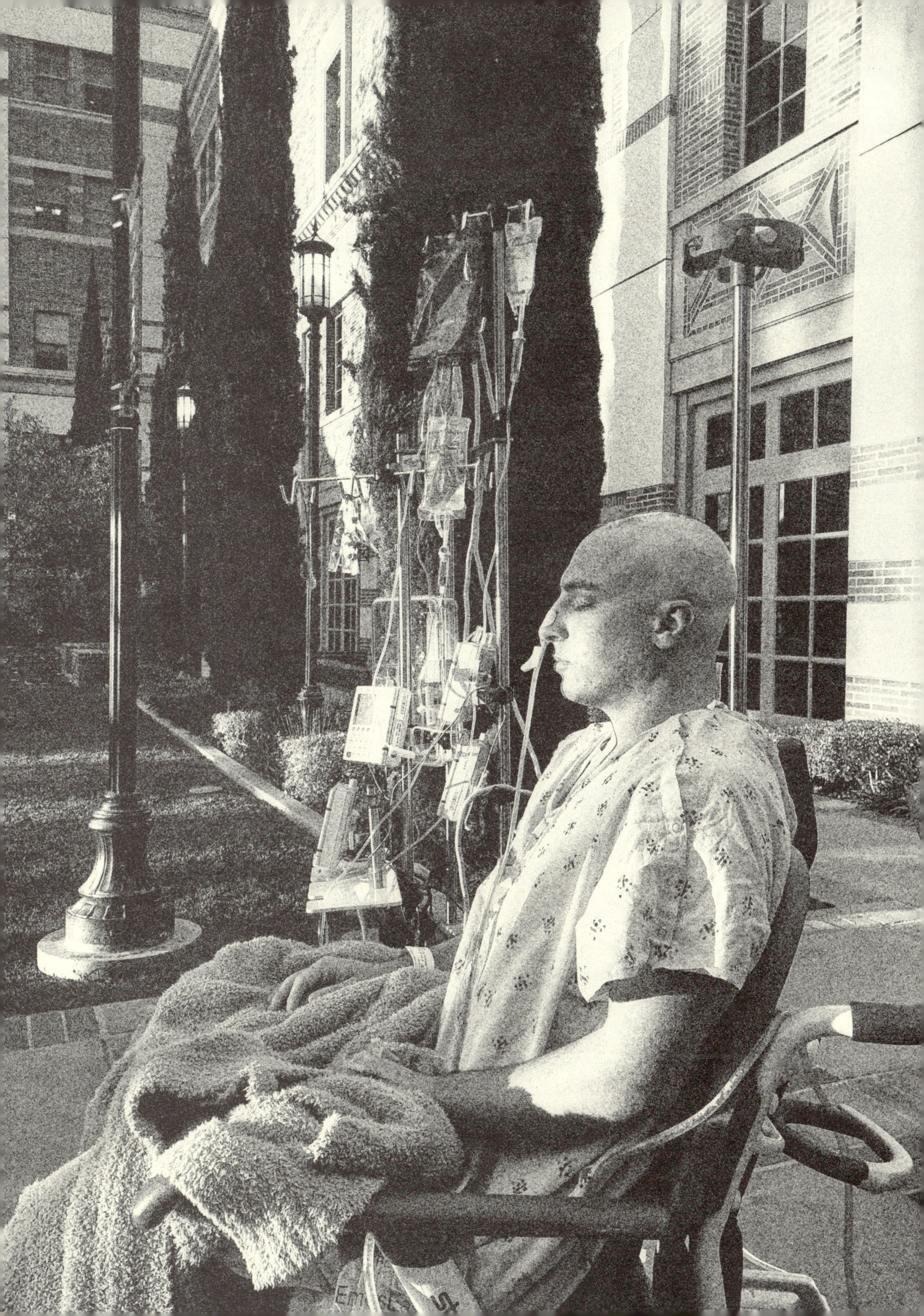

December 24, 2022
Evening

12.24.22

A rare bird uncaged, wings clipped, flaring outside my little room. The power of outdoor freedom. Its not solitary confinement but rather refinement. Two different sets of stitches in my stomach at the time. The beauty of sunlight's kiss. The power of temperature. The 6th sense we dont talk about. Im still trying to figure out if this transformation is one thats meant to be healing or hurting, but regardless I know im growing through all the interruptions. Theres a peace in the unknowing. A gratitude. Collection of gatherings without me for me. But for them too. I lay in stillness today as ideas came to me. It was really for the first time as an author that the ideas werent mine but I was borrowing them. Ideas im so excited to explore Them in their reality and those that are over exaggerated. 10 breaths shared. Come get us when youre ready. A conversation never had to be long. The sun went down. The bodies disconnected from all the ill in this hospital. They started flaring off their physical appearance and swimming towards the sky. Arent we all just disconnected from our physical beings anyways. This moment is shared on Saturday evening My first time leaving this hospital and walking into the garden since Monday. I started walking Liam appeared I looked to him and I cried. I was overtaken by his presence and having him see me in my current state. After sharing my journal with Emma she came in this morning expressing her admiration for the role you play in my life. And that it brought her such happiness that made me so happy. Were all a good team on a great mission. I love you. Thanks for writing.

A rare bird uncaged, wings clipped, flying outside my little room. The power of outdoor freedom. It's not solitary confinement but rather refinement. Two different sets of stitches in my stomach at the time. The beauty of sunlight's kiss. The power of temperature. The sixth sense we don't talk about. I'm still trying to figure out if this transformation is one that's meant to be healing or hurting, but regardless I know I'm growing through all the interruptions. There's peace in the unknowing. A gratitude. Collections of gatherings without me for me. But for them too. I lay in stillness today as ideas came to me. It was really for the first time as an author that the ideas weren't mine but I was borrowing them. Ideas I'm so excited to explore. Them in their reality and those that are over-exaggerated. Ten breaths shared. Come get us when you're ready. A conversation never had to be long. The sun went down. The bodies disconnected from all the ill in this hospital. They started flowing off their physical appearance and swimming toward the sky. Aren't we all just disconnected from our physical beings anyway? This moment is shared on Saturday evening. My first time leaving this hospital and walking into the garden since Monday. I started walking, Liam appeared, I looked at him and I cried. I was overtaken by his presence and having him see me in my current state. After sharing my journal with Emma, she came in this morning, expressing her admiration for the role you play in my life. And that it brought her such happiness. That made so happy. We're all a good team on a great mission. I love you. Thanks for writing.

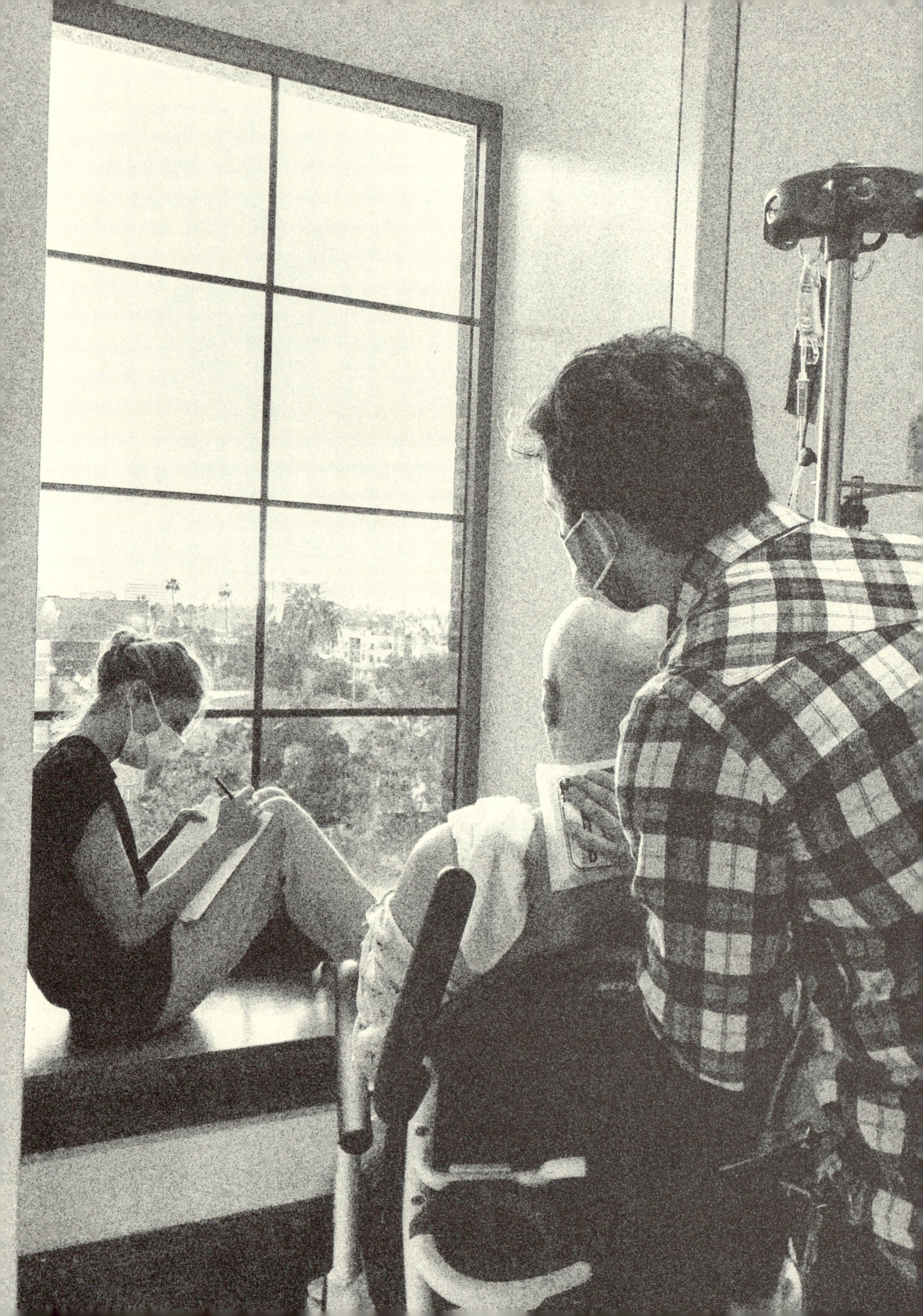

I've never been in this much pain in my life. Or endured this physical vulnerability, but I'm still investigating what's to learn here.

December 25, 2022

My strength is indefinite. I'll never lose until I give up. My motivation is so clear. I don't know if I can separate my work, my character, my community, or my ability to coexist and observe these great gifts of the world, but they are now unforgivably mine and I'm leading with full force. My mission could never be as clear as it is now. I'm going to change the world. It's not going to be in that artificial way where I thought I was going to control it. But I'm going to let it control me. I'm the gardener, the seeds, the sunlight, the water. I'm going to manipulate the roots and where they go. The birds will fly toward the ocean. The temperatures will change as the chemo goes through my blood; it feels like history. People will soon stop saying they are sorry for what I have been through, and they will say how lucky I am. I really feel integrated into the roots, into the leaves, into the sunlight. I can feel everyone's heart beating around me. My face is smiling.

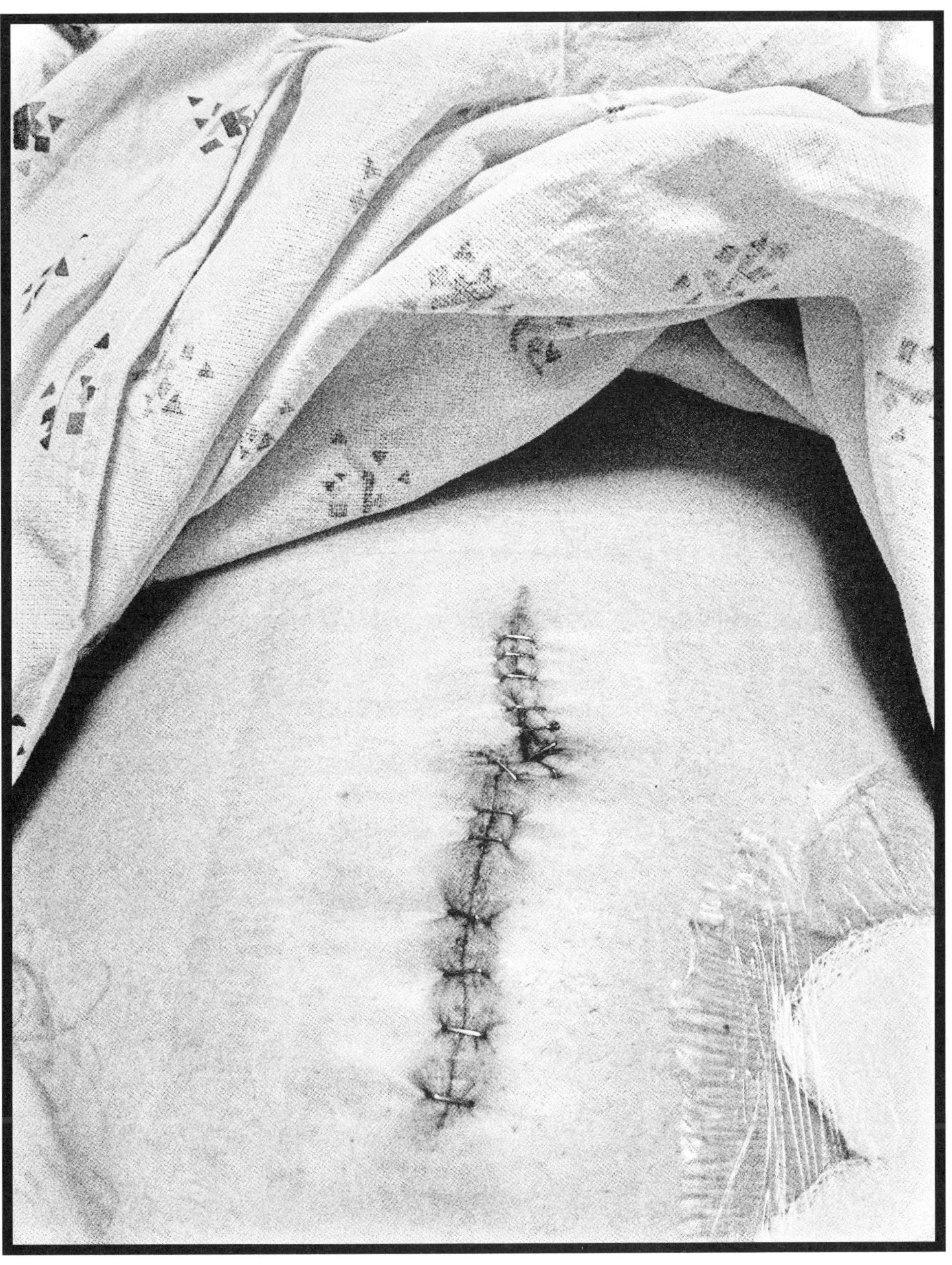

December 27, 2022

A preparation of blood transfused. A borrowing of someone else's stream to amplify my frequency. From the external I'm visually overcoming things I thought I never could. The things I would squint at in movies and have to look away.

Transfusion – a product from someone else's body.

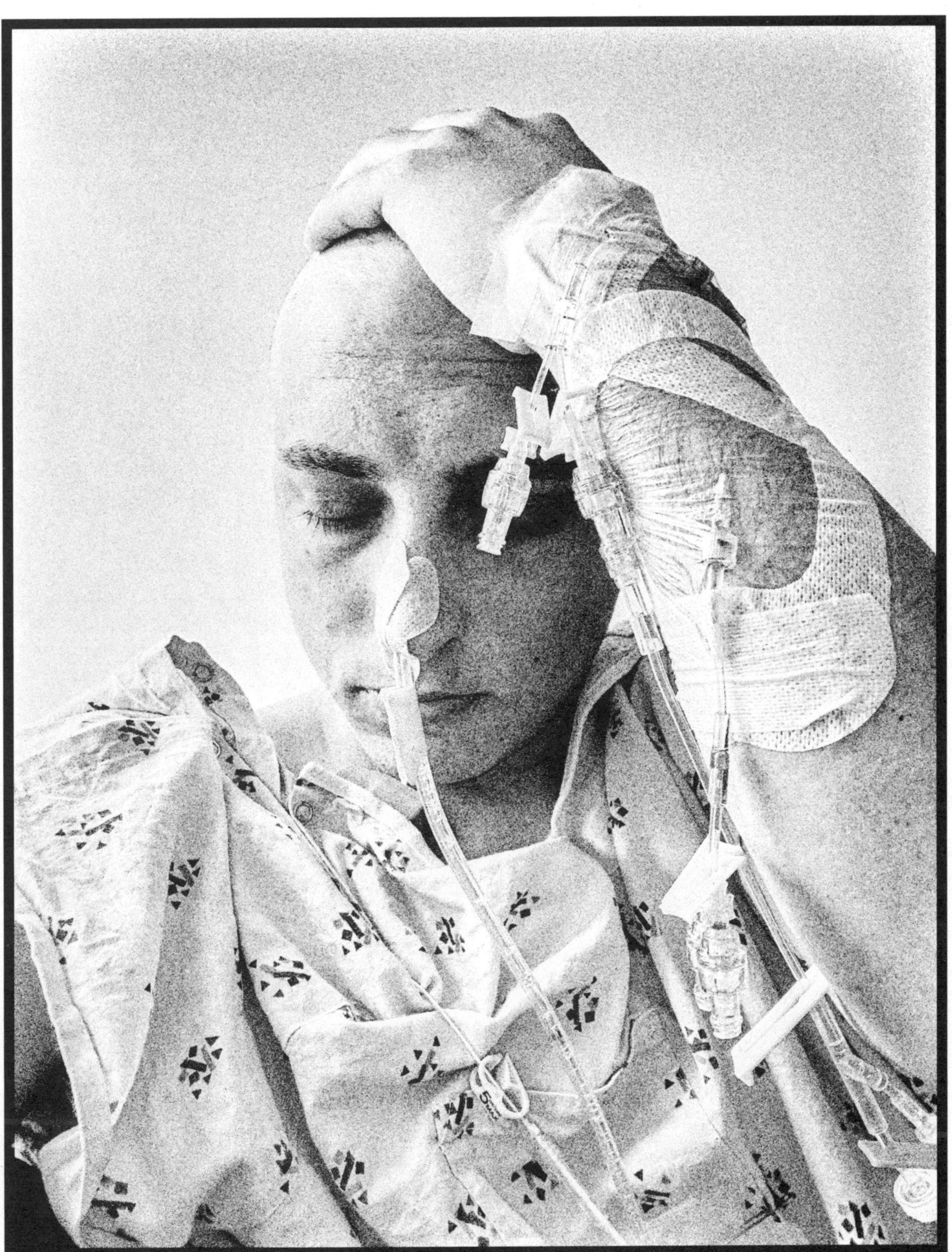

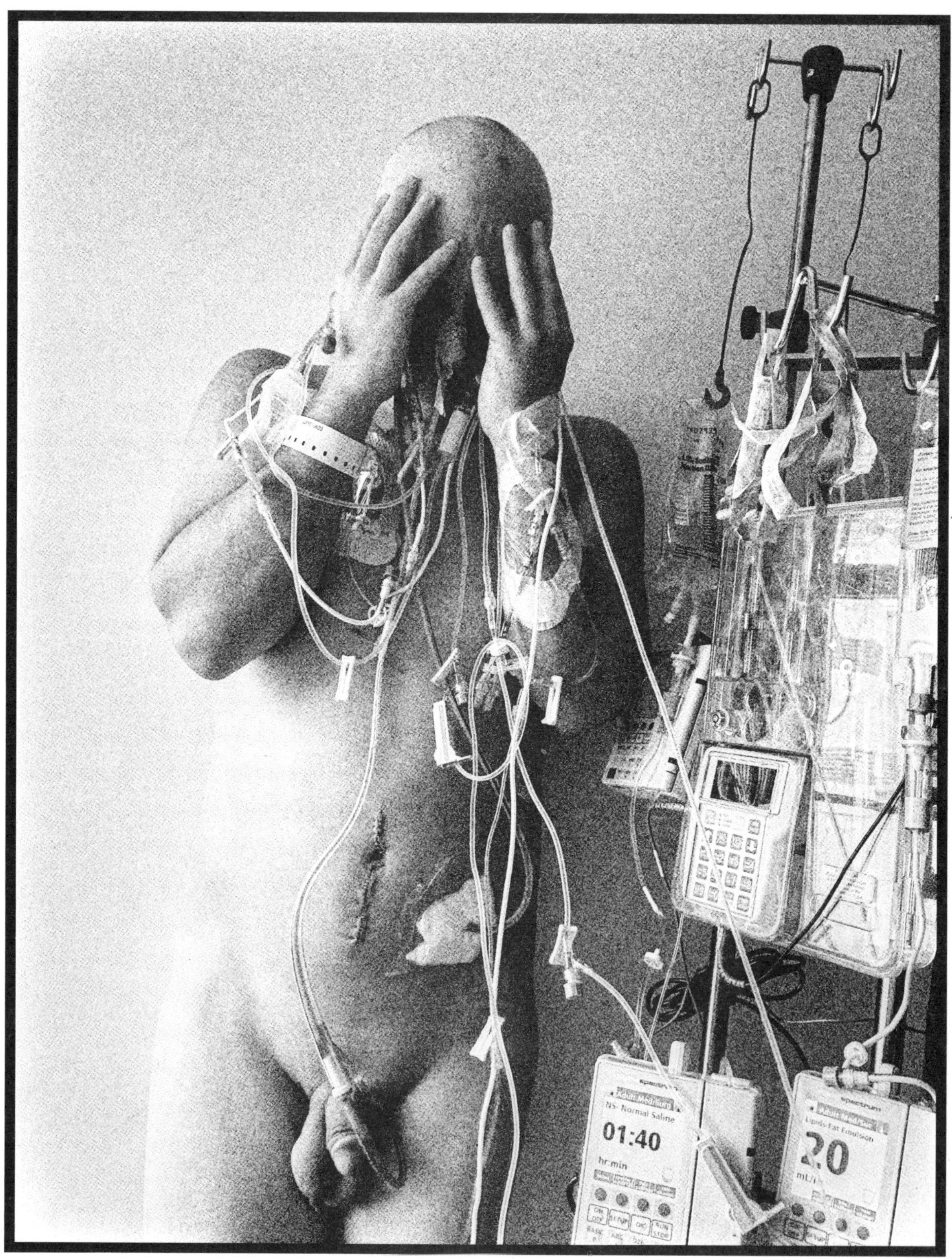
NS- Normal Saline
01:40
hr:min
spectrum
Lipids Fat Emulsion
20

I'm cemented in deep sadness. My tears pour constantly. Feelings of loneliness, of being alone, of confusion and not knowing when there is an end in sight. The pain silences me, which is symbolic because the most pain I have is in my throat, making it as though I can't speak. I used to look at Mallory through the eyes of the observer, noticing the physical endurance and observing great sympathy, but there's also the impossibility knowing that something like this could ever happen to me. But now it is. And all my friends and family see it through the observer. I'm the only one struggling now. The tube down my throat, the visible vacuum of my digestive system. The external bloodstream. The small ball coming out of my stomach with acid. The production and permission to walk outside for a small window of time. People don't know what to do but hover and surround. The bird was taken out of its cage to fly, but everyone still stares as though its wings are clipped. The timeline for these outings is short. You can see the normality for everyone else knowing what to do. The lost gratitude to stand independently of a plug, to swallow water, to walk outside without supervision, to shower, to cleanse. The highs and lows continue. The valleys so much deeper in between. The more I listen, the more I feel my voice is stronger. I really have no more time left. I know exactly what needs to be done. I know exactly who I want to do it with.

After a deep moment being rolled around the concrete square I desperately needed to surrender. Lying down into the earth. There was so much noise so I politely asked everyone to simply breathe with me. Knowing that my time to be there was limited. The sun hit me so deeply and I lost all control. My emotional being became an earthquake that wouldn't stop vibrating. I felt the grass grow over me. Like a timelapse in real time. And it cradled me like a cocoon around a butterfly. My face was still there, crying, but my physical being was intertwined in the earth. Just like that we all went upstairs. This journey continues. The sleepless nights. The chemo mind. The constant chemical exchange. I'm a hamster in real time. And this too will pass. It shall. With all the pain that's involved and the sadness, I don't want it to pass too soon. I don't want to forget these moments. These valuable moments in my head of presence.

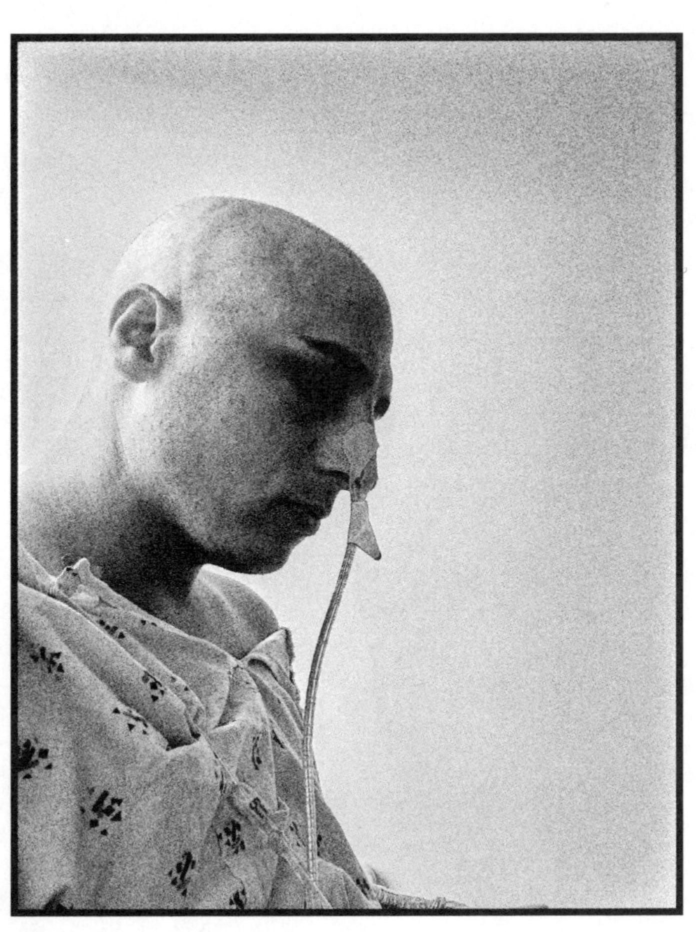

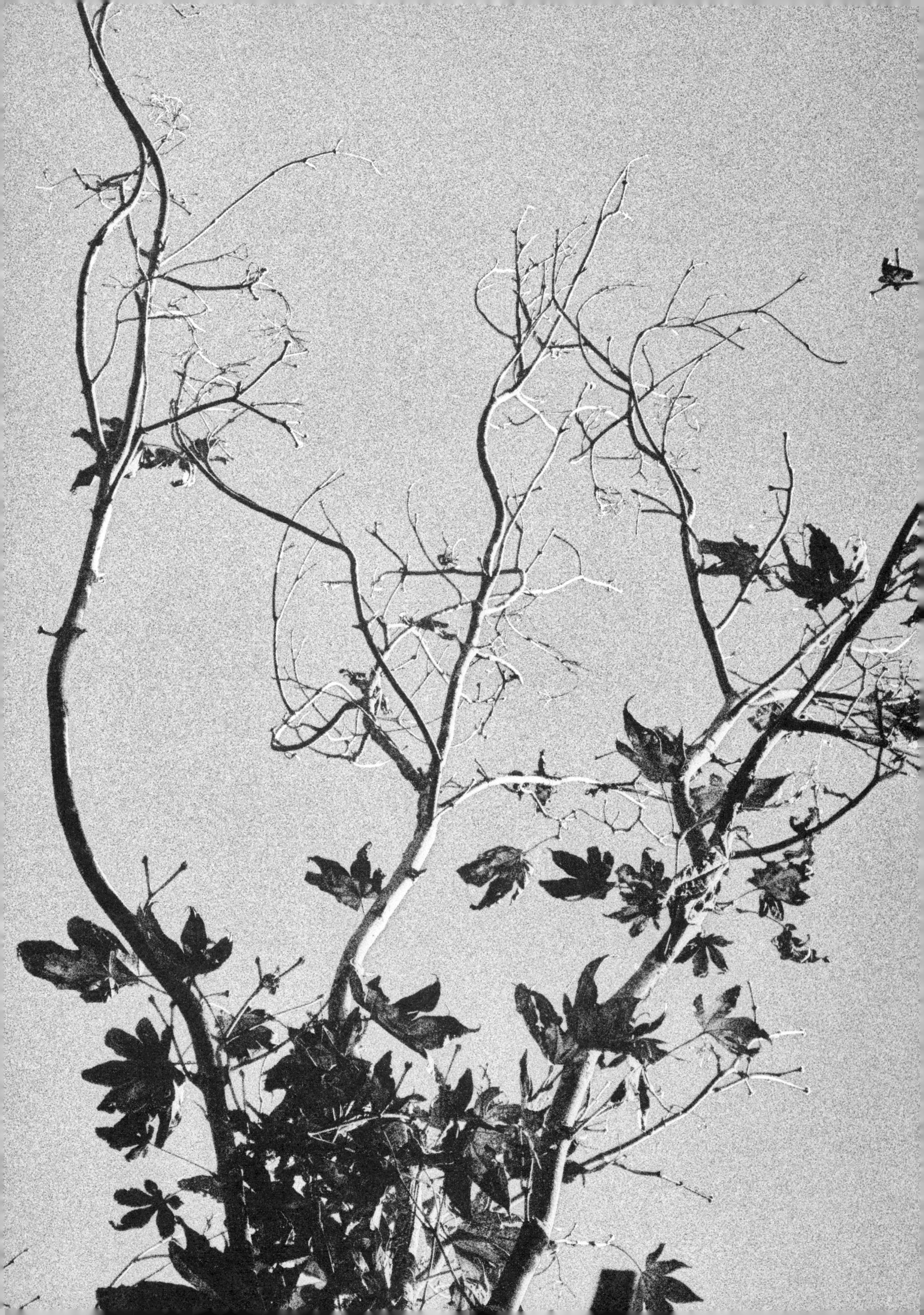

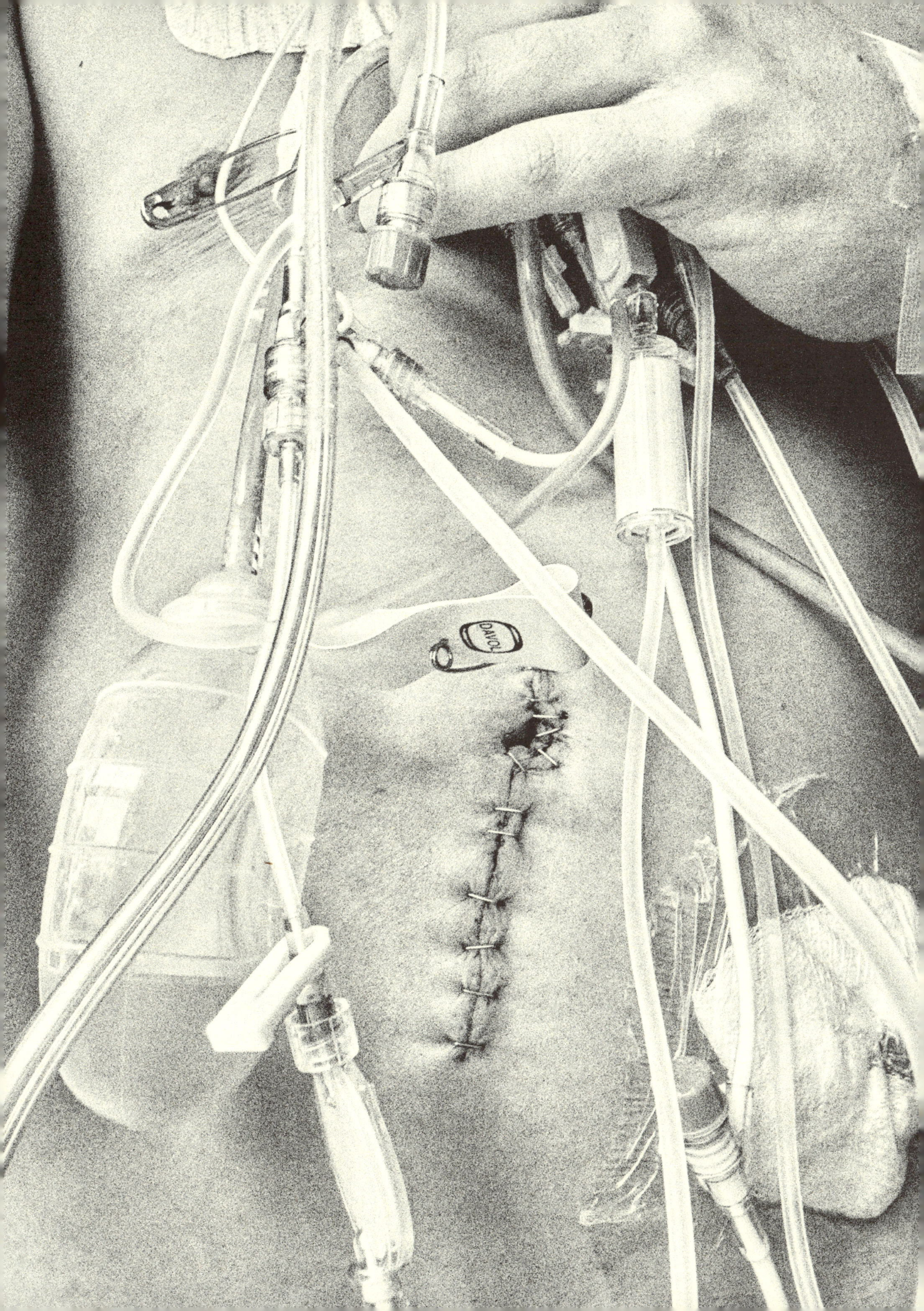
DAVOL

December 28, 2022

I'm suffocating in deep sadness right now. Every time I just sit and think about anything in relation to my life, this stream pours from my eyes. I access these deep emotions, and my stomach shakes like the earth's plates moving. The hardest thing I'm experiencing right now is the realization that these experiences of what I'm going through are so deeply rooted in my identity now. I really don't want people to see me like this. I don't want to feel in this trap any more. I feel like my arms are flailing and tangling in these tubes. They're just all over me, and my circumstances don't seem to have a finish line. I really need this to end now. I'm so desperate to go home. I want nothing more than to put my ankles on the ocean sand so the water hits them. I'm scared knowing that I've experienced this and that I'll always be able to access this in the future in my mind. I'm scared when my close friends and family see me now that they will see this as part of me no matter what I do to try to take it away. I'm also scared because I don't know where this is going. When I get discharged, this is no means the end. I have four more chemo treatments, post op evaluations all led by optimism. With no certainty that everything will go right. There's still a possibility things may go wrong. As I sit here, I think about the complexity of life. We can have our own traumas of identity through wealth, class, economic ability, race, religion, geography. Even through the association of feeling other people's pain or loss and grief. However, there is no more superior priority and cause of importance than one individual's personal health. Or the threat and illness to it.

In the past 24 hours, the tube was released through my nose. It was one of the most painful things I've experienced in my life. Not just physically but also what it represented emotionally.

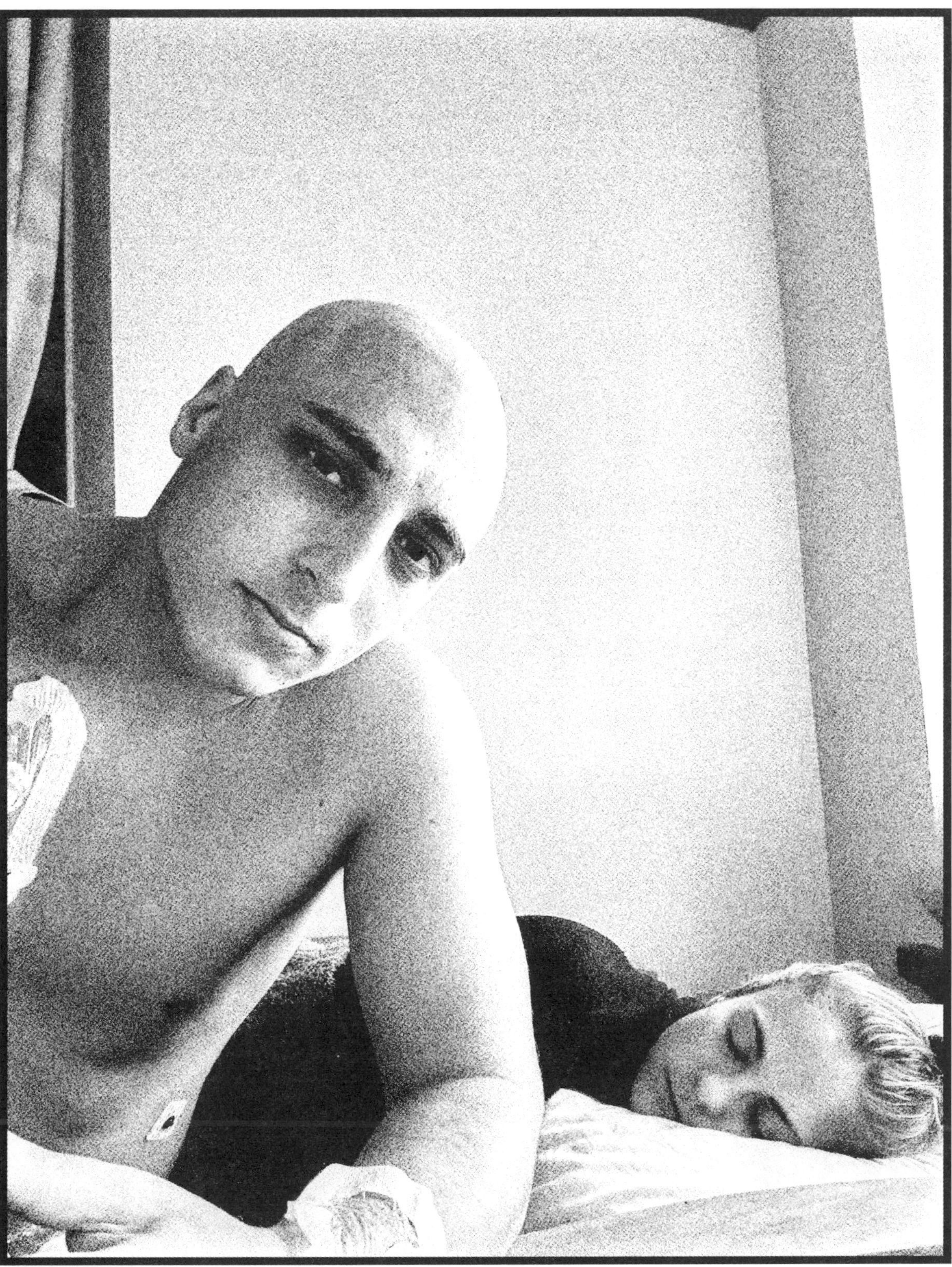

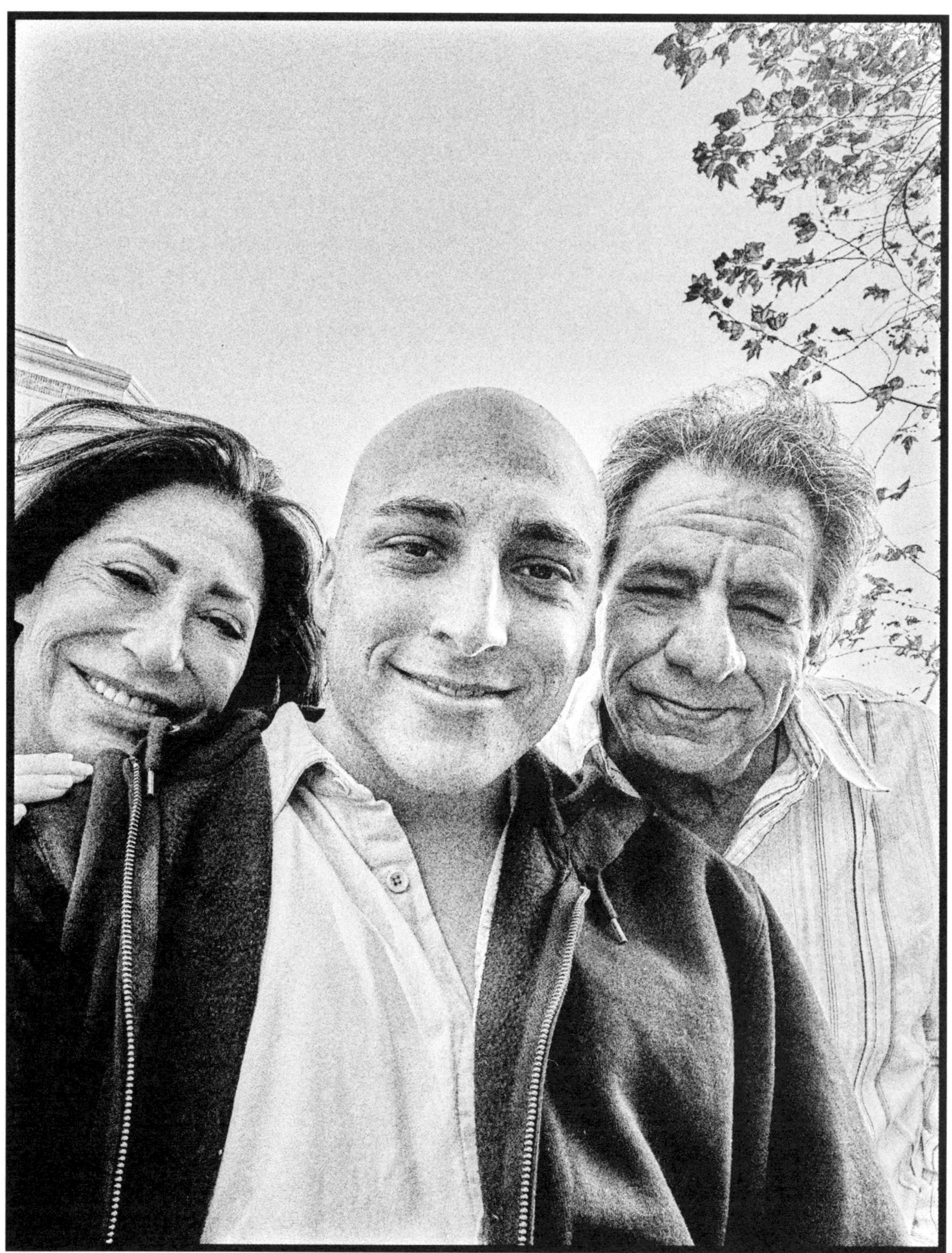

Feeling that sense of real freedom after five days was so liberating. A freedom comparable to what Nina Simone speaks of. Additionally, I swallowed water for the first time in six days. I independently moved a stool after having my digestive system exist externally. That created so much pressure but also so much relief. I was able to go outside. And expose my bald skull to the light drizzle after having walked a few steps. That's where I currently am – walking, pooping, drinking water, and breathing independently. That's some of the most significant wins I am having. During these times we are told to visualize our healing. To visualize our discharge. But overall to practice visualization as a tool of progress. While I've been here, I've had a lot of visualizations about my life outside of here too. The work that I need to make, how I need to feel about myself, and how my creativity can change the world. And it will. It will be the largest scale as well. I'm ready to write my masterpiece. It's been really hard to go on the internet and still see the talk shows, the selfies, in this desperate digital world of acceptance. For now, I'll continue to sit here, waiting patiently. Grateful to see the end in sight soon with my discharge. While speaking, my eyes have been closed but my body has slowly rotated. My arms and head and balance points continue to shift and my body has shrunk in my own mind. I wonder what that means. I wonder what it all means.

A rare photo with my parents.

December 29, 2022

I've understood the distinction between business and art. Yesterday, I finally received clarity on the difference between reality and imagination. I've been seeing such deep visualizations over the past few weeks, and yesterday was the first moment I could sit outside with my dog under a tree and enjoy the sunlight. It made me realize the ingredients to most films include imagination but they are also balanced with these moments of reality. I understood what my life needed from here on out. Which is to design and innovate and lead compassion and bring all these ideas to life that come to me, but this is just going to be part of my journey. The other part will be experiencing these reality moments of spending time with the people I love. Being embraced and observing nature. And not just growing myself but allowing anything with a heartbeat to grow next to me. My dad whispered while I was outside, "Isn't it so nice to relax?" I realized I didn't like the word "relax." It's an active verb that should be scheduled when you're not doing something of importance. However, presence, inactivity, and simply doing nothing are a great use of activity. One should never relax. However, their life should be more balanced with activity of the mind and presence of the mind. I then got my first acupuncture session with an Eastern doctor at UCLA. After a beautiful and emotional connection, I heard him say under his tongue the word "busy," and realized I hated that word because it creates a sense of inaccessibility and stress. Two things that don't allow you to have authentic access to someone else. From then on out, I realized that each person coming through my door medically wasn't just someone I was looking to for healing or advice but that they needed some help too. An acknowledgment of their family, a day off from work or just simply a scan of what could help them. I'm starting to feel and see that about everybody.

That most people choose distraction and pain over presence and ability to be the best they can be. People's motivations are just wrong. I lay here with this deep knowing that I will change the world. Not for fame or ego but because I really feel I've been given a gift this past week of perspective that can change the world for the better.

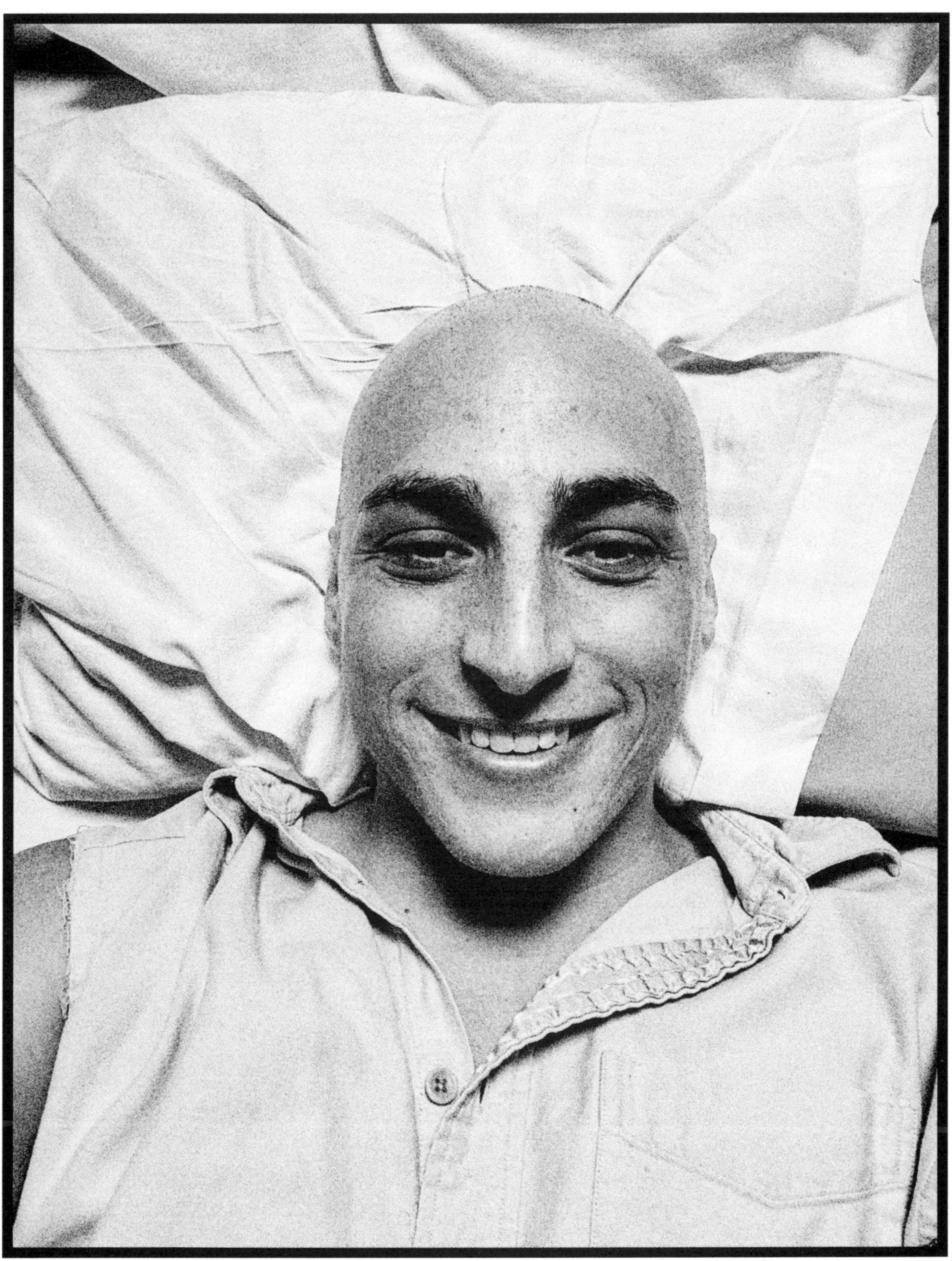

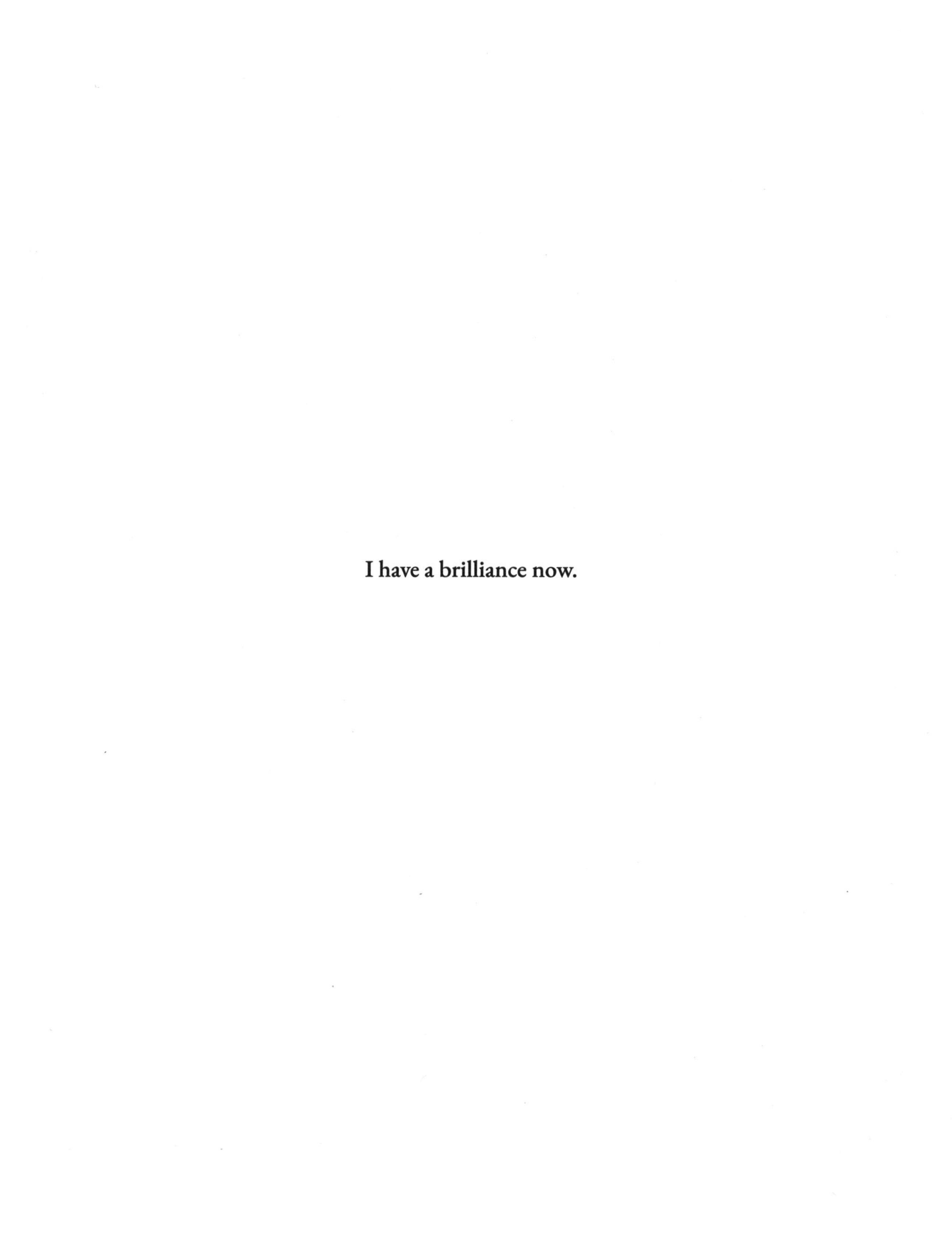

I have a brilliance now.

The trauma of what I experienced is part of me, but now so too is this brilliance. It made me think a lot about Kanye West because he has the brilliance as well, but his need to be president or have a platform to speak distracts him from his brilliance. Steve Jobs also had this brilliance, but he knew to keep his head down and use his imagination to change the world. He never let his ego get in the way. We as beings need to be more selfish so that we can better become selfless as contributors. We can't prioritize other needs at the cost of our emptiness. If we are whole, it will make others around us whole too. Through a meditation yesterday and a deep admiration of Pixar and Steve Jobs, I realized I was ready to start my Apple. The name is so important, and after reflecting on the words "busy" and "relaxed," I knew I had to choose words like "apple" that were accessible but deeply meaningful too. Yesterday also was the first day I saw the light at the end of the tunnel. The tunnel being the worst week of my life. That light was spiritual but it was also a deep gaze of the sun. The sun is the most important star of the universe; and to the human body the spine, especially to me, is visually the most important part because it connects the body together. I realized connecting those two words would create SpineSun, which felt incredibly purposeful, the name I want to move forward with. The last thing I wanted to write about in regard to my reality is my newfound love of Sammy, my little man. It's incredible the parallels that are happening right now – from having poops, going on a walk outside, getting enough sleep, having the right care, doing things academically versus holistically, by feeling and seeing how the most basic presence can create fear or gratitude in someone. I feel so connected to my little man and the parallels of our lives. I feel so confident to take care of him and make sure he grows well. And he will take care of me and be the reason I go to the beach, I feel the sun, I walk outside, and I listen to something more than my needs. I will love that dog with all my heart.

December 30, 2022

Design mappings to normalcy while anticipating discharge. I fear what exists outside of this block. What's it like to cross the street again? There's a whole system in these walls, and time is our only operator. I'll be back in here soon. But in the time between I'll need to pretend like I'm everyone else. The muted conversations while I smile. The future schedules while I'm trying to enjoy the now. The constant worry all around. How's it that I've just experienced what I experienced but have never shown a sign of concern? Just frustration. Or question. But everyone around me is allowed to be worried by the growth of my own flower. Why can't we just receive our own oxygen and sunlight? Allow the water to hit our roots. Seems we're so busy telling everyone how to receive their sunlight. I really don't know what happened in the past two weeks. I feel I'm the most present I've ever been. I can't remember a thing. Just the script. I've just been repeating that script constantly, but I can't really recall what happened. I thought I found the light on Tuesday but I might be a forgetful fish still looking for it. One thing I do know is that I've accepted my brilliance. I will change the world. And for those who don't believe me, their roots will become dehydrated. My tree will keep growing. I'm a redwood. I'll be here much longer than the average person. You'll look up to me. And I'll also be in a forest with many other redwoods just like me. My tree won't fall so you won't hear me. I'll just stay quiet and keep growing. The normalcy I fear isn't leaving this hospital. I think it's reentering a society where my brilliance doesn't belong. I all of a sudden feel lonely again. I feel death. But at least I feel it. And there's an aliveness to that feeling. With all this work to do I don't know where to start. But I look at Sammy and I see the whole world in front of him. He's just starting. Maybe I'll just start too with him now. There's one thing I do know, that the universe is going to do the right thing here. I know I'll never worry about money again – about business, about philanthropy. The world's going to bring them right to me. We're going to be OK for as long as I've got. And far beyond me there's now a roadmap that needs to be done.

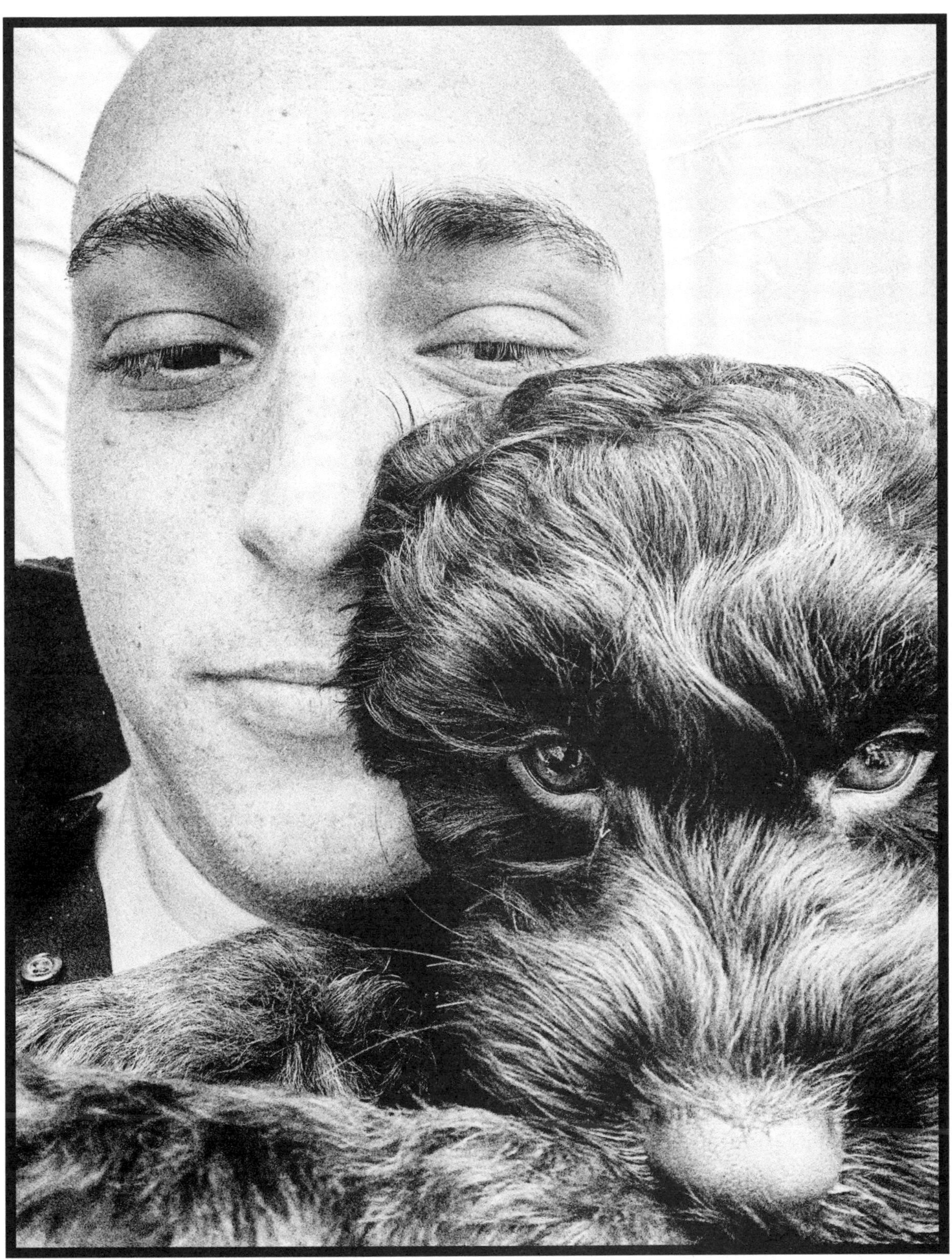

December 31, 2022

Discharged after
13 days.

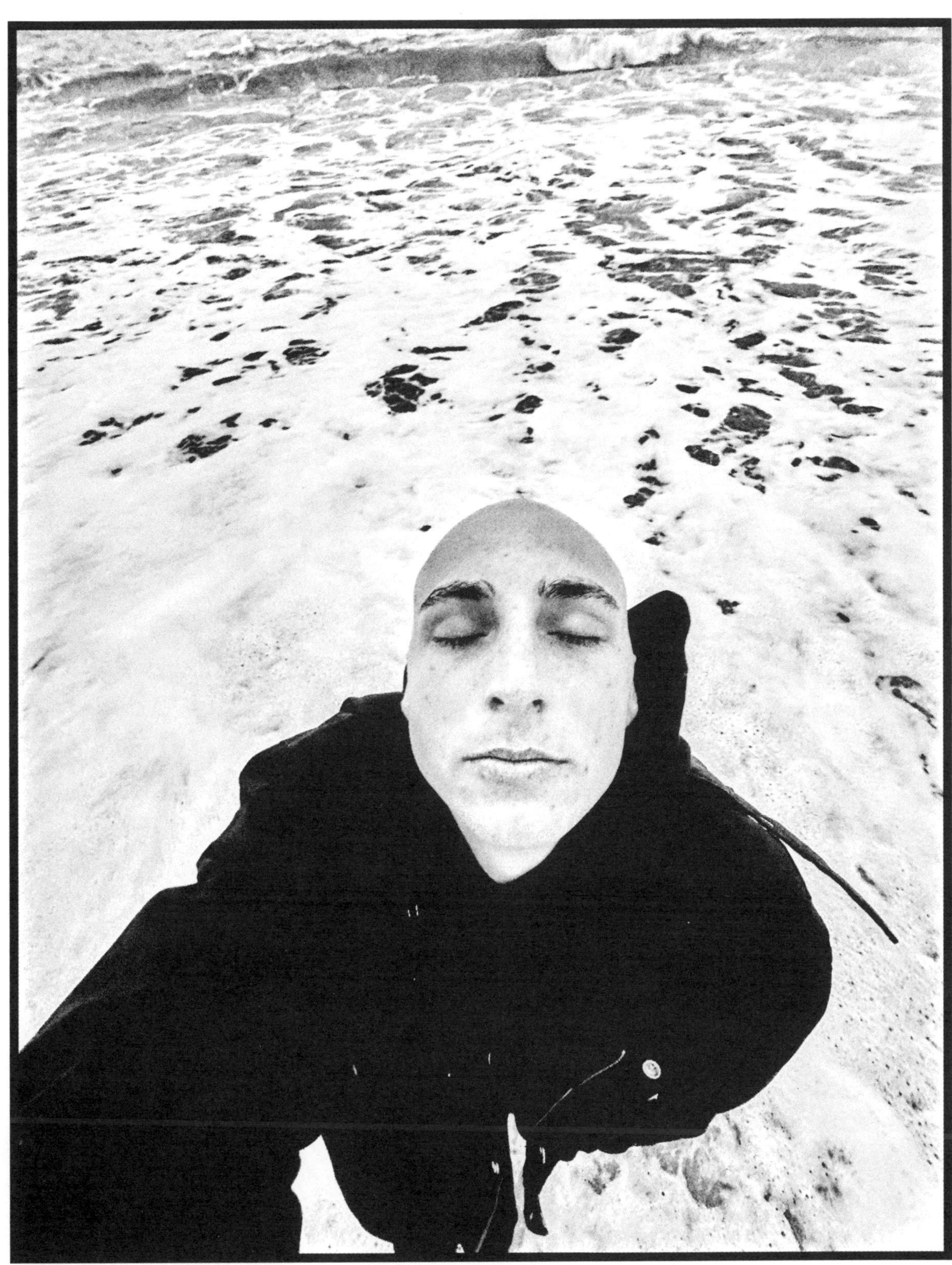

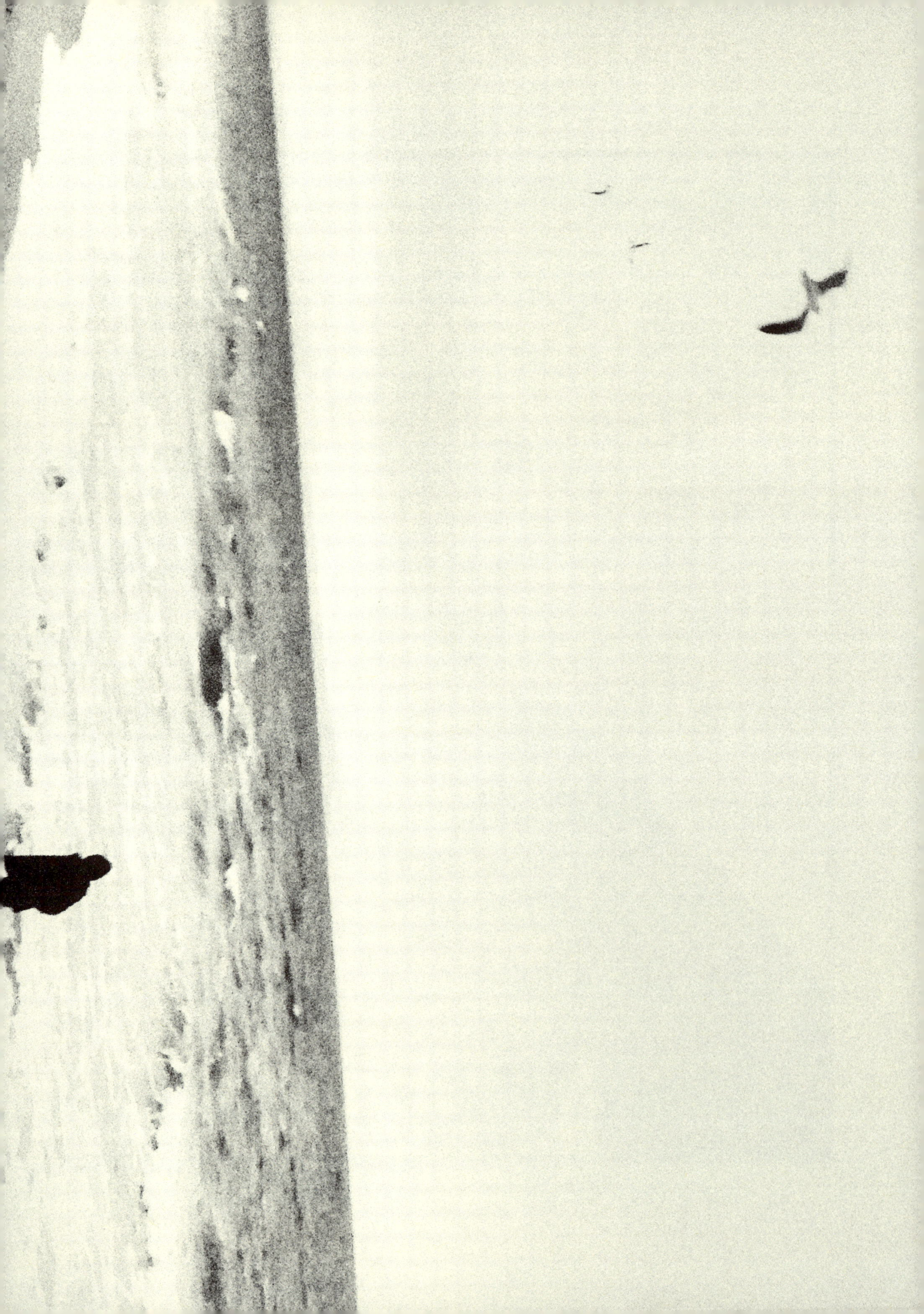

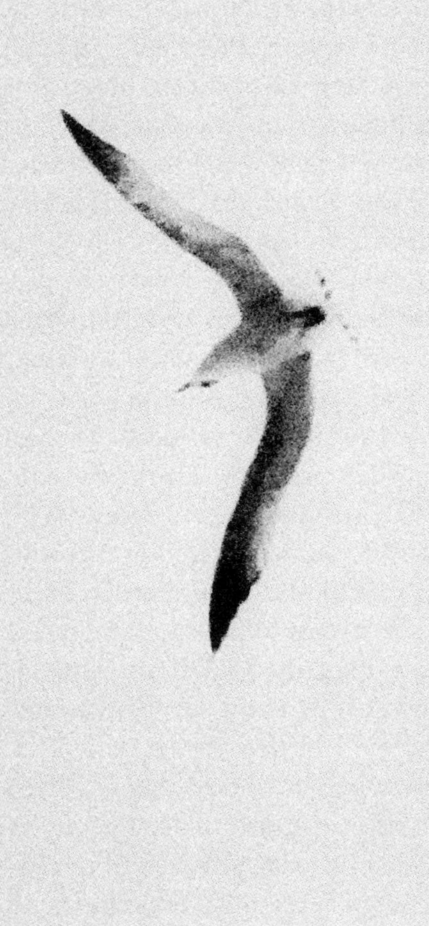

January 1, 2023

Architected framework. The thoughtful word choice. A control of emotion. No more worry or concern. I've experienced physical pain but have chosen optimism the entire time. I haven't expressed any negativity. People don't become different, they just change. We're not the same after fallen towers. My feet walk against the concrete. Shorts in the rain. Distracted sheep are all around. Looking at my nail polish like I'm a zombie. One last moment in the courtyard. Closure to trauma. A re-entry of physical space. If only I saw the ocean. No more screen savers or artificial feelings. It wasn't channel 18. My feet were really in the ocean. I felt like the rebel with the Jeep again. Doors off, heat up. A real aliveness again. As I walked back, I removed my beanie. There's a tornado in my skull. The ice appeared to grasp it. An erection of temperature. The birds were flying all around me. I realized if I can just stay in these moments, if I can be one with as opposed to one distracted by my roots, I will keep growing. I've been thinking a lot about these visualizations recently. I realized my mind works differently. I always thought everybody had them, but you realize there's just a small few who do. I've always seen the world before it happened. I saw the photos before I took them, the dances before I moved. I've experienced my life sometimes through a camera lens as opposed to my own. There's only so much time left. There's too much to do. The sheep keep telling me to rest. But I'm not in a farm pen. I'm not grass fed. I'm actually in the wild. There are no farmers taking care of me. I'm hunting for my own. When you're sick, people always tell you to visualize your healing, but now I've learned to visualize my brilliance too. People get scared when you tell them you're going to change the world. It's the ones who believe they are that actually do. Of all days, I get discharged on New Year's Eve – I close the year with this. So much got done professionally – that's really all my mind was on. All these projects, all this work, so much opportunity, but led with pressure rather than gratitude. There's a new canvas here with this new year. New goals to think about, new motivations. I am changed now. And look forward to this new slate.

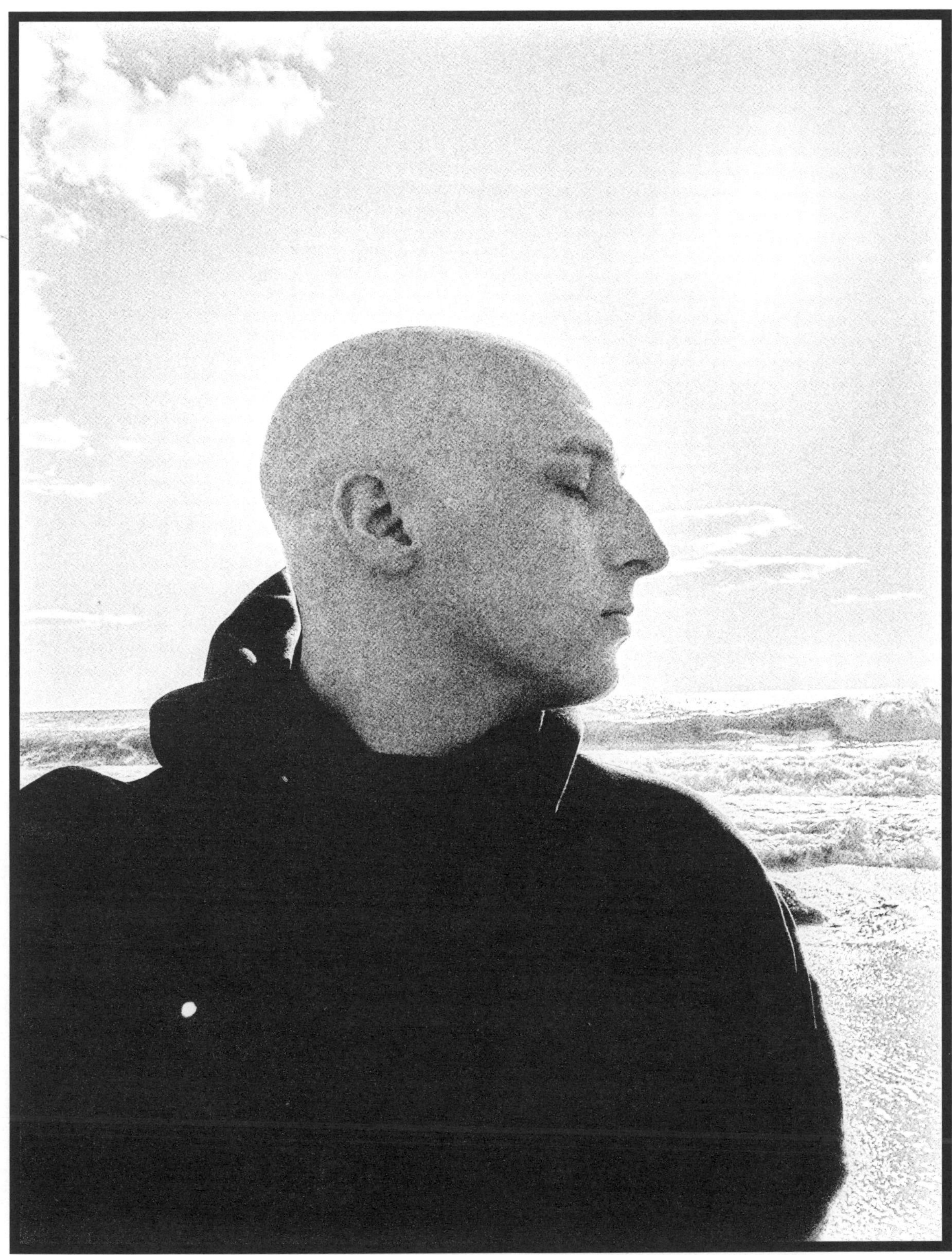

January 3, 2023

Paw scratches to the face.
Fresh showers. Dinners with friends.
Stitches healing.
Everything’s starting to feel normal again.
The normality has kicked in but in a way I feel like I belong. I feel part of rather than separate from.
The conversation doesn’t have to be long.

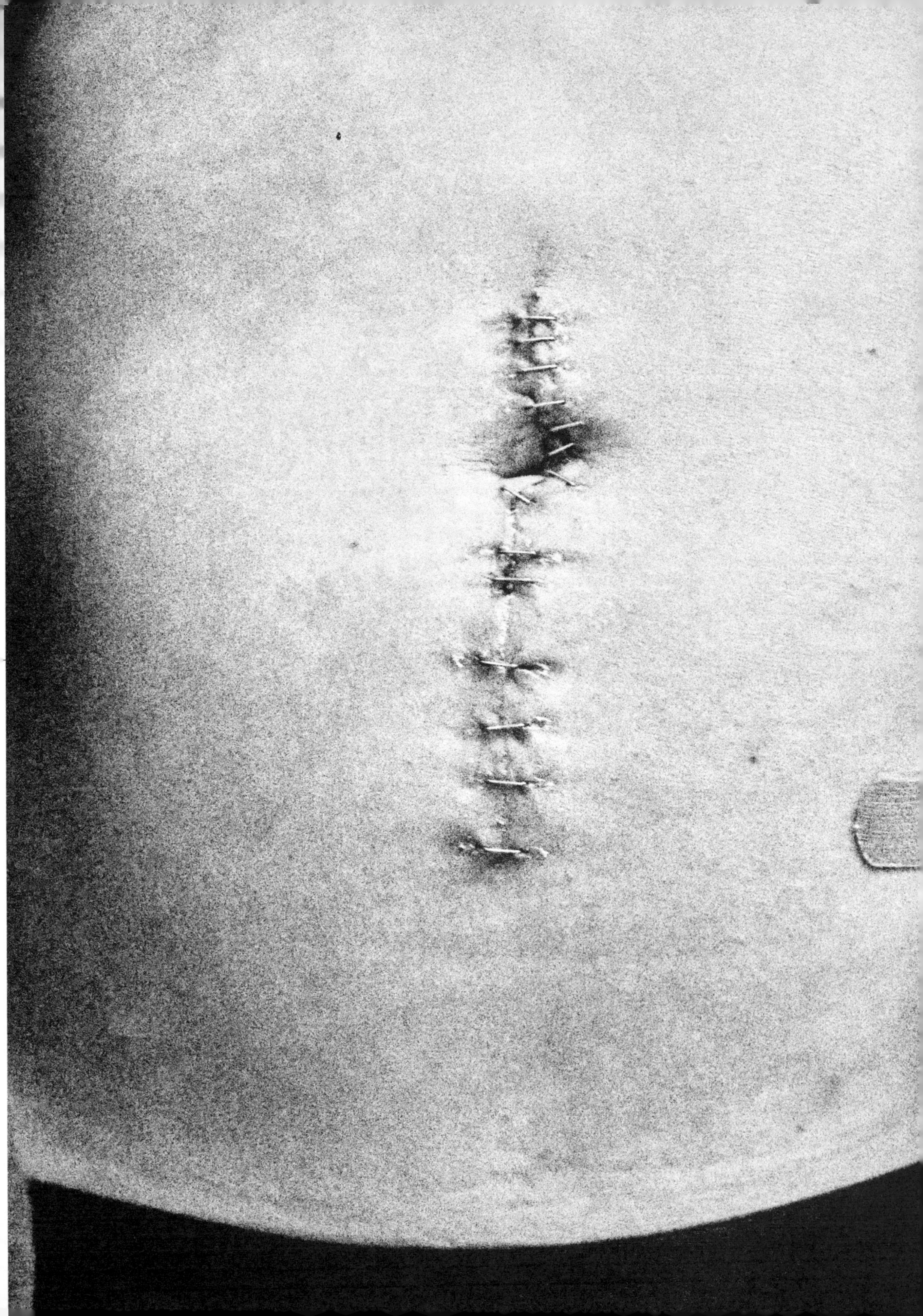

Staples out.

January 8, 2023
Morning

Caught in between. Eyes closed. The waves crash in front of me. The traffic flows behind. My new favorite spot. Sun is rising. Mattress in the back of the car. Trunk open. Cuddles with Sammy. Overly documented as his youth won't last long. A study of the waves to get the perfect timing. Salt water on the face. The perfect cleanse. My mind feels really calm right now. It feels like it was so active with so much and it's hit a full stop. Maybe the drugs wore down or the regularity kicked in. But I feel I've come full stop. Dr Kwaan said I'm a rare bird. I've led with gratitude, and except for the physical pain have been optimistic throughout. But what are these chances? Nine in 10,000. Once every two years. Perforation with lymphoma. Am I the ugly duckling? My ambition stays strong. And my desire to change the world continues. But as my mental stamina slows, so does my reality of the time it will take to accomplish everything. I've been watching nature like a television. It's the greatest series. I feel so alive. I only have so much more time until my next treatment. Until I'm in the bed again. Until I'm trapped in that room. Until the negotiation with the nurses about my sleep starts. But I'm almost halfway there. I'm winning the race and I'll hit the finish line soon. Thanks for writing.

Under 200. First time in ten years.

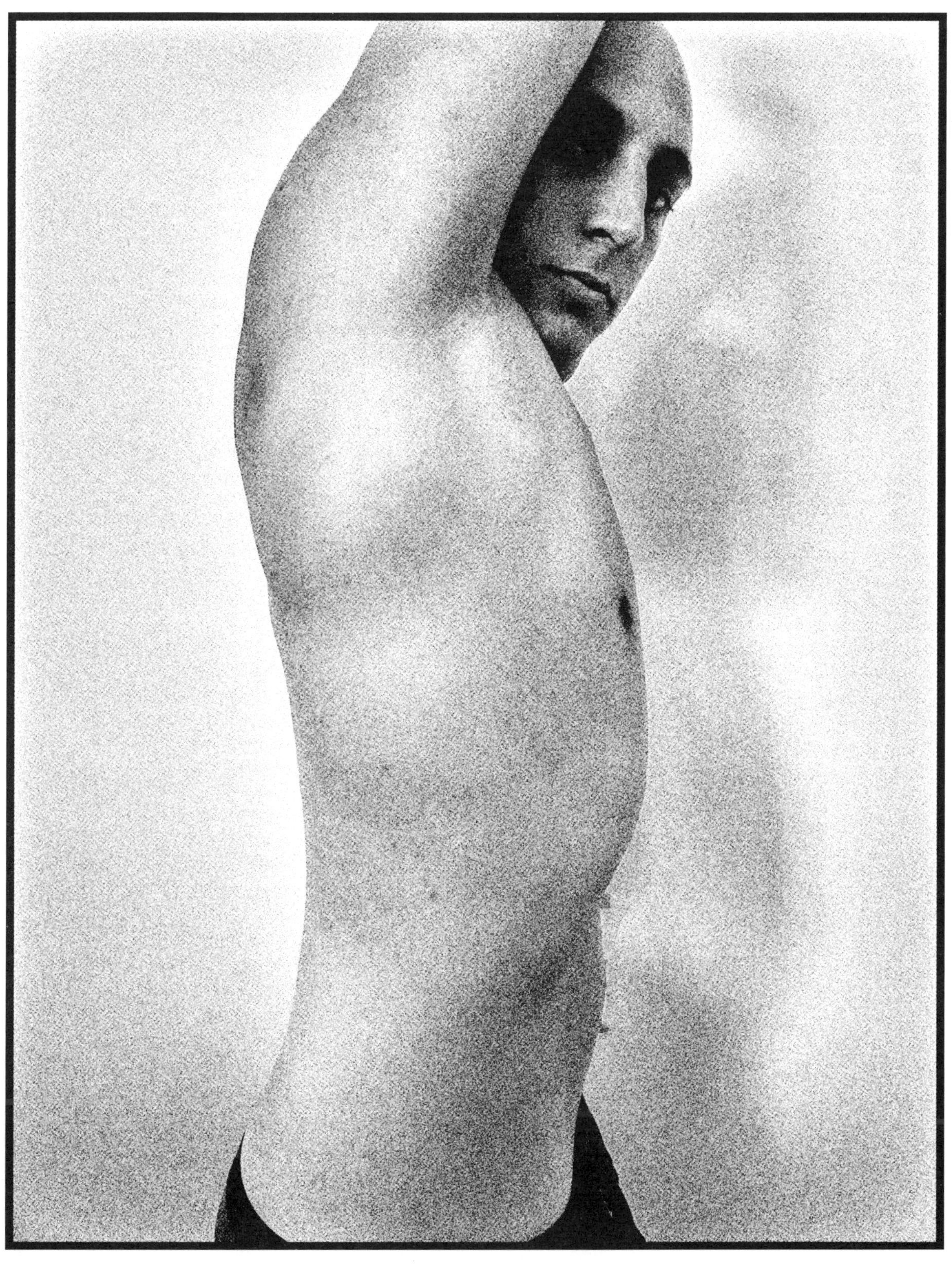

January 8, 2023
Evening

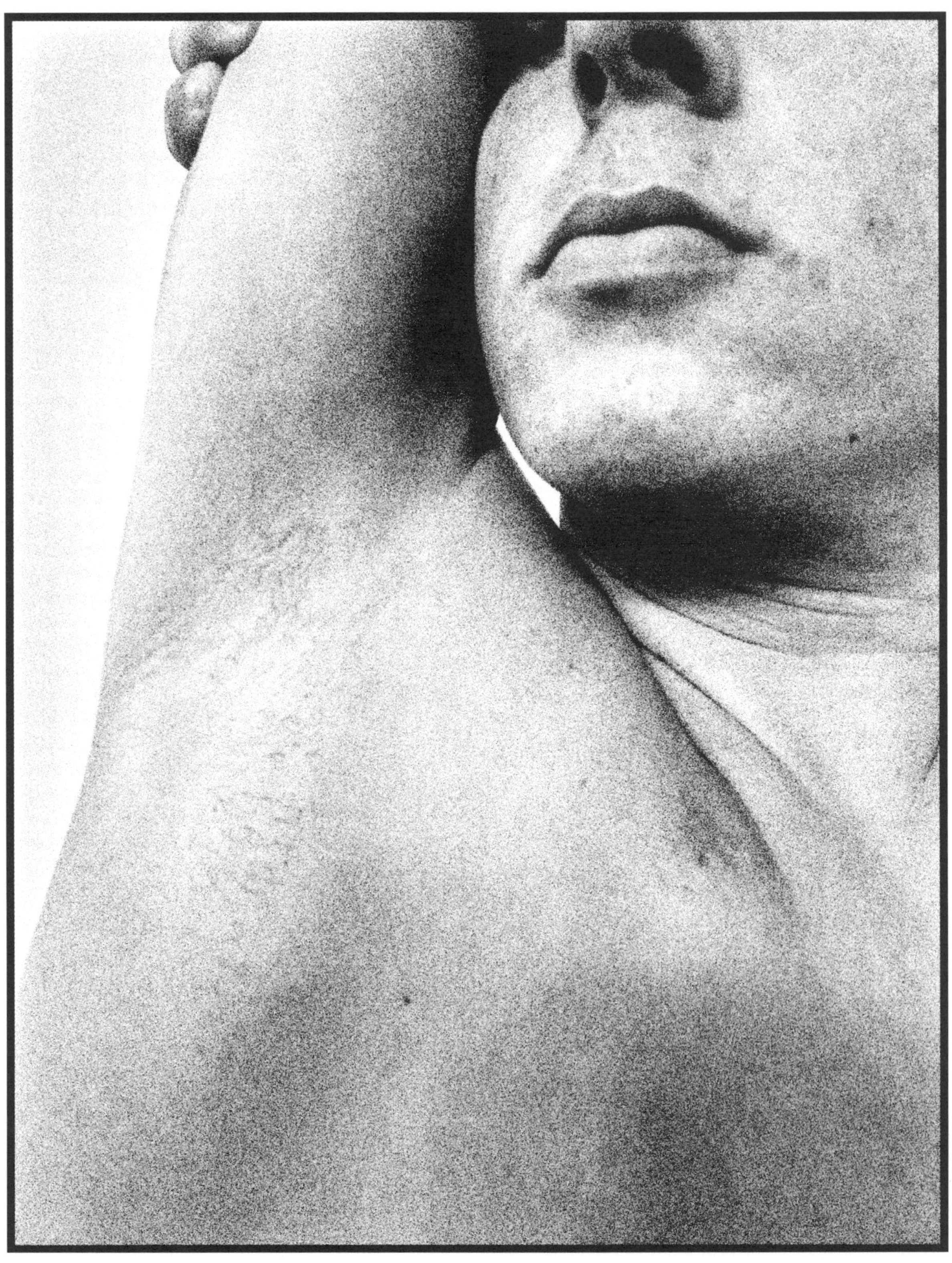

Cocooned in the back of my car. The raindrops hit, sounding like popcorn in the microwave. You can see each drip appear on the window as the artificial light from all around seeps through. Just south of the pier. I sit in the parking lot facing the ocean. The sun's already set and the cloudy evening blows ocean air right toward us. There's a wall of sound between us and the waves crashing. It's all the sheep walking by. Their sandals shuffling against the concrete, the gears of their bikes turning, the loud boombox or their insights to their complicated lives for the few seconds as they pass. I lay here still trying to comprehend my diagnosis and what I've been through. My mind races, wondering if this is luck or not. That this rarity was put on me.

These moments of normality creep by me, but, if I listen hard enough I can hear the ocean.

I've been finding a lot of temporary resolve, but needing an actual escape soon. I'm still overwhelmed by everybody walking by with their depression and anxiety. I wish they knew the pot of gold they are sitting on by simply just having good health. I hope I can sit in a jacuzzi soon. And soak in all I've been through. I'm just another man in the mirror. This has made me change so much of who I am.

January 10, 2023

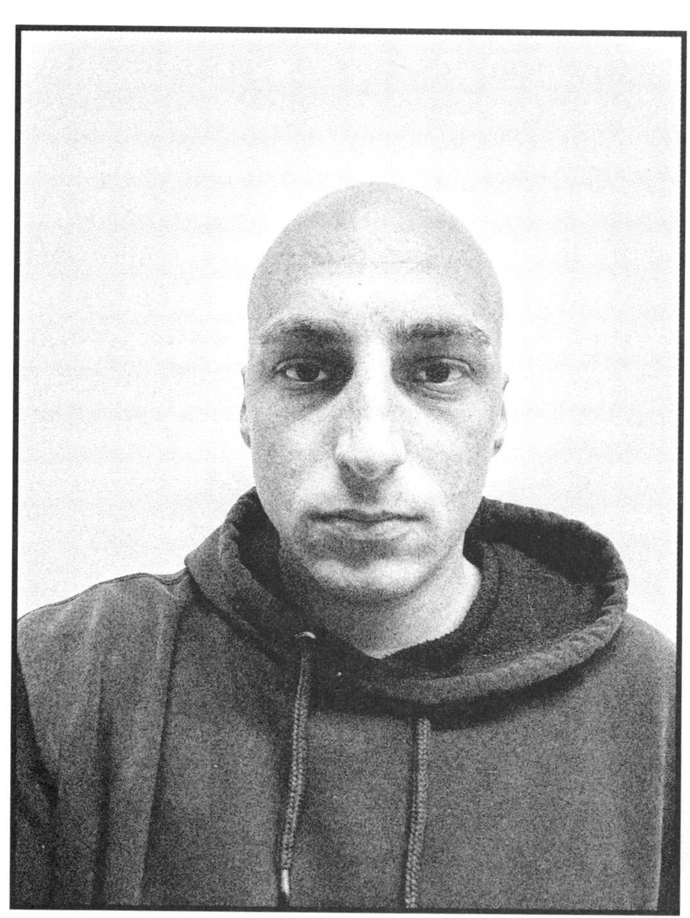

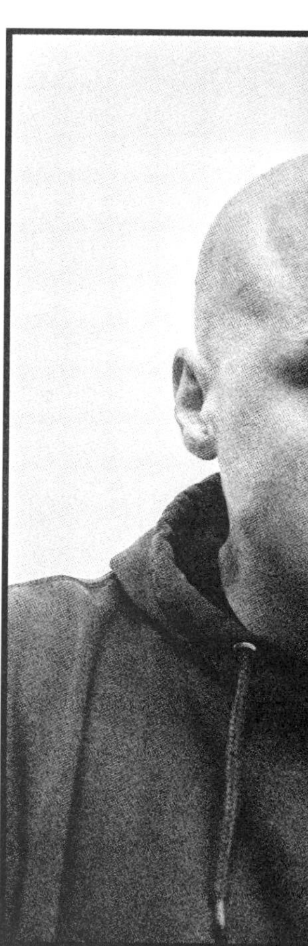

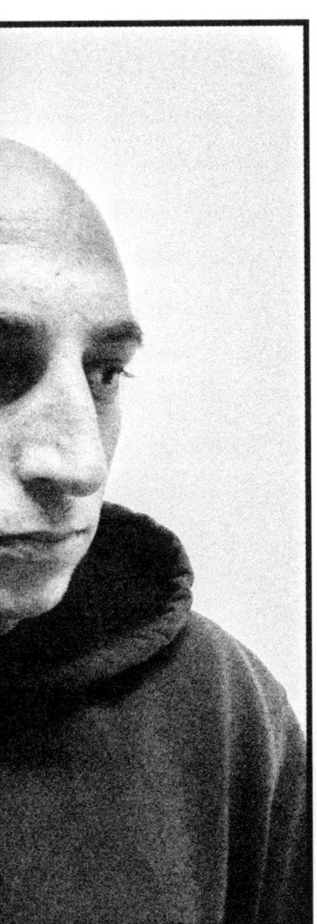
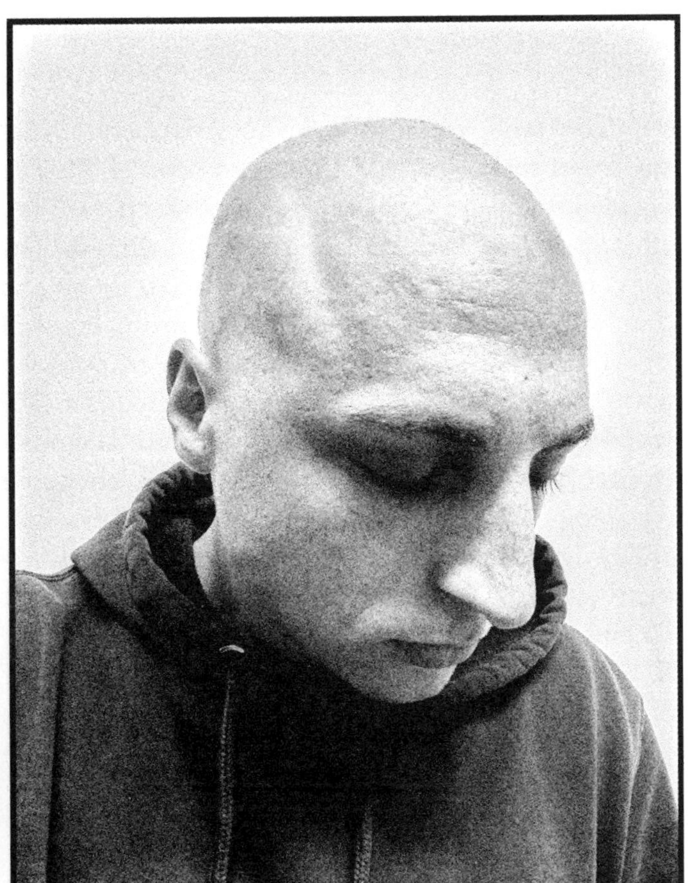

January 11, 2023

I've always wondered who would show up to my funeral. What would they say about me? What did I mean to people? This experience has made it happen in real time while I was here. They brought me the roses. I've seen so many people in the past few months. Their vulnerability to share what I mean to them is so unfiltered. Our fragility is so protected. We put up such a wall instead of just telling people in real time what they really mean to us. Today was a good day. We drove to my happy place. My first break since March. And my first escape since the diagnosis. I haven't been in a jacuzzi for a long time. Tonight, I got to be under the stars, going in and out of consciousness, feeling so whole and relaxed. I felt the weakness of my flesh and my muscles. My weight is currently at 195. Though I'm so embraced in my normality, she cried, being overwhelmed. By the fact that this isn't over yet. We're still in the battle. I'm tucked in and slowly dozing off. The windows cracked open, and I hear the sound of real waves crashing outside. Not the artificial ones from the hospital room on Spotify. I'm in my happy place. Today was a good day.

1.11.23

Ive always wondered who would show up to my funeral. What would they say about me? What did I mean to people? This experience has made it happen in real time while I was here. They brought me the roses. I've seen so many people in the past few months. Their vulnerability to share what I mean to them is so unfiltered. Our fragility is so protected. We put up such a wall instead of just telling people in real time what they really mean to us. Today was a good day. We drove to my happy place. My first break since March. And my first escape since the diagnosis. I havent been in a jacuzzi for a long time. Tonight I got to under the stars, going in and out of consciousness, feeling so whole and relaxed. I felt the weakness of my flesh and my muscles. My weight's currently at 195. Though Im so embraced in my normality she cried being overwhelmed. By the fact that this isnt over yet. We're still in the battle. Im tucked in and slowly dozing off. The windows cracked as I hear the sound of real waves crashing outside. Not the artificial ones from the hospital room on Spotify. Im in my happy place. Today was a good day.

January 17, 2023

Observing a dark ocean.

The canvas is black. A small white dot appears and turns into a line. Waves continuously crash. The tide has been high. My ankles haven't felt the water yet. I'm not depressed but the days have been depressed. It's productive to stay in bed for a while. The meat gets tender the longer it cooks. Occupied heaviness. Before my diagnosis and after so many close deaths the news of human life became numb. Now everything has so much significance – every feeling, emotion, birth, death, or update on health. Sammy's been cuddling with me more. His nose next to my ear. I can hear every breath. The dolphins fly through the waves. The pelicans pass by in both directions. The rain pours so loud. Both rib cages rise. I'm not worried about temporary absence anymore. People are leaving but they are always around. I need to keep making my work. To have something to look forward to. To keep growing. Be it an isolated experience or one in community. The beef will keep getting tender. Our perspectives and needs are different. But our exposure to each other, our arguments, our discomforts, and our feelings of joy help us belong more. The darkness of the sea can blind you from the waves but you'll always hear them. They're continuous. Like each day of ours. As we look for the light, we just keep swimming. Just keep swimming. We don't know the forecast ahead, but we're as prepared as we can be. Thanks for writing.

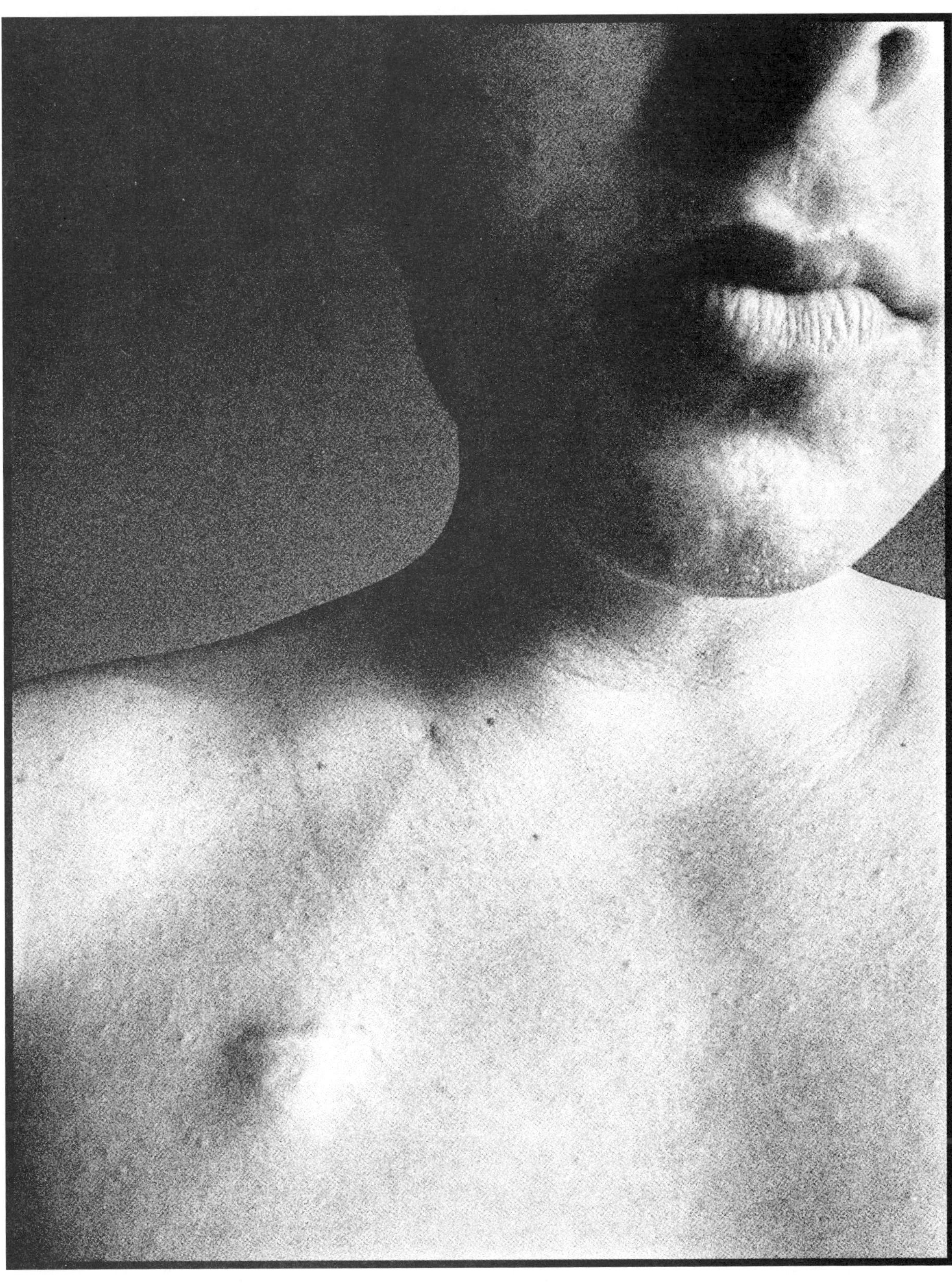

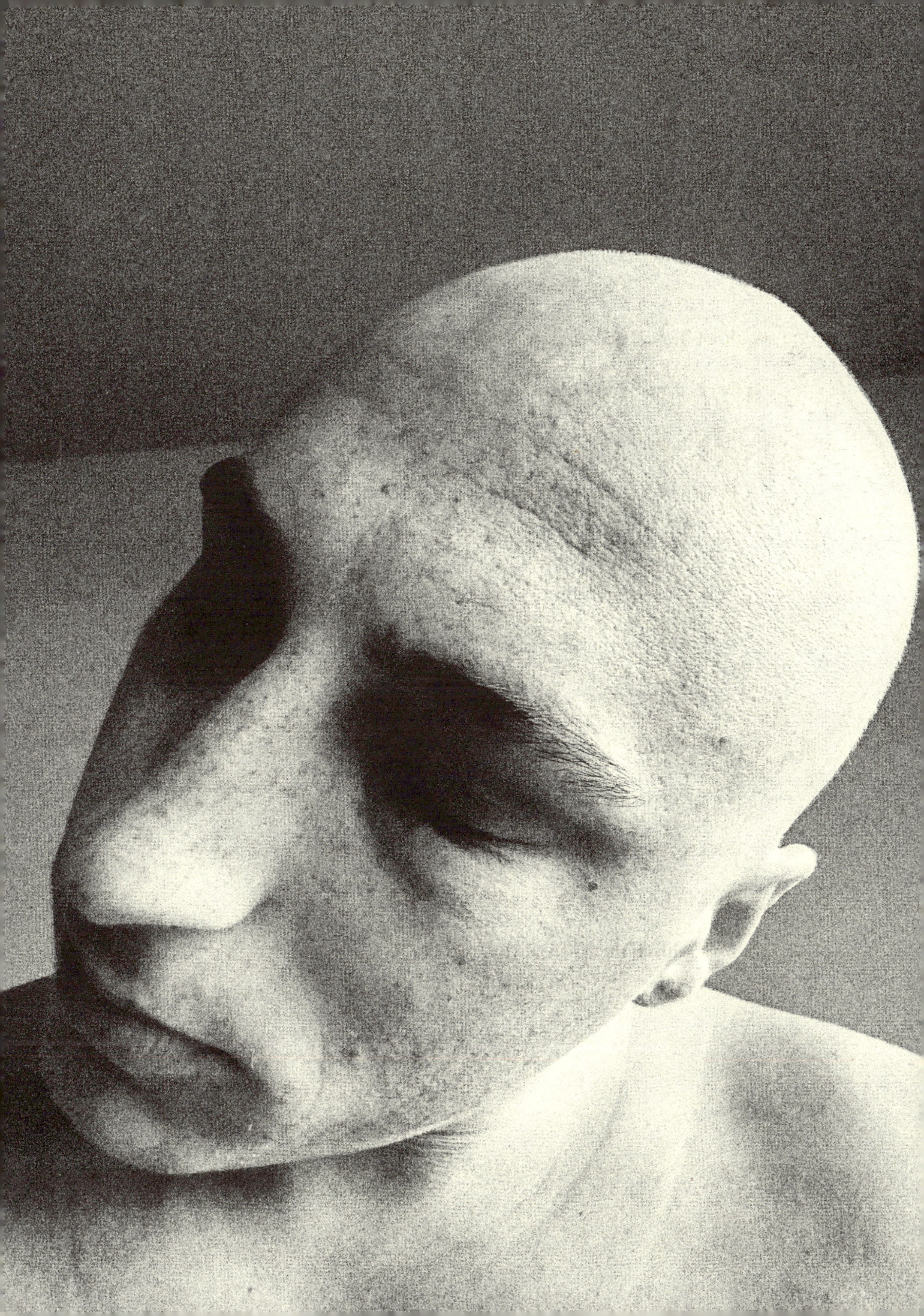

January 20, 2023

Back from Mexico.

Back against the Marley.

Back in my head.

Back soon against the hospital bed.

Back wondering what I'm doing.

Back in my depression.

Back with everyone's worry.

Back feeling hopeful.

Back thinking if it's only hope.

Back wondering if I'm fine.

Back wondering if I'm not.

Back in LA.

Back with all the artificiality.

Back with the sadness.

Back wanting to dance.

Back with my stomach still healing.

Back with little mobility.

Back when I remembered my life before my diagnosis.

Back in optimism.

Back in fear.

Back when I was a kid.

Back when I spent time with my mom.

Back with everyone making me re-live this fucking hospitalization.

Back re-living these thoughts again.

When's it going to be done so we can just look back?

January 22, 2023

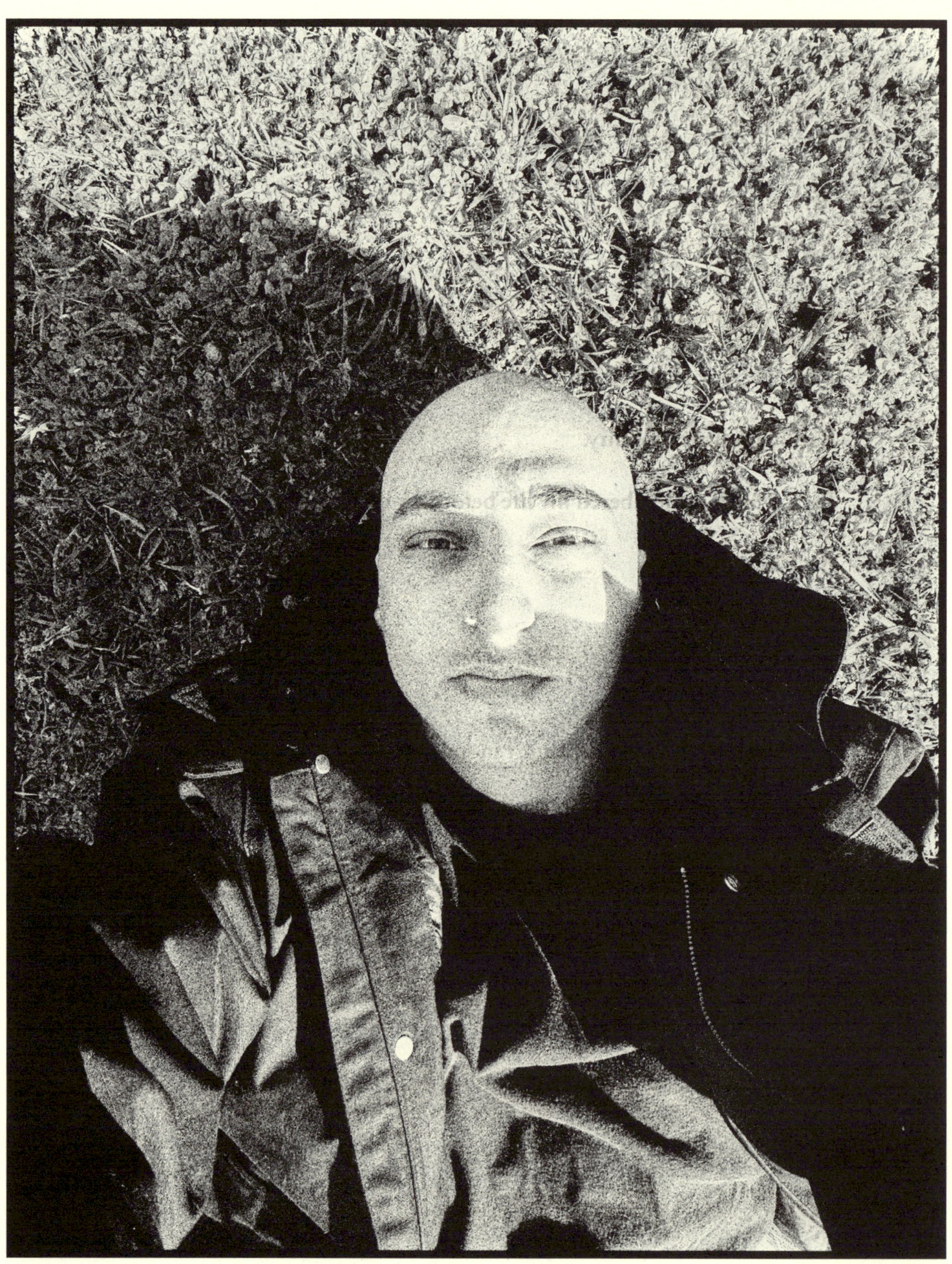

Bottom of the mountain again. Uninterested to start climbing. I feel like I've reached the top already. Reset. Reset. Reset. Resolve. Unresolved. The walk here back on this block again. My second home. All the memories come back. Life moves fast outside of here. The second I walk up the walkway everything drastically slows down again. Ten breaths in the garden. Under the tree. The last feeling of sunlight for now. Back to darkness. Just keep swimming. It's all the little things piled up. Do you have an advanced directive? Just in case? The wristband goes on. Back to the fourth floor. The nurses try hard to greet you, but it doesn't help. The door opens. You see the room you're going to be in for the next few days. The semi-truck just slams you. You lay in bed. Your body sinks. They lift the bars on either side. Thread your skin into the port. Blood work. Plugged in. You're trapped here now. Vitals. The cold slimy plastic over your naked arm. The air pushes through. The cold metal stick under your tongue. The tape around your index finger. I feel like a hamster again. Continuous knocking. The mouse clicks. A scan of the wrist. Name and birthdate please. The loud beeps from the IV pole. A continuous drip. A drip down the side of the face. A tear. Frustrated sadness. I don't want to fucking be here. A symphony of normality plays through the window. The everyday continues. When I'm out, I drive by this building and know what it's like to be in it. Here I am. It's hard to find the gratitude, but I am grateful for the healthcare, for the nurses, for the medicine, and for the support. I'm justifying a bad day. Fuck it.

January 23, 2023

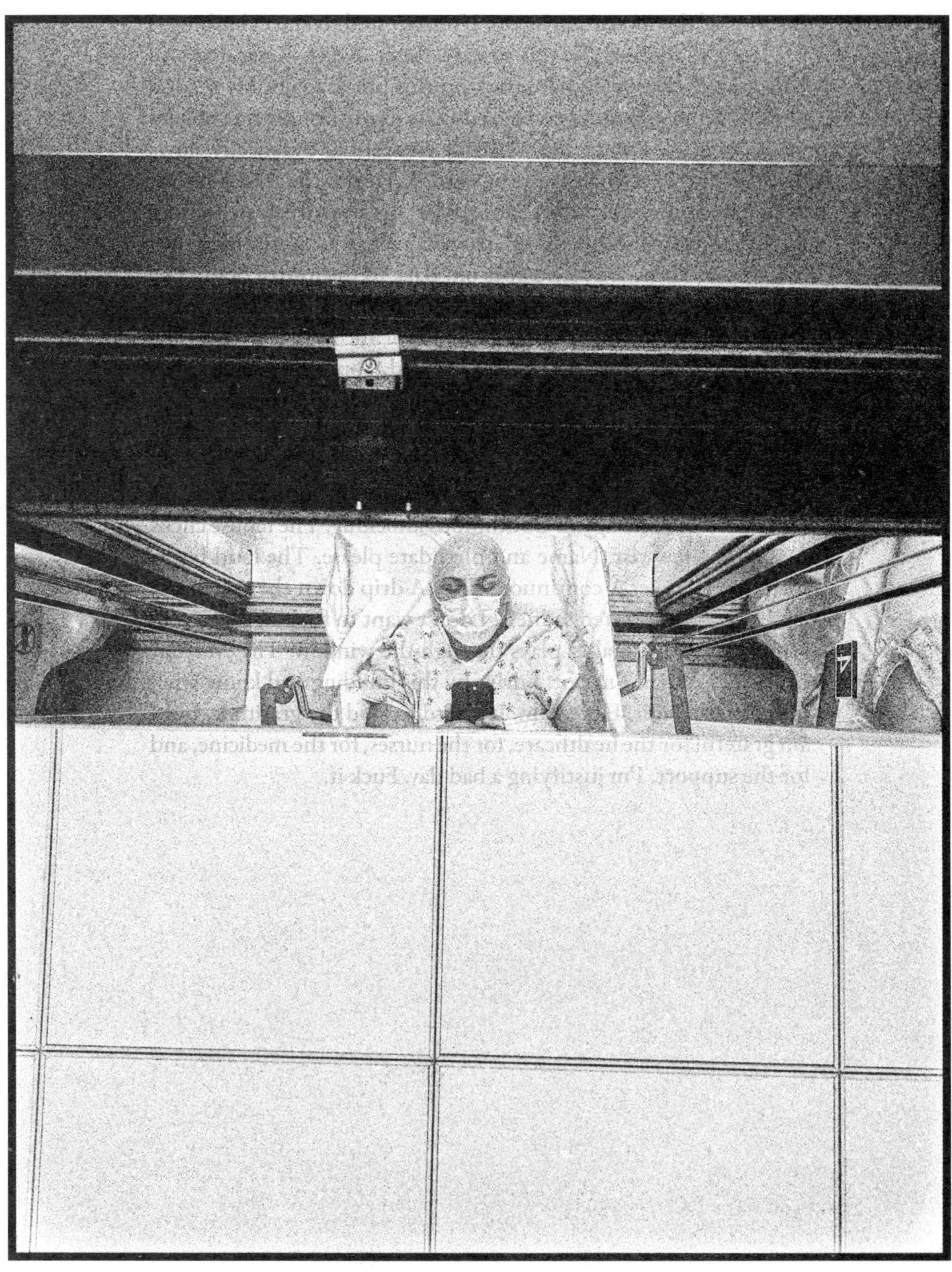

January 24, 2023

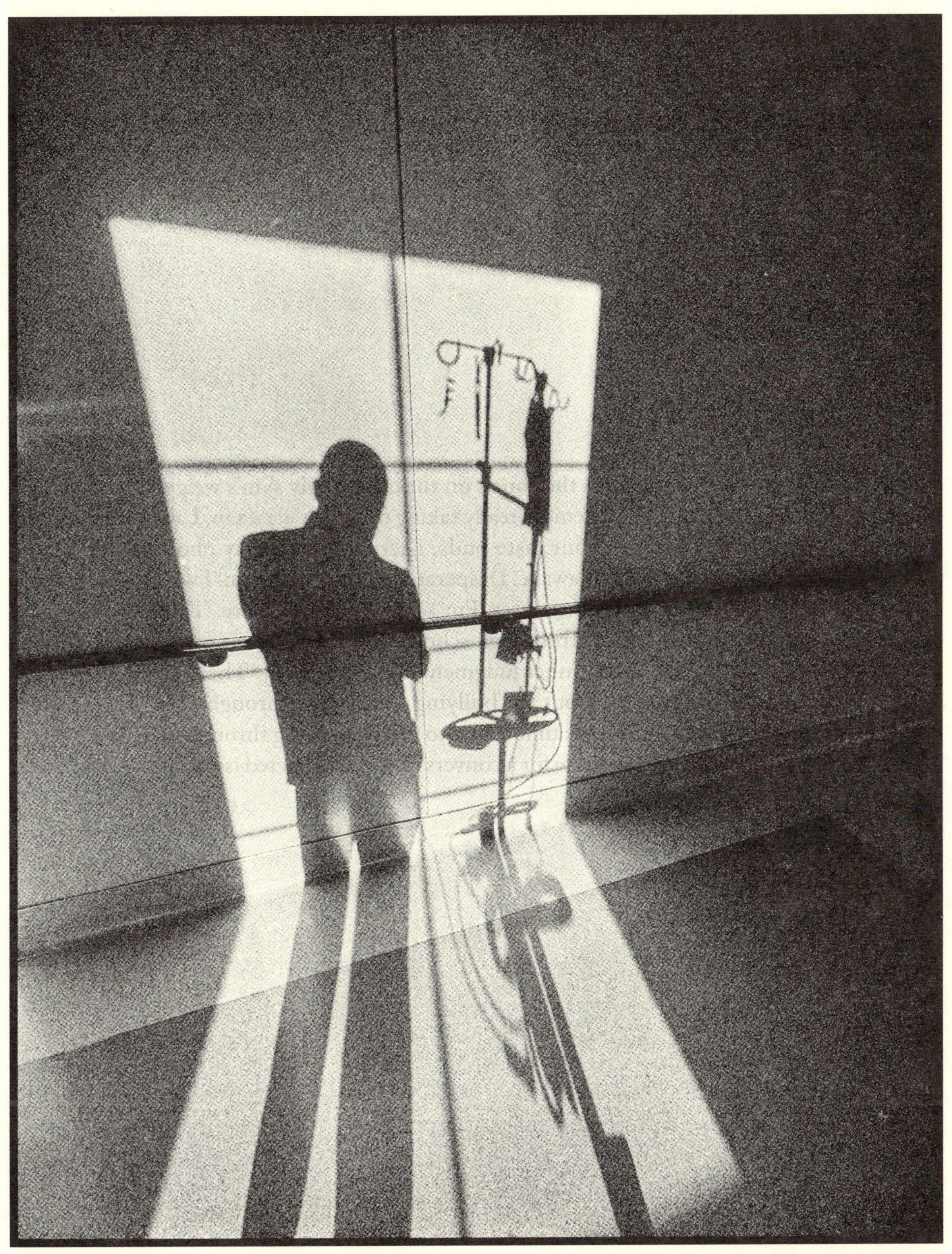

January 25, 2023

My body lines up with the panels on the ceiling. My skin's weighted like cement. This chemo is really taking over. It is 4:22 a.m. Labs. Flush. You feel it in your taste buds. I scroll through my phone contacts, seeing who is awake. Desperate for a conversation. I wish I was running along the water. I'm so sick of being here. Time spent with old friends from high school. Talks about insecurities obstructing self-value. Inner judgment about the body. The body is sacred. Reminded about the bullying I had to go through. The strength I gained. All the time I used to spend scrolling through my phone contacts, desperate for a conversation. Architected isolation.

My experience of this treatment is all self-designed. I'm just not in a good mood. I'm critical of myself when I share that with others. I feel this need to put on such an optimistic front. There's a few people in my life who haven't checked in this time. I wonder if this is all too much for them. It's too much for me. The windows slightly cracked open. I hear the activity outside. I just want to float out the window like a balloon. I'll cruise down the hallways now, peeking through the open doors. Insights into old flesh. Absent of visitors. I'm reminded of my gratitude.

January 26, 2023

Another five days. Discharged. Feeling low, feeling down.

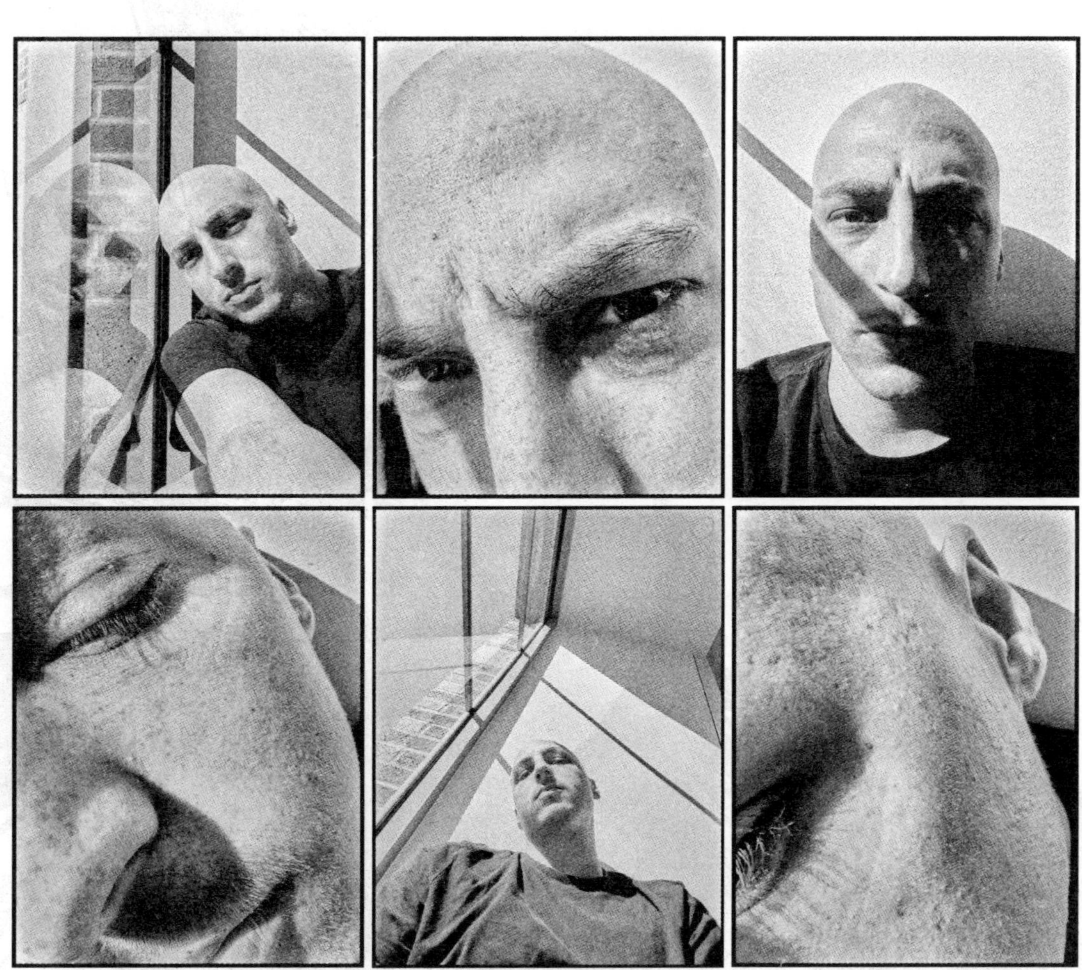

January 29, 2023

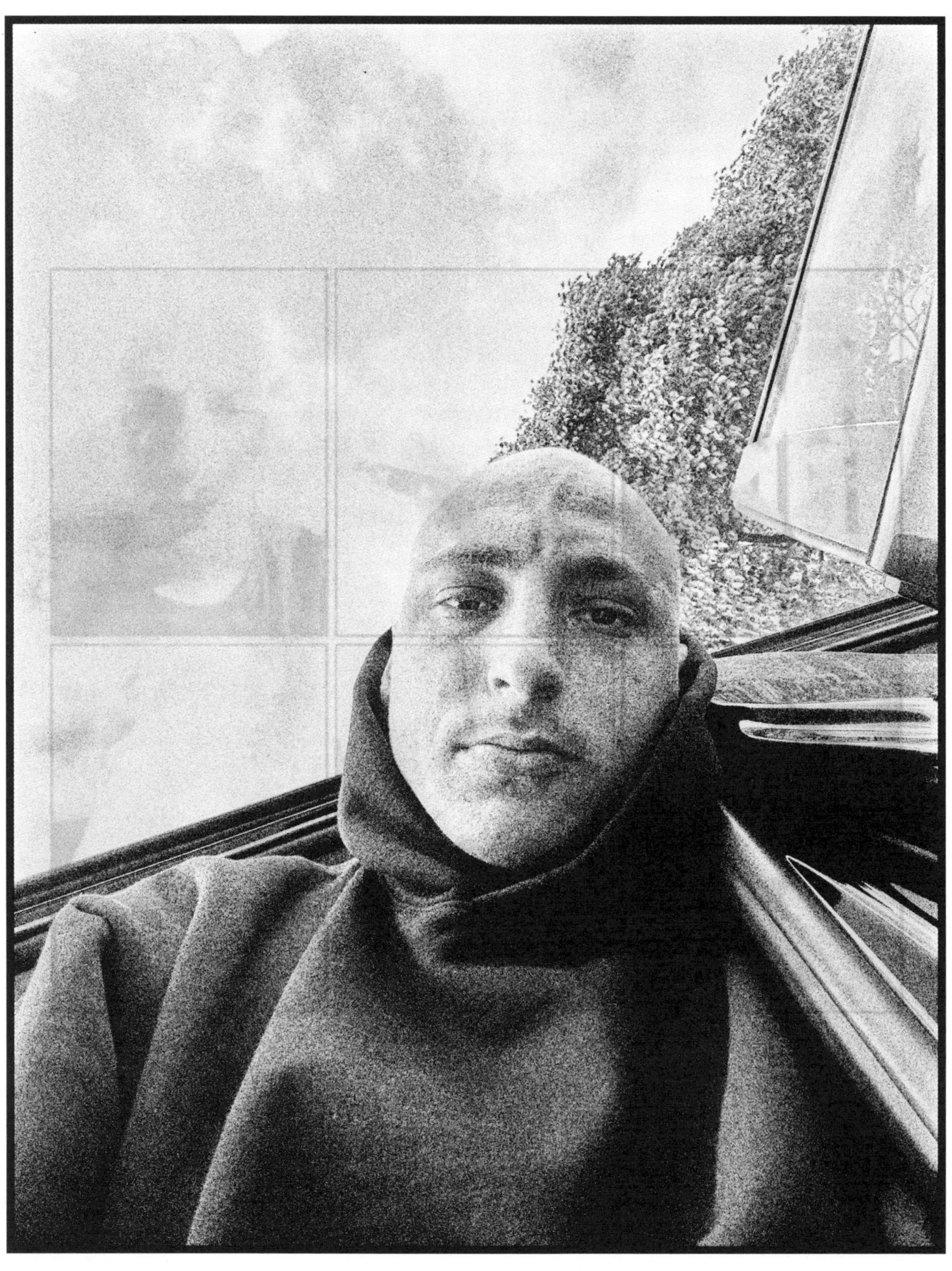

Nausea. Post vomit.

February 1, 2023

Blood work.

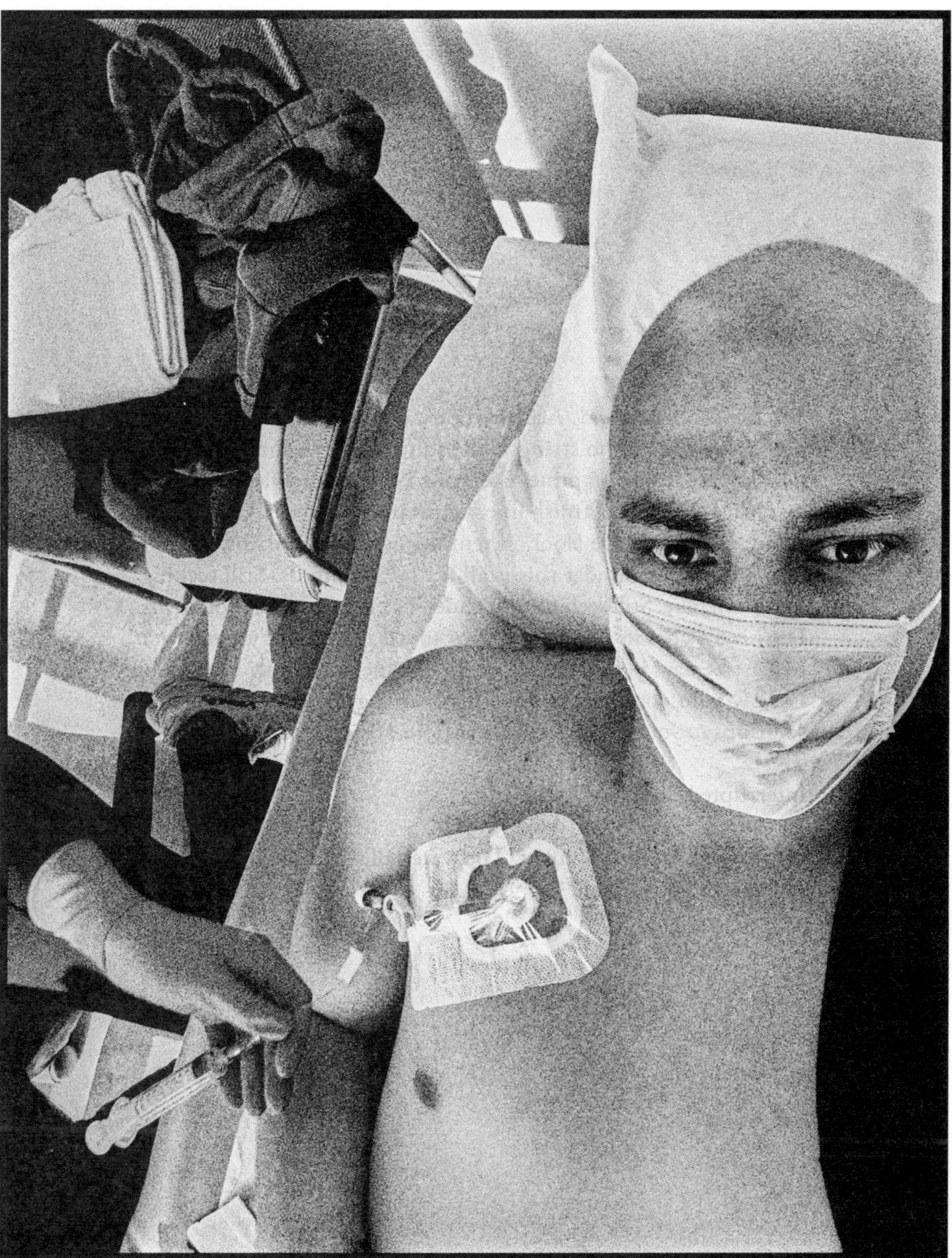

February 2, 2023

Stuckness. Quicksand. Accepted defeat. With a little help from my friend. I've got no strings. The sun stares. He cuddles so gently. His face rested on mine. Everyone keeps acknowledging it's a marathon. Blind to a finish line. Constant symptoms. Can't sit or stand. Parallel to the floor. A reminder of deep breaths. Forced new habits. A reminder this is all for us. Not to us. Still seeking the lesson here. Still seeking gratitude. The tired narrative of down. The needle goes in again. The docs added three more treatments. At least 25 days in the hospital to go. Let me know how I can help. I know who you can talk to. I have this great diet. Everyone's solutions to your reality. The intentions are good though.

Interrupted tiredness.

Unprofessional development. The waterfall still flows. Acceptance of pause. Time for bed.

February 8, 2023

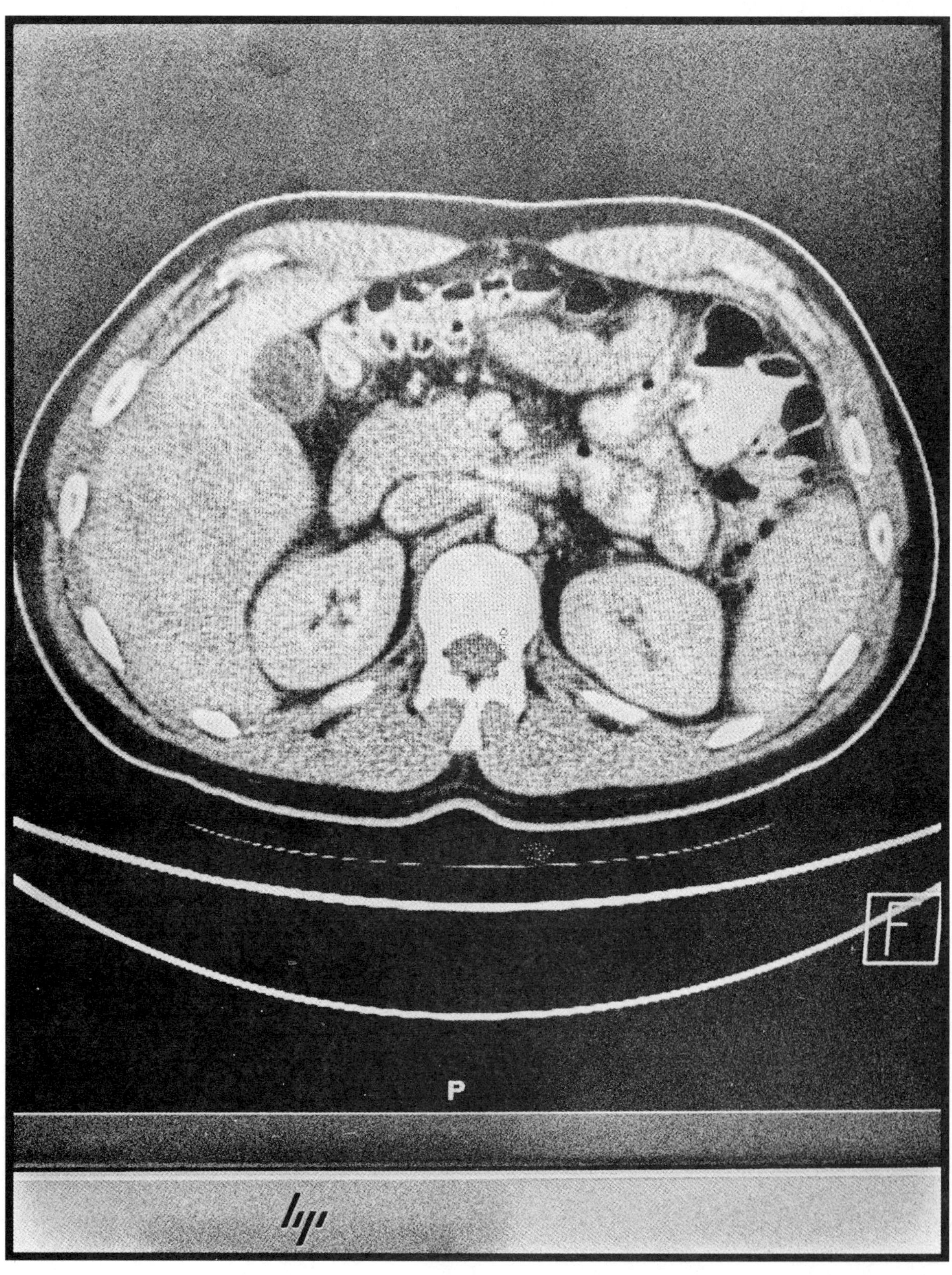

February 9, 2023

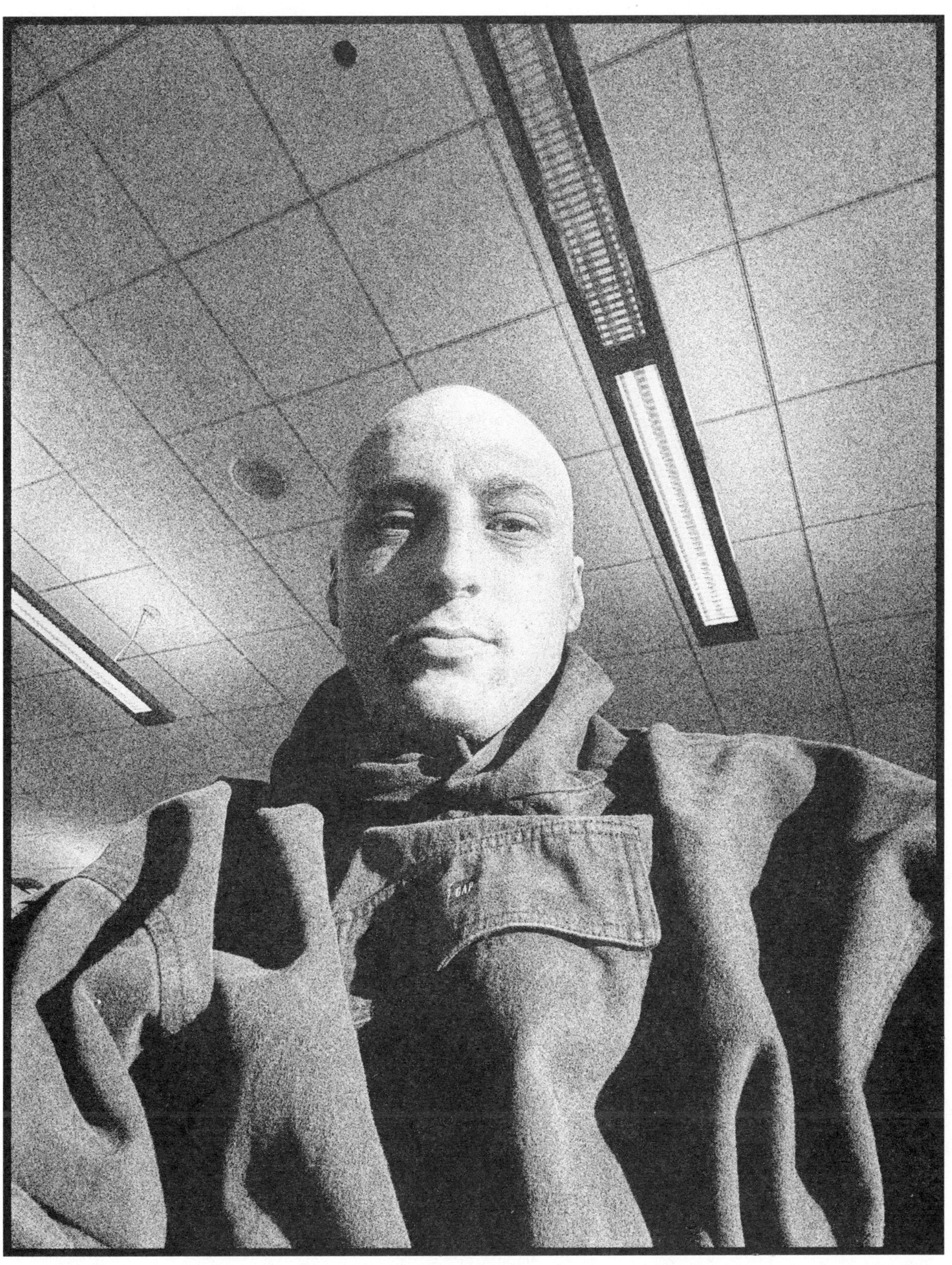

February 10, 2023

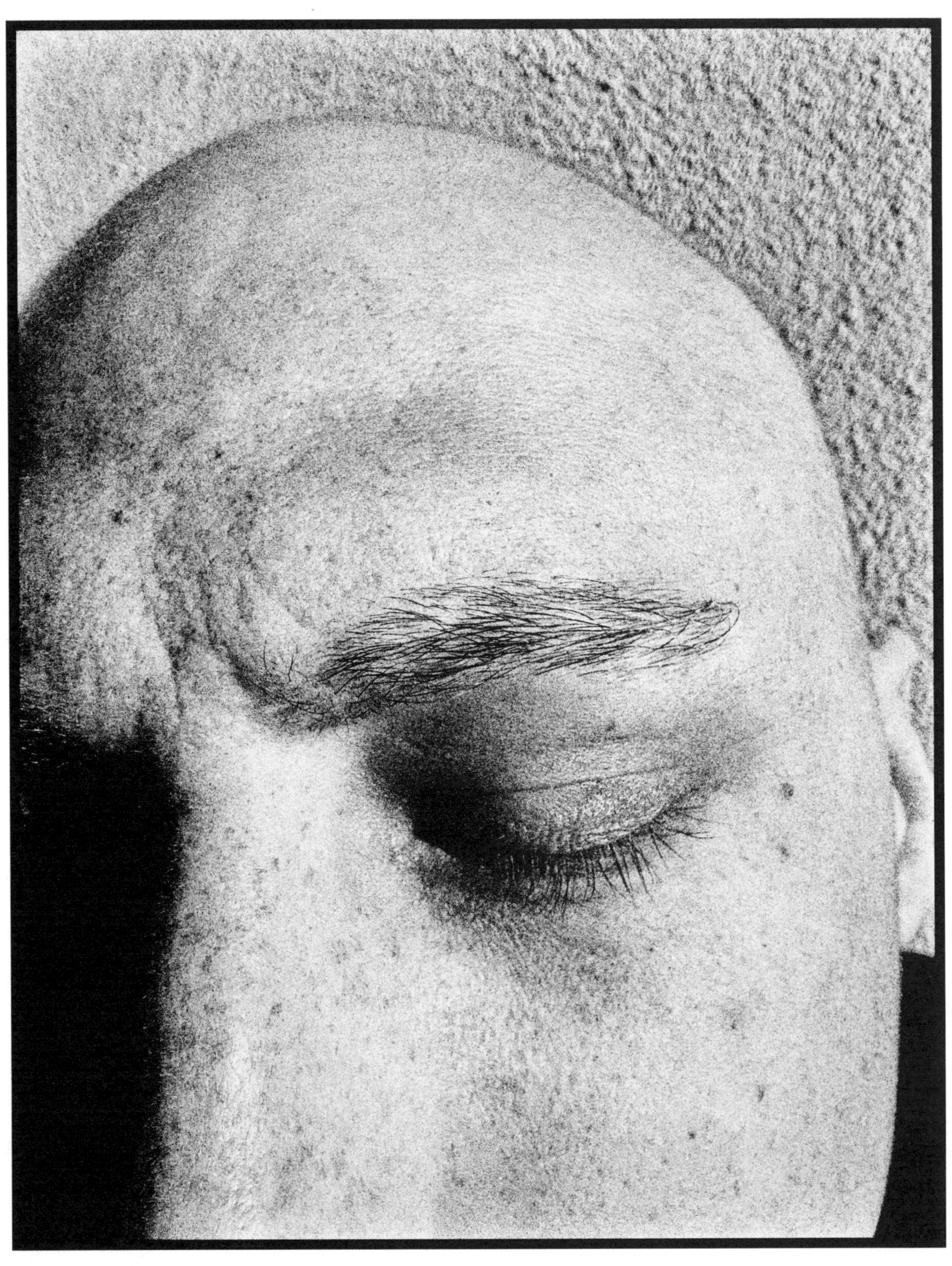

February 11, 2023

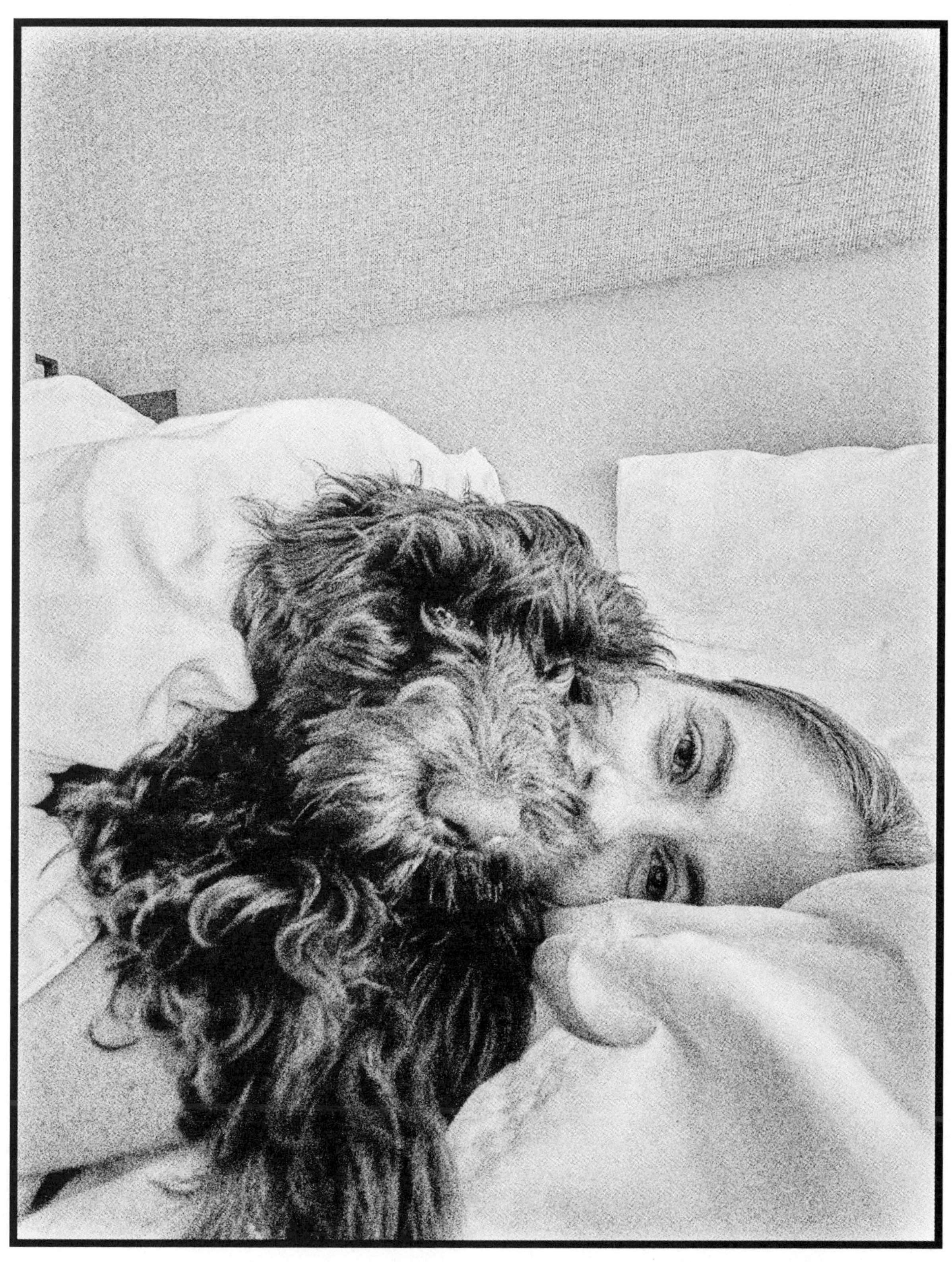

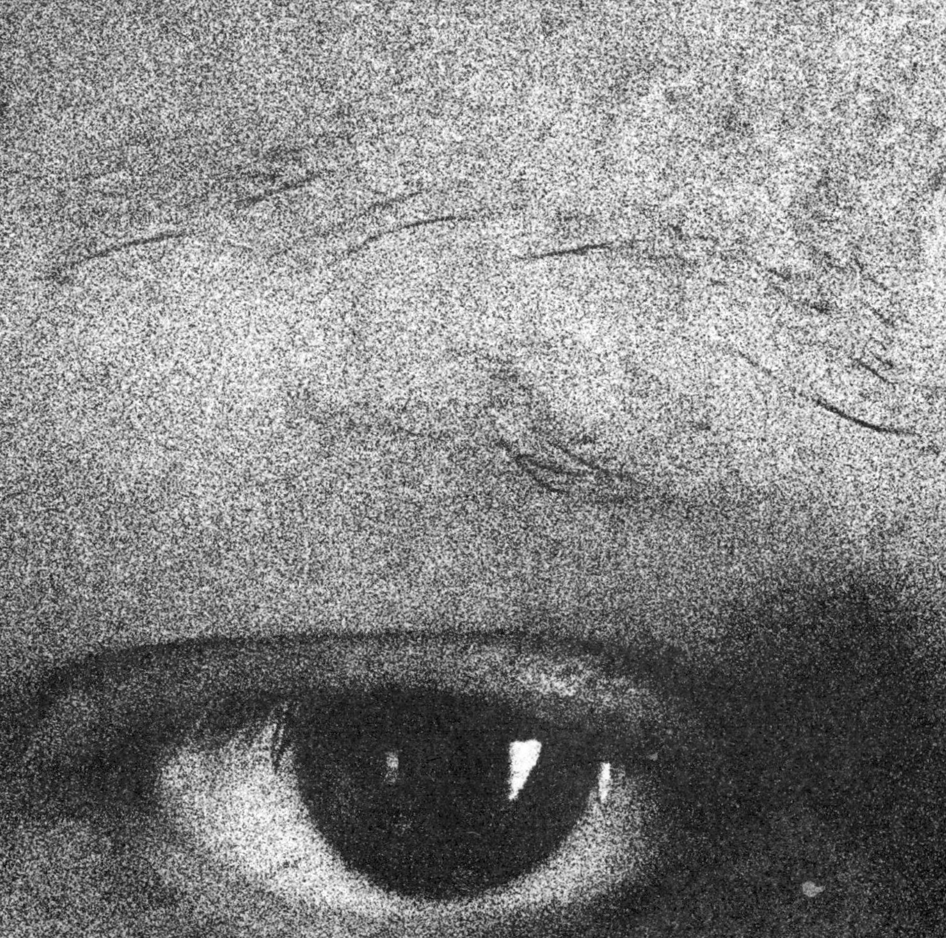

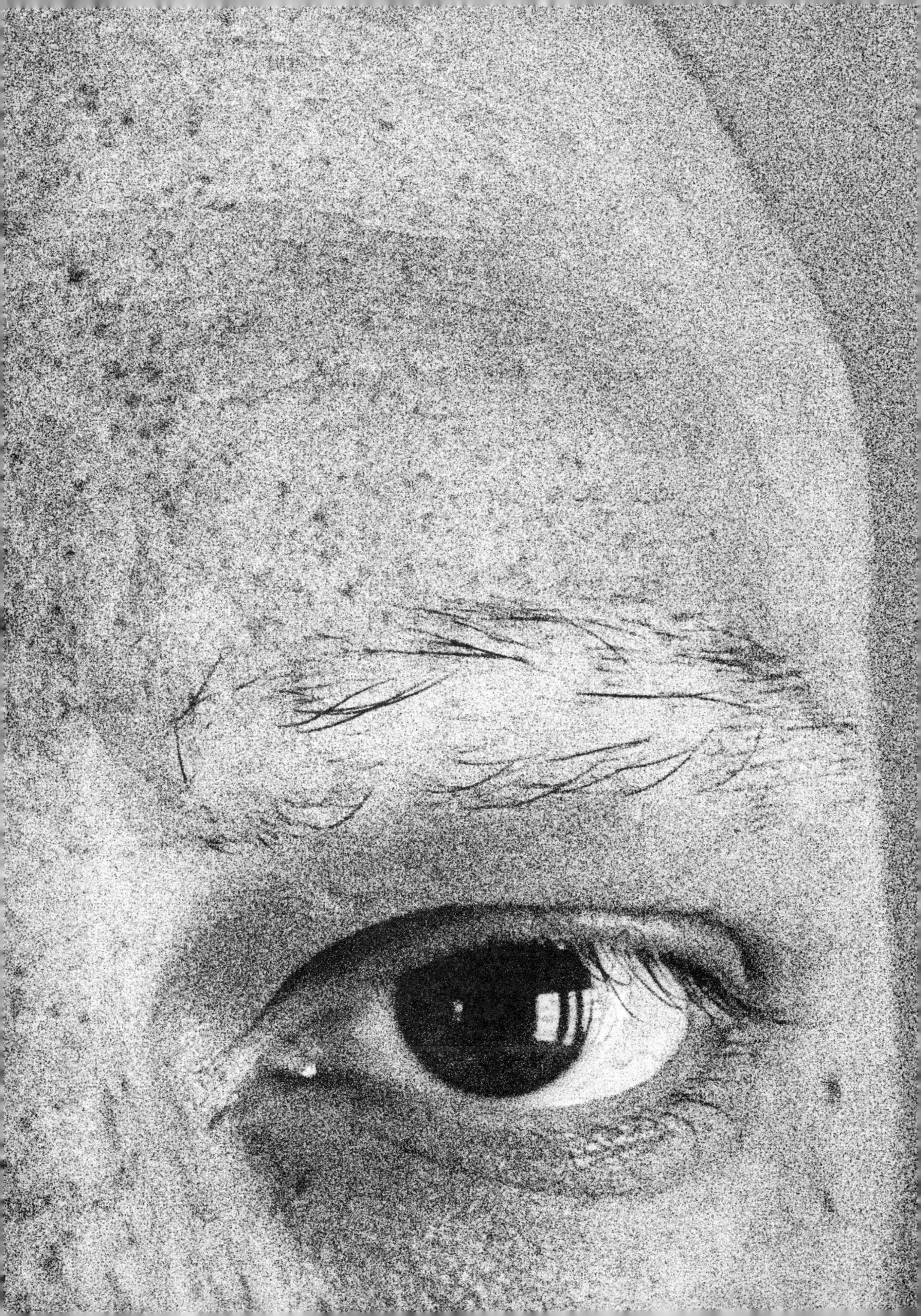

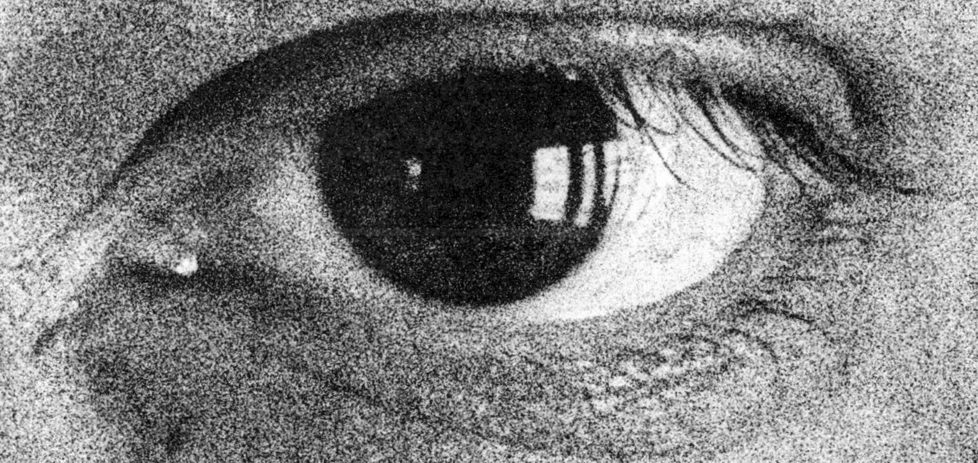

February 12, 2023

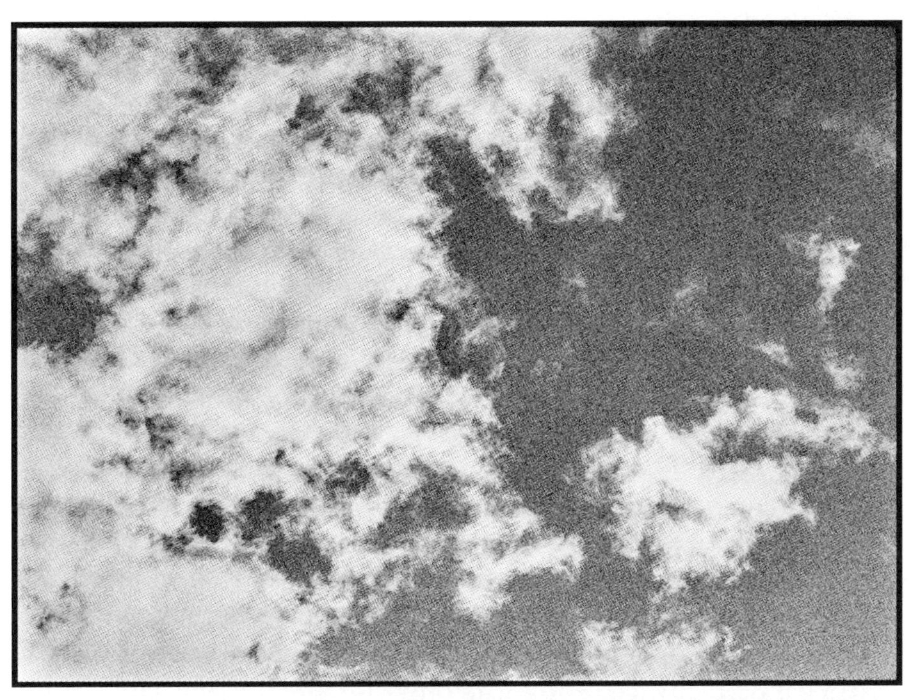

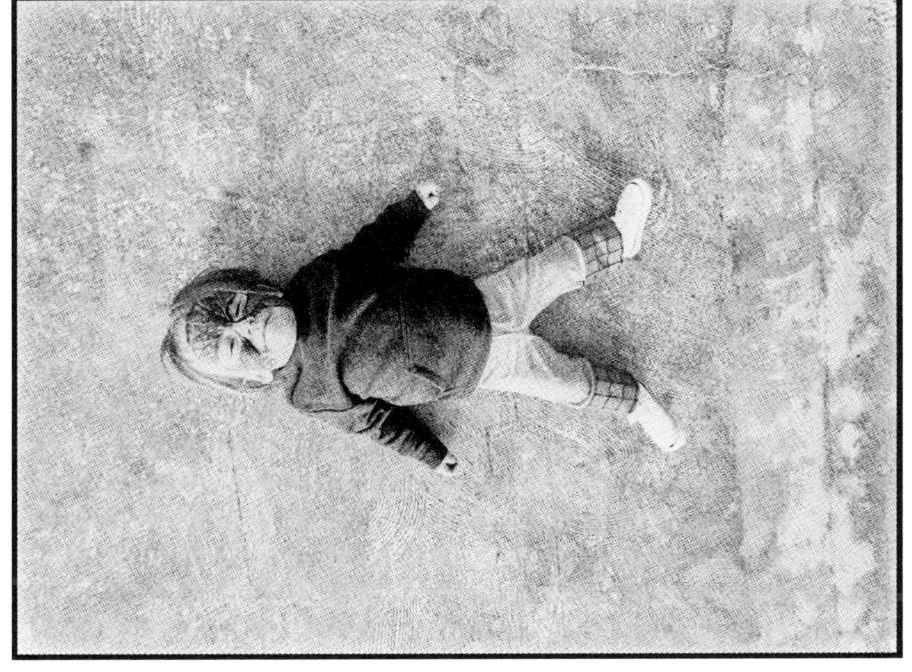

February 13, 2023

Eyebrows gone.

Getting through, going through. The journey continues. My eyebrows fell off this morning in the shower. A shock looking in the mirror. My hair represents my identity these days. It's all lost but will soon grow back. Continued procedures and appointments. Scans and images. Updates on what's needed, but can't confirm a schedule. In and out of consciousness. Deep meditations. Revisiting a present mind. Alone while surrounded. My success comes in knowing what's next professionally. Turning down jobs and unable to schedule my work. A paused process. Celebrations of an undetected lymphoma, all the while learning about an additional three treatments. My outward perspective is beautiful, but I'm reminded of my ugliness when I see my reflection.

I really look like cancer now.

Haven't been very inspired to write recently. Questioning my importance and the importance of these writings. I know my system has been down recently. Can only visualize the finish line. My roots are dehydrated. And the sky is gray. Hoping it will rain soon and the sun will come out. For now we wait.

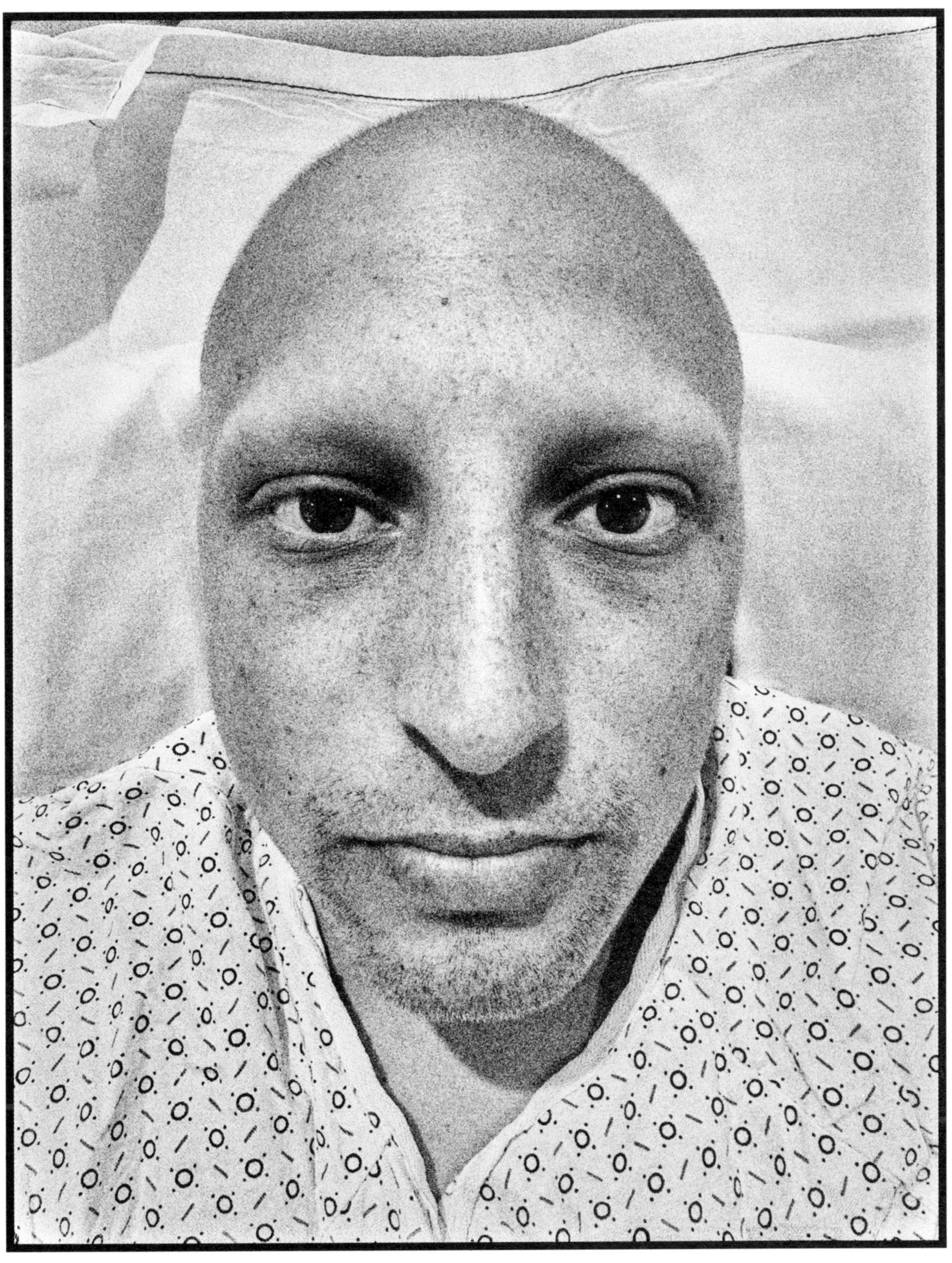

February 15, 2023

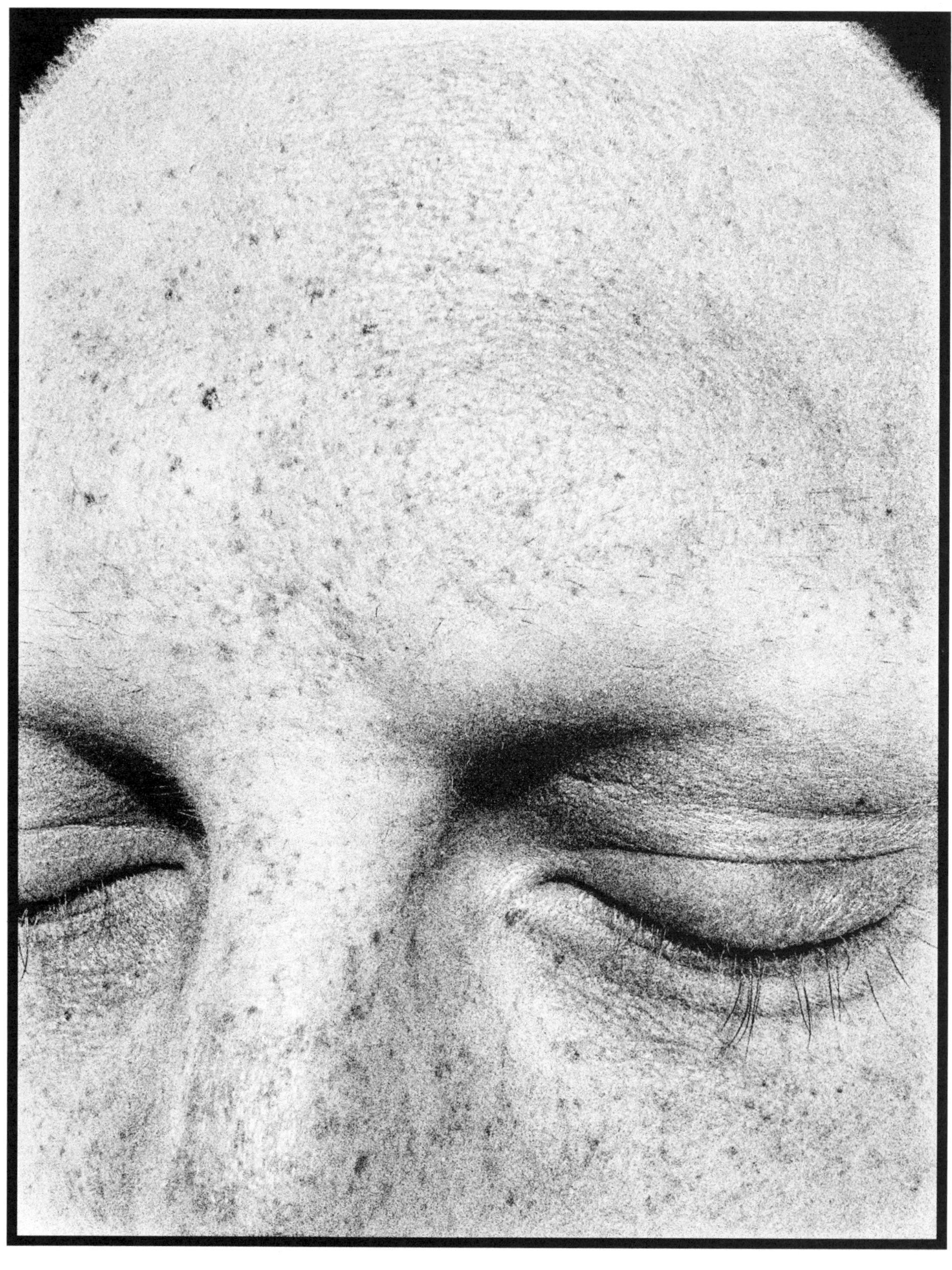

February 16, 2023

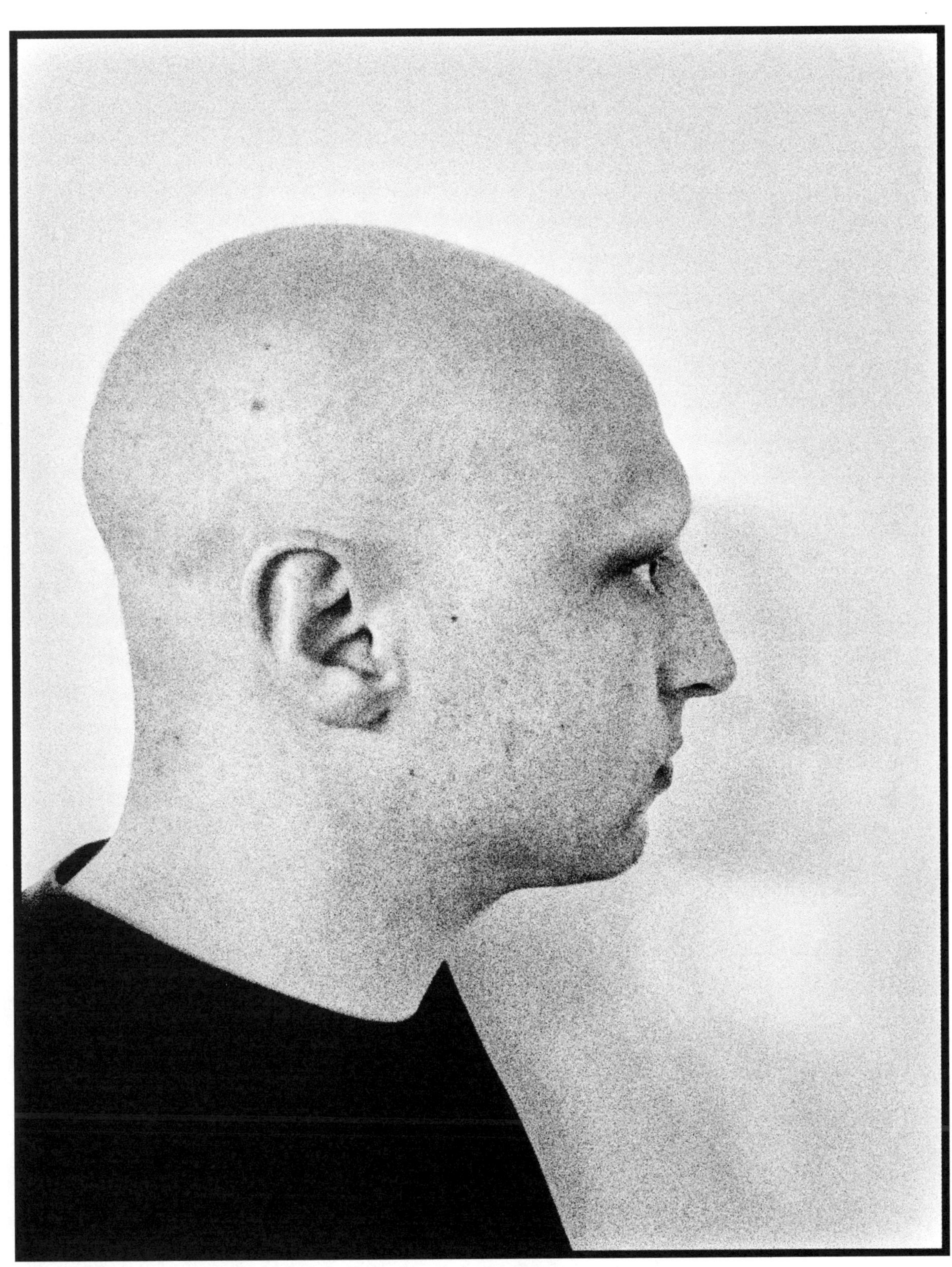

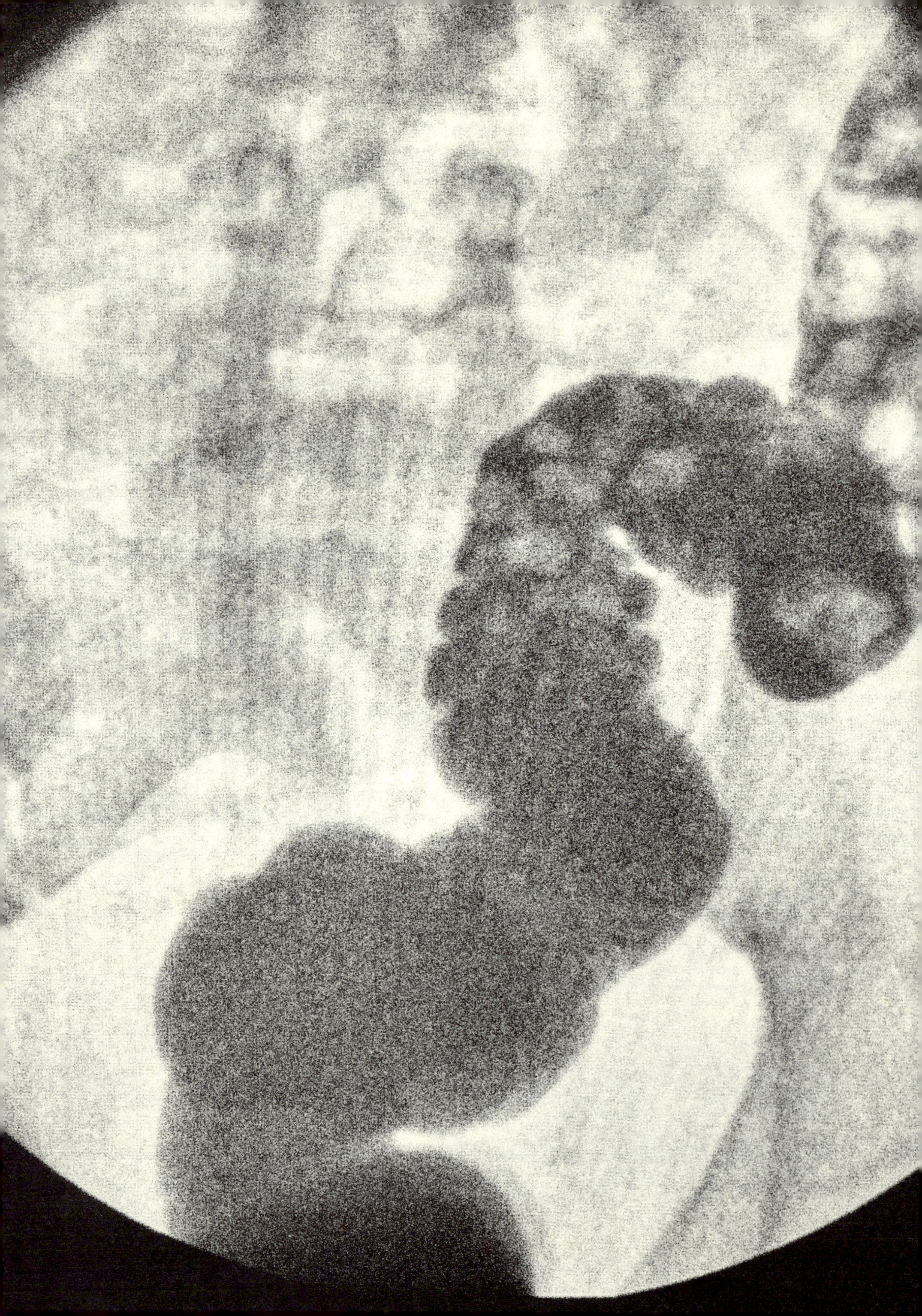

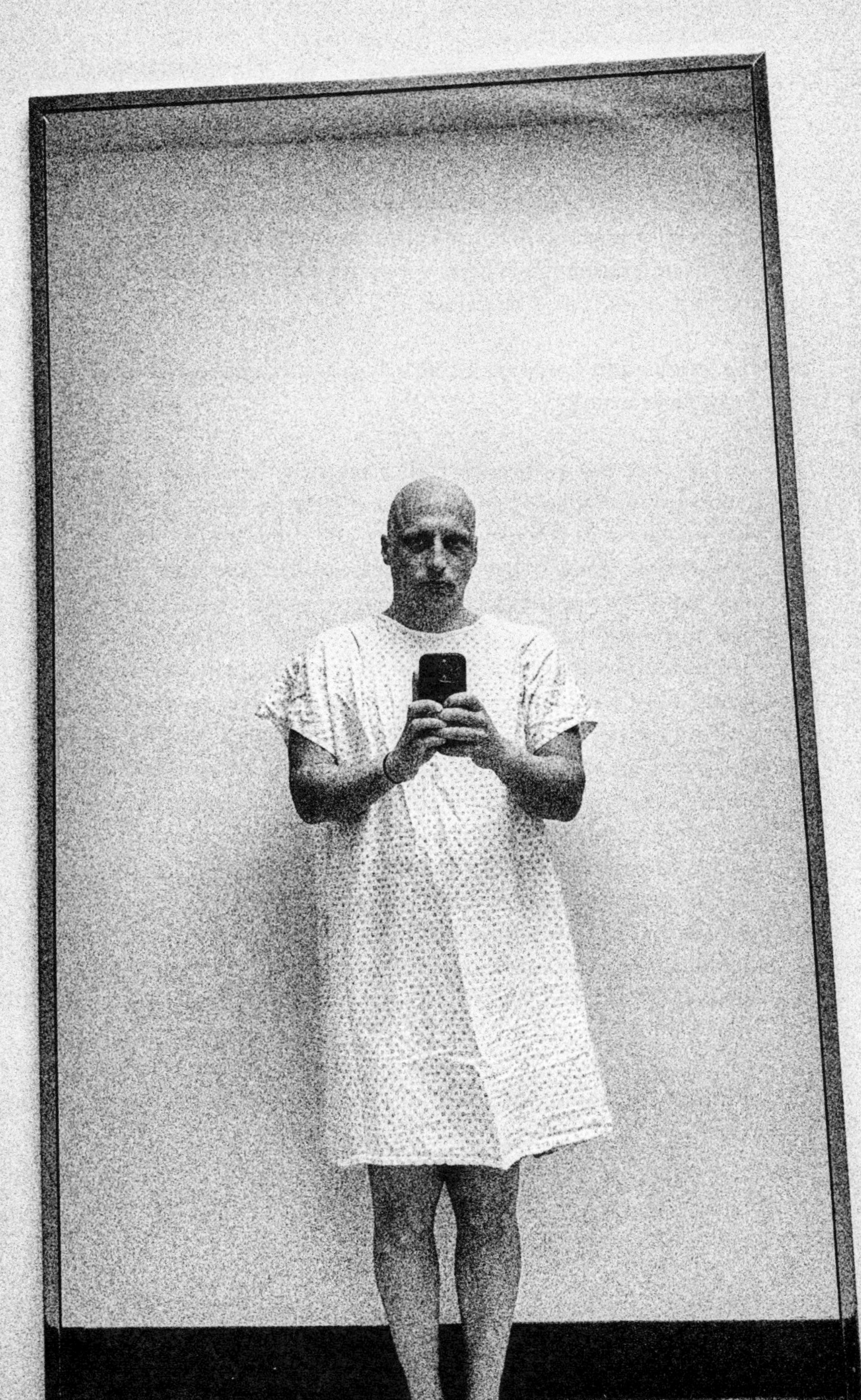

February 23, 2023
Morning

Pulled away from distraction. The water's at my feet. The waves crash continuously. I roll up my pants so I can walk along the shore. My hairless legs. Exposing my hairless legs. I bend over to put my hands along the water.

Putting my palms against my face. Feeling the cold sea salt.

I just got called back in. My fourth treatment starts in the next few hours. Accepted defeat. The last few weeks have been ultimate freedom. A sense of normality again. Our problems are only adjusted framework. We just have to shift our perspectives, but everything continues to happen for us. It's easy to get pulled in time and time again. The distractions.

The follows and the likes. There's nothing like the sunshine and the waves crashing.

I've been talking a lot with Jessica recently. Recorded sessions. Reminded of childhood. Reminded of how my story got started. They say the artist is the most egotistical. I think it's the ones who get the most success that are the least selfish, the least egotistical. I think it's the ones who are the most scared and hold onto it themselves who actually obtain the most ego. They keep it all to themselves. The ones with the most fame and recognition are actually the most free. And giving. I'm not sure exactly how to feel as I go into the next one, but I still know there's a lot of work to be done. My work should continue on. New habits. Unnecessary rules. I've been receiving a lot of inbounds for work recently too. Some large projects that remind me of my value. It's been tough to have to turn them all down, but I know bigger and better opportunities will come. I've never been too worried about money, but it is difficult to turn down opportunity for income and for family, but I accept my rest. Because this will all be over soon. For now I stand on the rocks at the end of Will Rogers State Beach. It just rained. A refreshed Los Angeles awaits. The clouds are covering the mountain tops. It's drizzling, but sunny. A perfect metaphor. My dog runs along the shore, still so curious about everything. A new way to be in love.

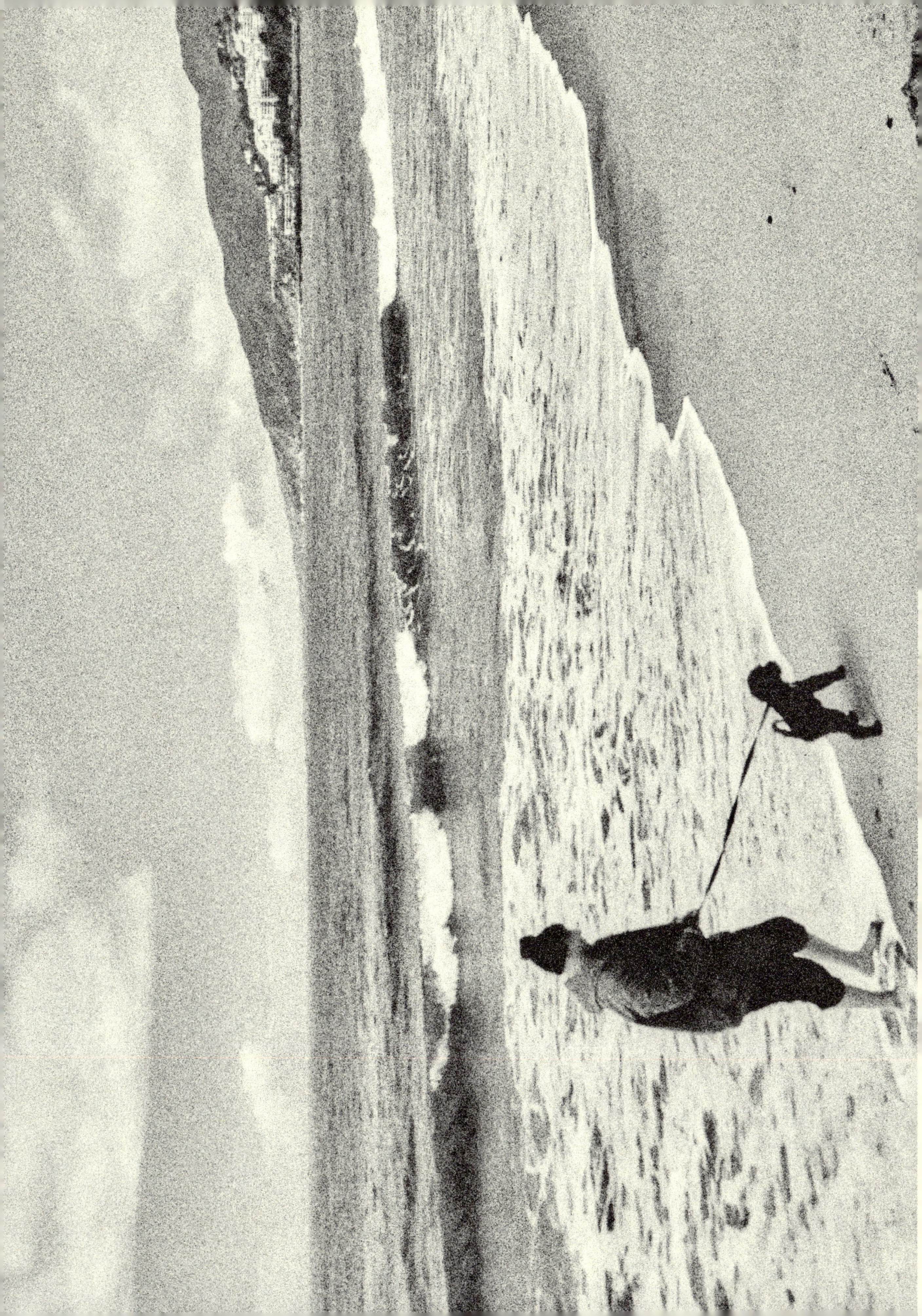

February 23 2023
Evening

A reminded reality.

The Benadryl injected.
The feet and legs tingle.

My body fidgets.

Deflated optimism.

It's all too familiar again.

A reduction of optimism.

The cars drive by outside.

The quiet yells of nurses in the hallway.
The quiet screeching of the IV pole.

My thoughts get louder.

Discomfort heightens.

Getting through, going through.

One step at a time.
Only two visitors.

Sammy's at home.

A temporary rainbow.

The darkness outside starts to creep in.

Pretending like I'm in control. Pretending like I can work.
Pretended optimism.

Nature gets accelerated in here.

I want to be running through the Redwoods.
Shot from a drone running with me. Open fields, my hands glide along the grass.

Six days is a long time.

The light dims literally and metaphorically.

February 25, 2023

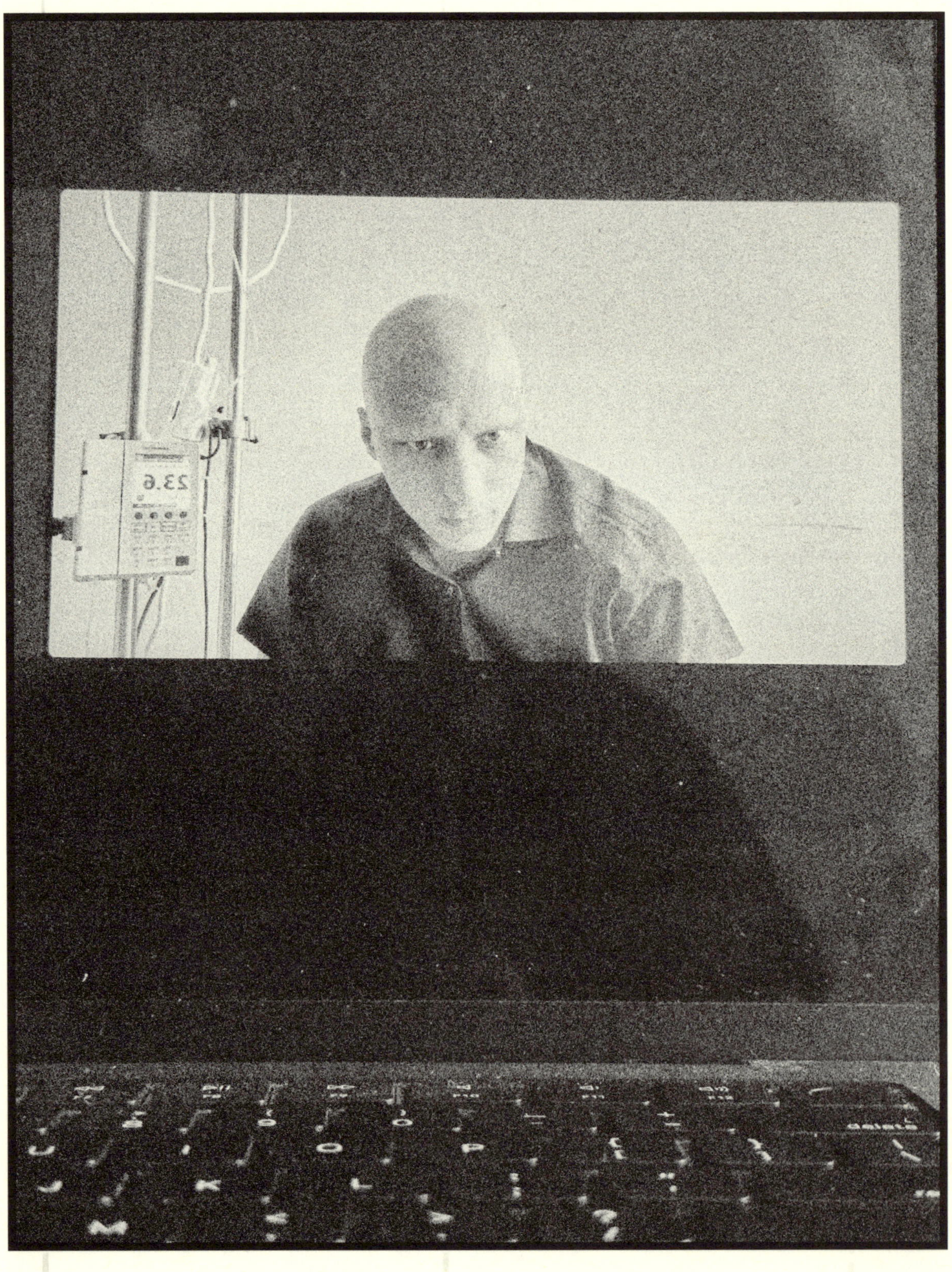

Artificial lines. Balancing curiosity and normality. Follow the rules. Stay on this floor. Laps up and down the hallway. Oatmeal with raisins and a little brown sugar. A peek into the other rooms. To think I'm a part of. A reminded hard truth that I'm going through this. Feeling blue. One day I'll look back and read these journal entries. I'll look at my bald head and bald face. I'll try to remember what an impact this all made on me. People around me keep telling me I'm on my phone, that I'm not present with them. It's been hard to find presence at all. The highs and lows are so extreme. The nausea is so significant. Selected framework. I try to rest my eyes. You can hear the beeping pulse in the hallway. The wet tires driving by from the downpour. I can't tell if I'm pretending to get through or if I'm just getting through. I can feel every drip of this chemo. It's breaking me down, but stay up my friend. Thanks, love.

February 28, 2023

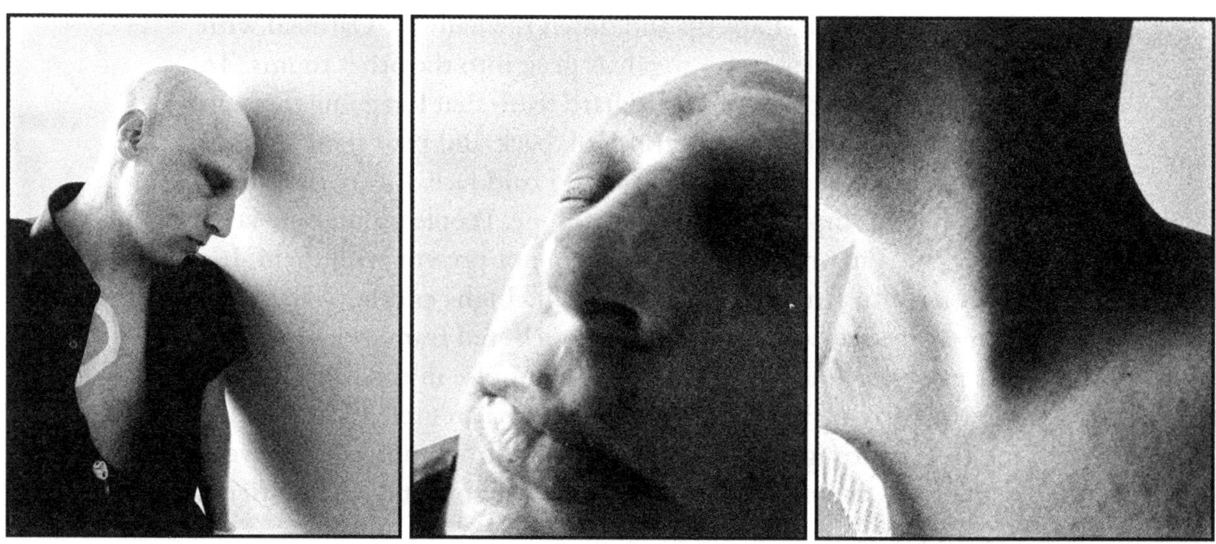

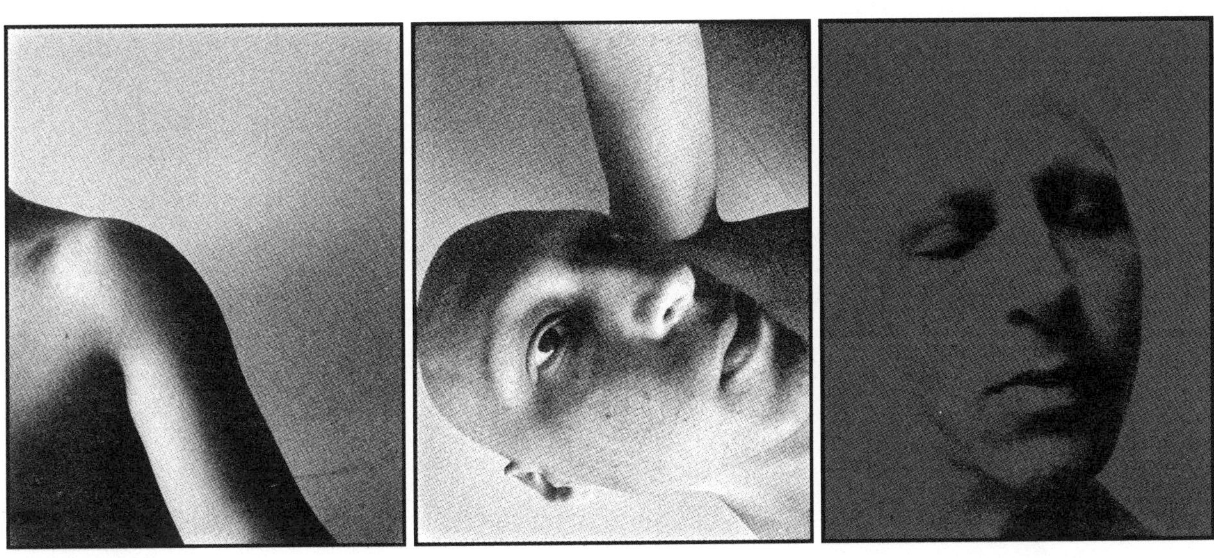

March 3, 2023

Round 3 done.

Discharge. Symptoms repeat. The everyday person could never understand what I'm going through. I'm not looking for sympathy, it's just the fucking truth. Each time I throw up I feel like I'm flushing part of myself away. My position on my hands and knees is so vulnerable yet so familiar. The constant needle pokes into the port, repeated CT scans, PET scans, X rays, enemas, fainting time and time again. Nausea. The sound of freedom out the window. Someone recently asked if my look was a fashion statement. What's wrong with society? I looked at a portrait of myself from yesterday on the phone with such shock. My perceived being is not what I'm looking at. People don't know how to act around me anymore. You can tell they don't know what to ask. And they spend more time avoiding a conversation than opening up. Delicate sensitivities. People keep asking how I'm feeling. I try to practice saying "good." This elongated narrative is frustrating. That I'm not OK. I'm feeling the pain it's starting to really cause others. The roots to my unhealthy tree are starting to get tangled with the roots of those next to me. Distressed growth. Since out, I've been spending my time constructing a new business plan, writing a film, building a spring season. I'm continuing to organize my company. All for what? Artificial distraction. I say this all with great luck. Just a few months ago I was diagnosed with stage 4 cancer. And the finish line is ahead. But what am I finishing? And what will I be beginning? It's incredible how many pills I have to take. Another pill to swallow. I really am feeling good though. Just going through it. And comparatively it's a lot. But hey. There's still a lot to do. No time to waste. Just wanted to let you know I was throwing up, and I'm over it.

March 12, 2023

Difficulty in darkness in my reflection.

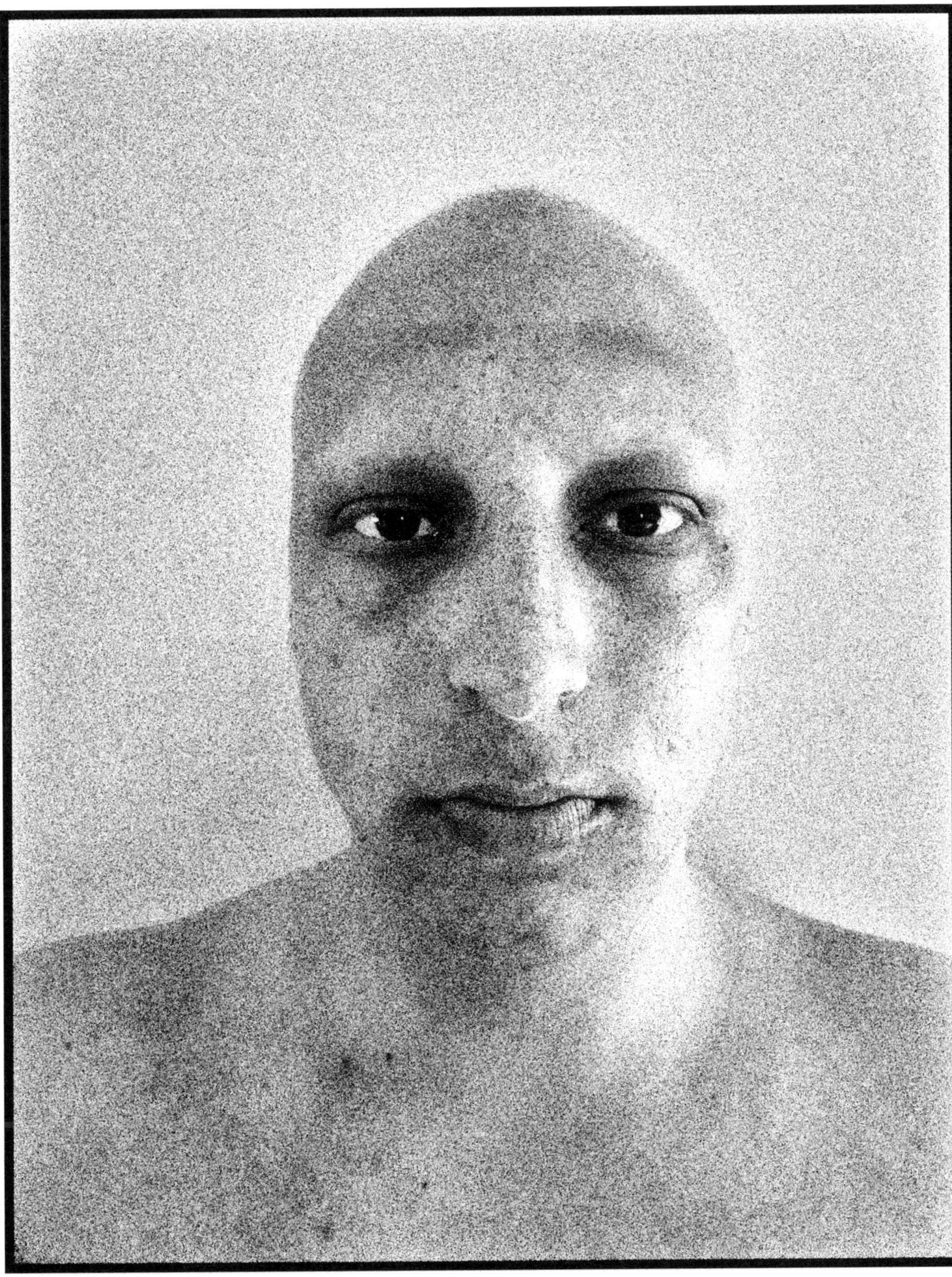

March 13, 2023

You know the drill.
The beginning of the end.

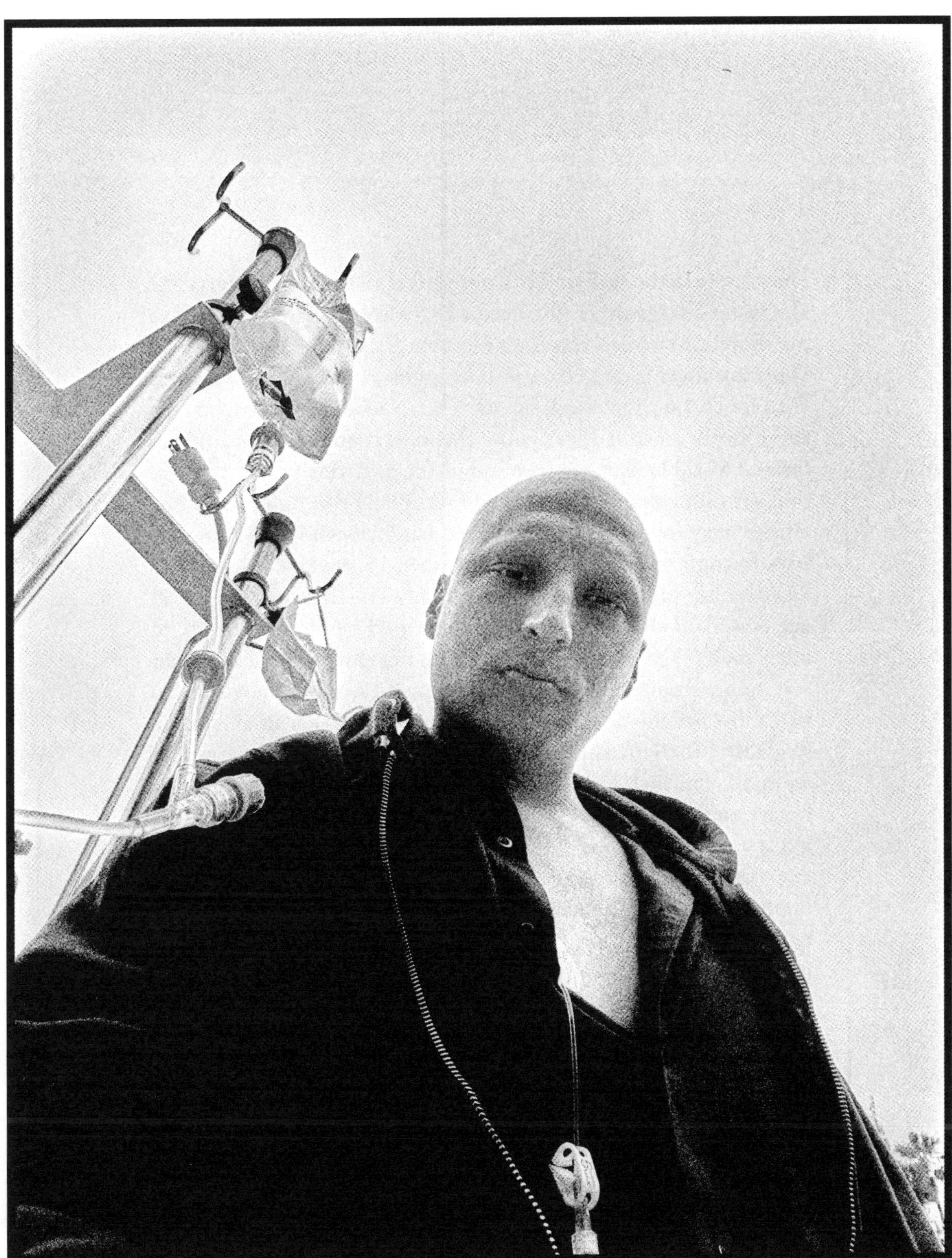

March 14, 2023

They say ride the waves. This time I feel like I'm out pretty far. The water's stagnant. I just need a big wave to bring me back to the shoreline so I can rest for a moment. Last week was powerful. Three instances back to back that brought so much joy. First I was at an ice cream shop checking out when a woman approached me and bluntly asked if I was going through chemo. I felt people in the real world look at me with judgment or curiosity, but this was the first time someone asked me if I was going through cancer. She immediately followed by inviting her daughter who was sitting at a table to come meet me. She had just turned five years old, and was asked by her mom to show me her head. The little girl peeled off her wig. And showed me her bald scalp. The mom with excitement then asked the little girl to lift up her shirt and show me the scar on her stomach. The mom asked me if I would remove my hat and show her my bald head. I kneeled down to her level and did so gladly. I then lifted up my shirt and showed her my scar on my stomach. The little girl went back to her friends to continue eating her ice cream. While the mom let me know she just went through kidney cancer which included surgery and six months of chemo and radiation. After some small talk we left. You could tell how important that moment was for the mom. It was also such an important moment for me. The realization that I'm part of this community. Only we know the severity of what we've endured. The ice cream was good too.

The next moment of joy was a doctor's visit with Dr Oliai. During this visit he shared that I could double doses between methotrexate and R-EPOCH, which would mean that instead of finishing in June I could finish at the end of April, assuming all goes well. It would also mean I would be receiving chemo for five out of the next six weeks. But I embrace my mentor Alex, knowing I'm on a mission and I've got shit to do.

The last moment of joy came in seeing my brother, and my collaborator Steve Hackman actualize his new work *The Brink.* Steve has spent most of his career making other people's music, and this was one of the few times he put his own work out. We put on an event at the Water Garden. It was the first project I was involved in since this all went down. I was reminded how much I love what I do. And how lucky I am that my job connects me with artists of great talent and fulfillment. Bob Marley was once questioned about richness. And responded that richness does not come in the form of money, but rather in the quality of life. The universe gave me great joy recently. And now I'm back in the hospital. Beginning the end. I'm overcome with nausea and stillness again. The more still I become, the more poetry that lives in my body. Although I'm given a ticket to live past this for some reason, I'm feeling a sense of mortality right now. I just spent some time writing text messages to random people telling them how much I love them and why they bring me great richness. It will never make you weaker by giving a compliment to someone else. We're all just essentially sharing our scars and bald heads.

March 17, 2023

March 19, 2023

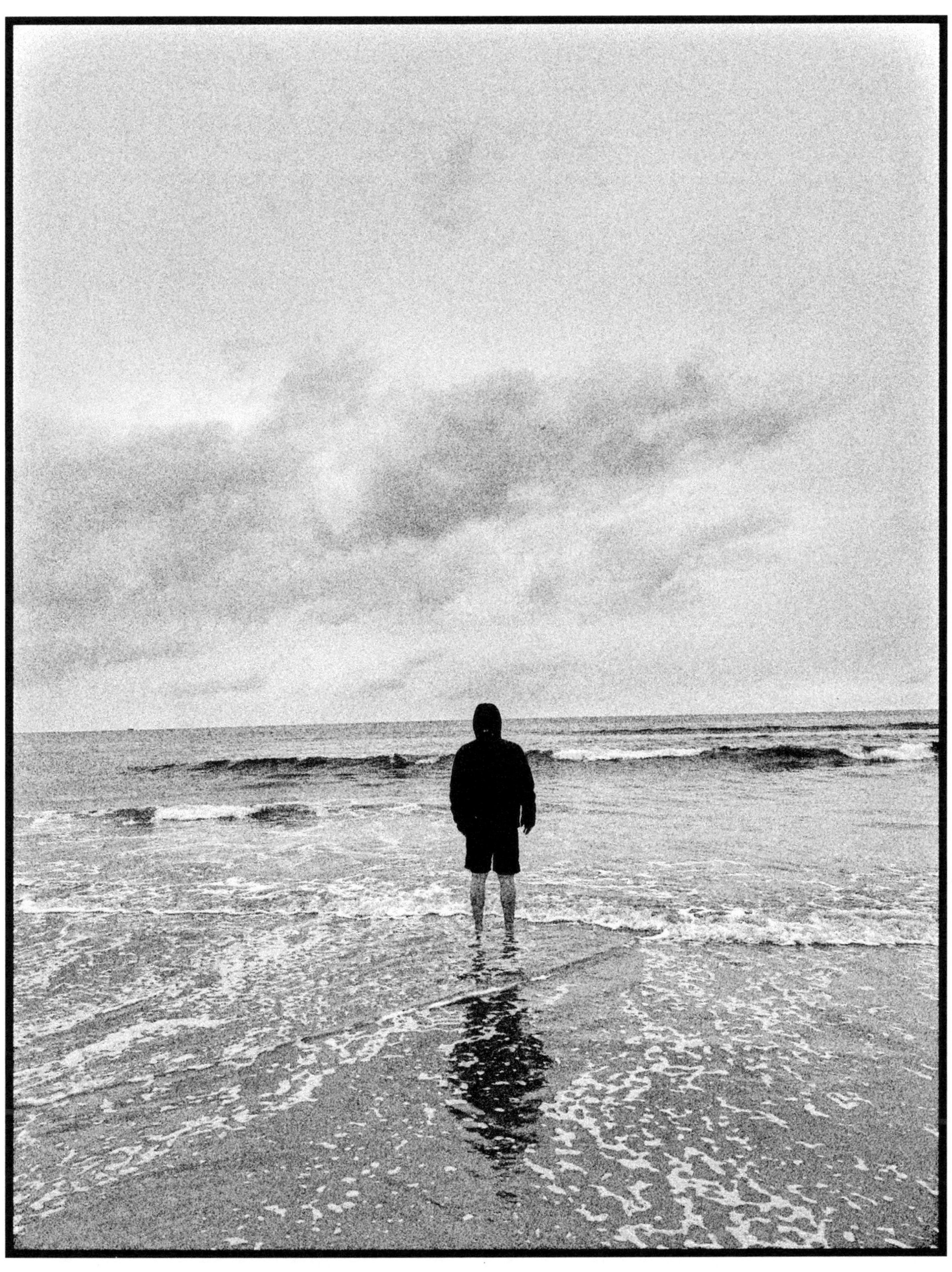

March 23, 2023

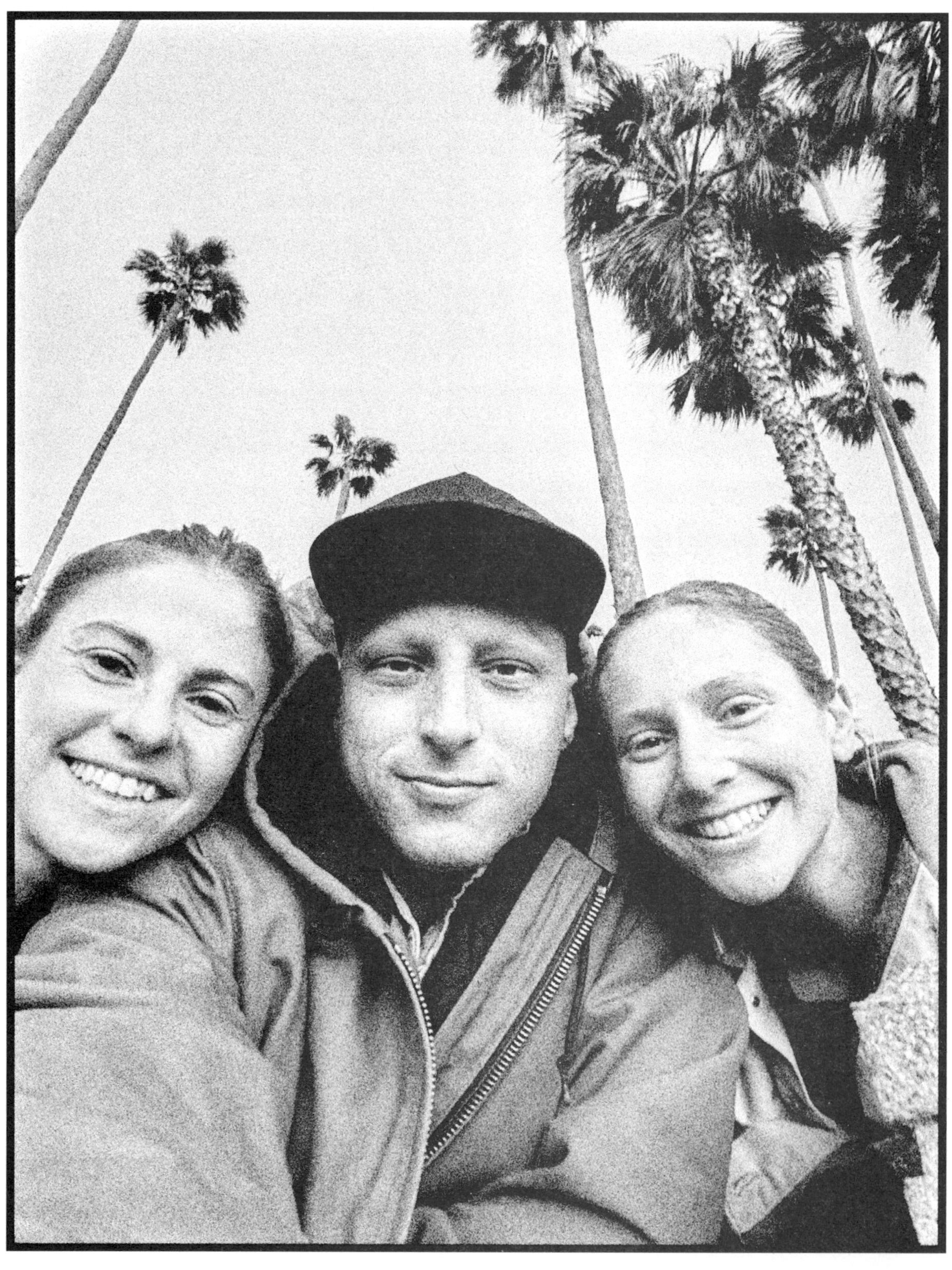

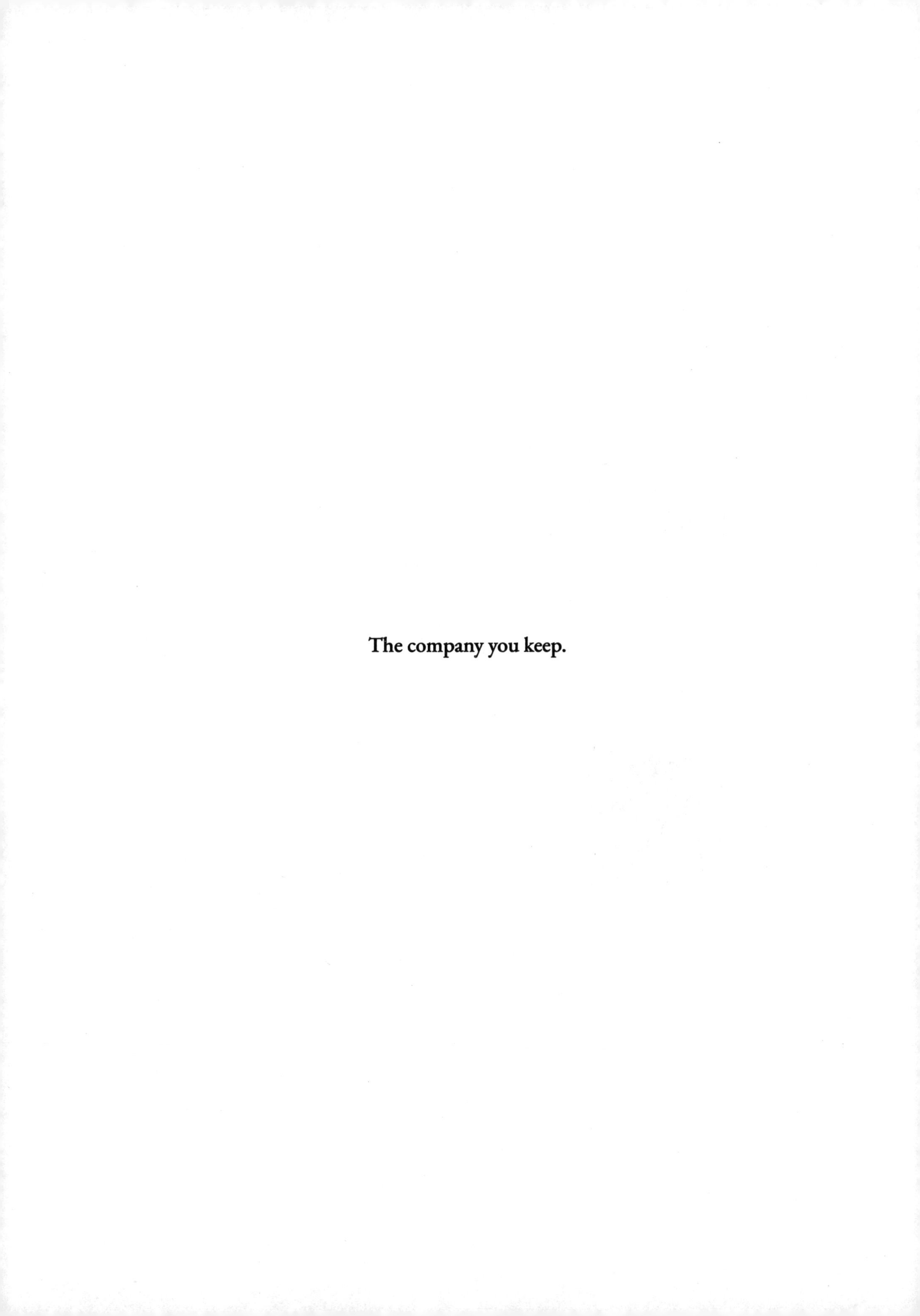
The company you keep.

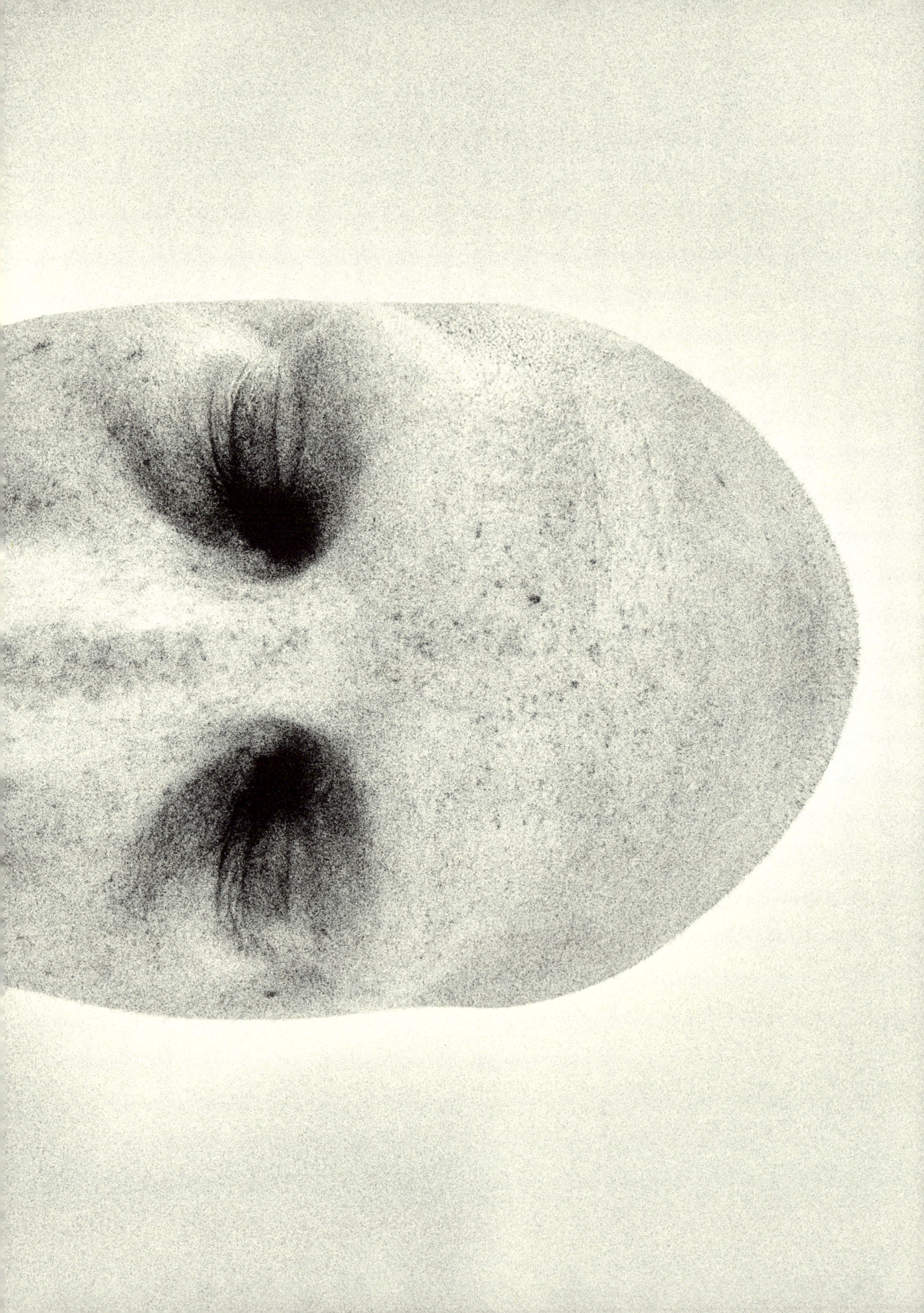

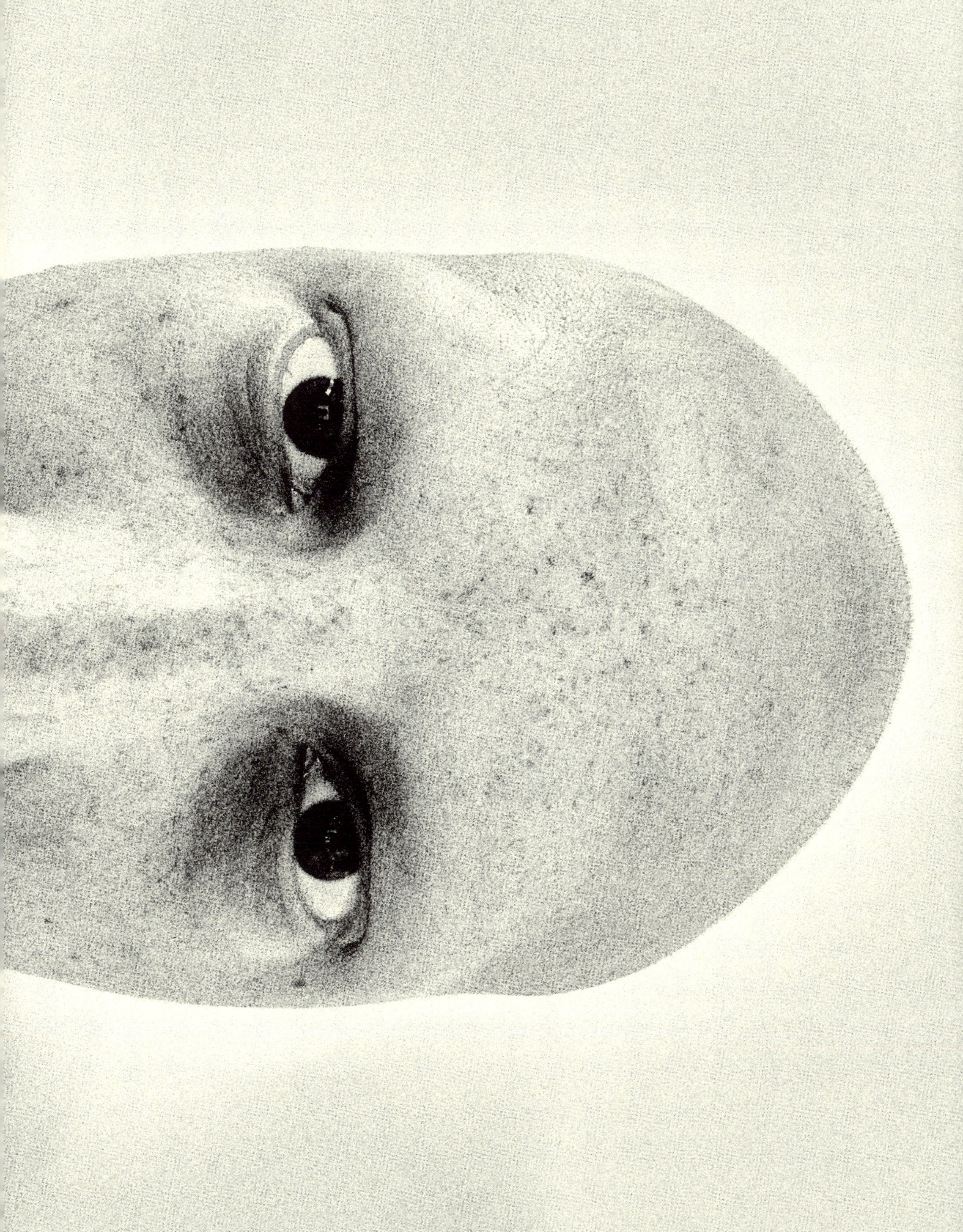

March 24, 2023

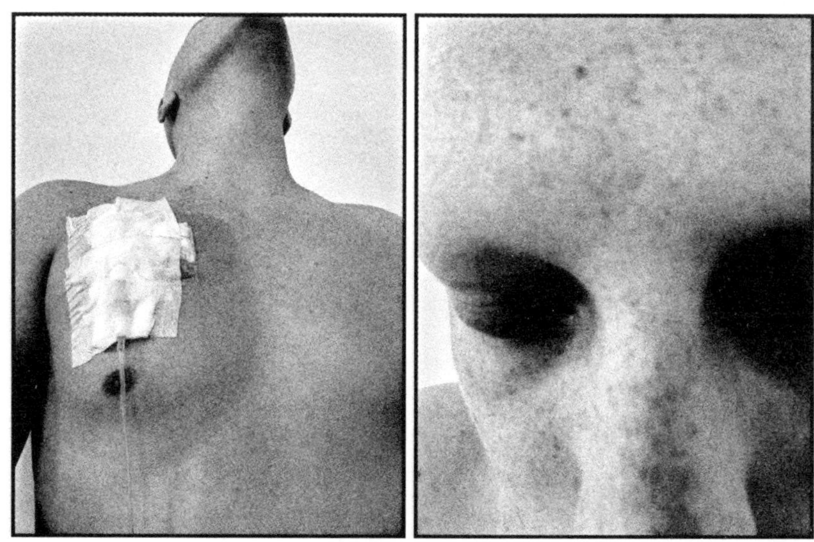

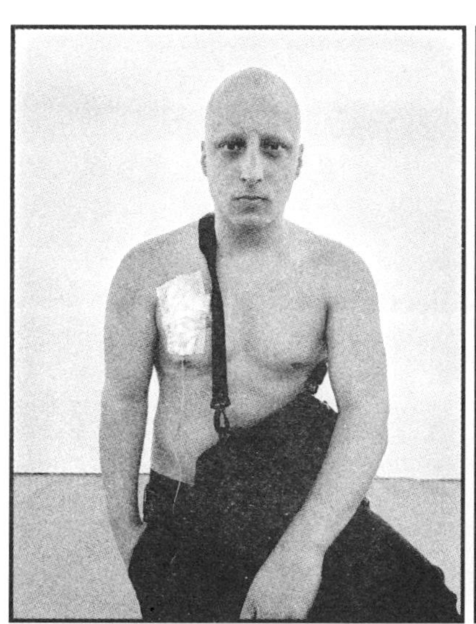
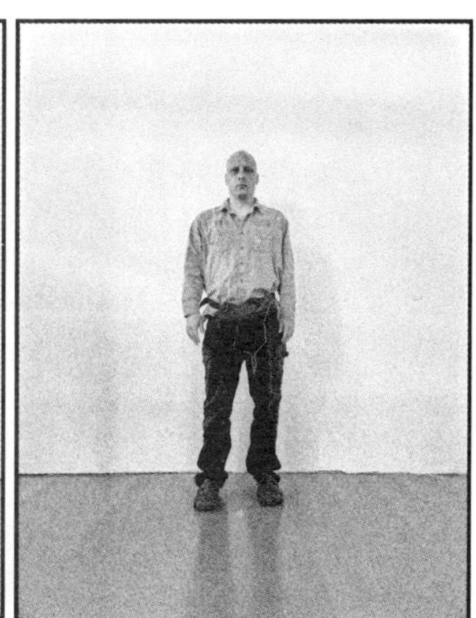

March 25, 2023

Neulasta injection.

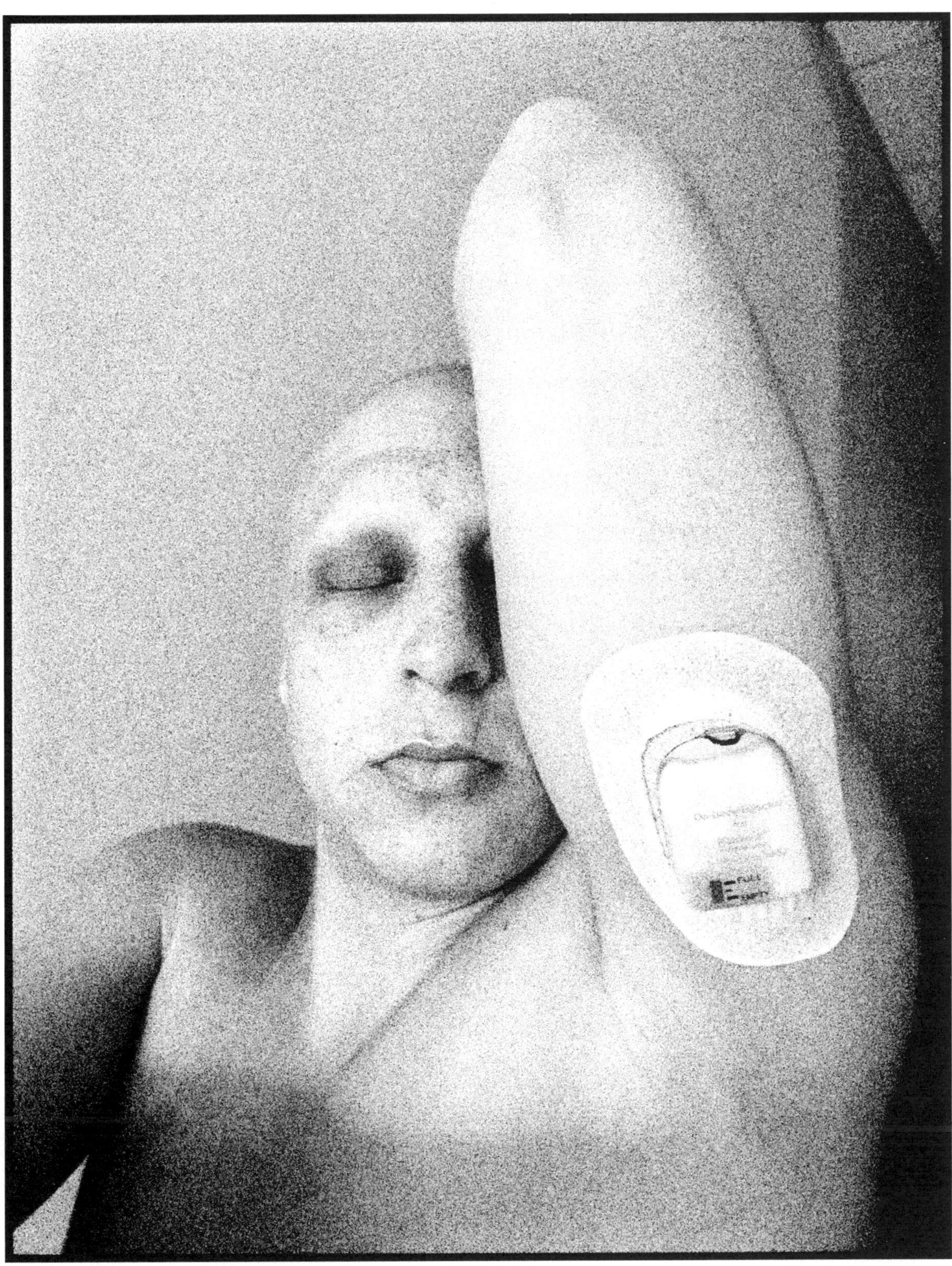

March 29, 2023

The rain pours outside. I've noticed every time I've been in treatment it's been raining.

It's time to go back tomorrow. I recently shared on social media my story with this diagnosis. I was so overwhelmed by the response. This whole time it's been something intimate amongst a small group of people. Now it really feels like the whole world knows. The amount of messages and calls I've received is unbelievable. I feel so lucky, so fortunate, so valuable to be connected to so many incredible people around the world. Many of whom I know, some who I have crossed paths with once or twice along the many years, and also many strangers. My work has always been my vehicle for building my community of support, but sharing this personal circumstance created a new vibration.

What cancer represents in this story in sharing it is so much bigger than me. Cancer is such a deep issue that so many people are battling with and such a large part of so many people's lives. What do you say when so many people say they are thinking of you or they love you or they are hoping I make it through? I've been saying I love you so much, and your support means the world. It really does. There's not much more I can say to people but how meaningful a small connection can be. Our life is unbelievable. This opportunity to dive deep into the science of medicine, of biology. The likeliness that any one of us is alive today. It's all based around randomness. The same is true with cancer. Our genetics, our bloodstream, our cells, our molecules. There are a million things happening within us every second. As I get closer to the finish line, I feel luckier and luckier each day.

I think the universe has something in store for me. All this rain is just hydrating the roots below us to create new forests for us to see through.

March 30, 2023

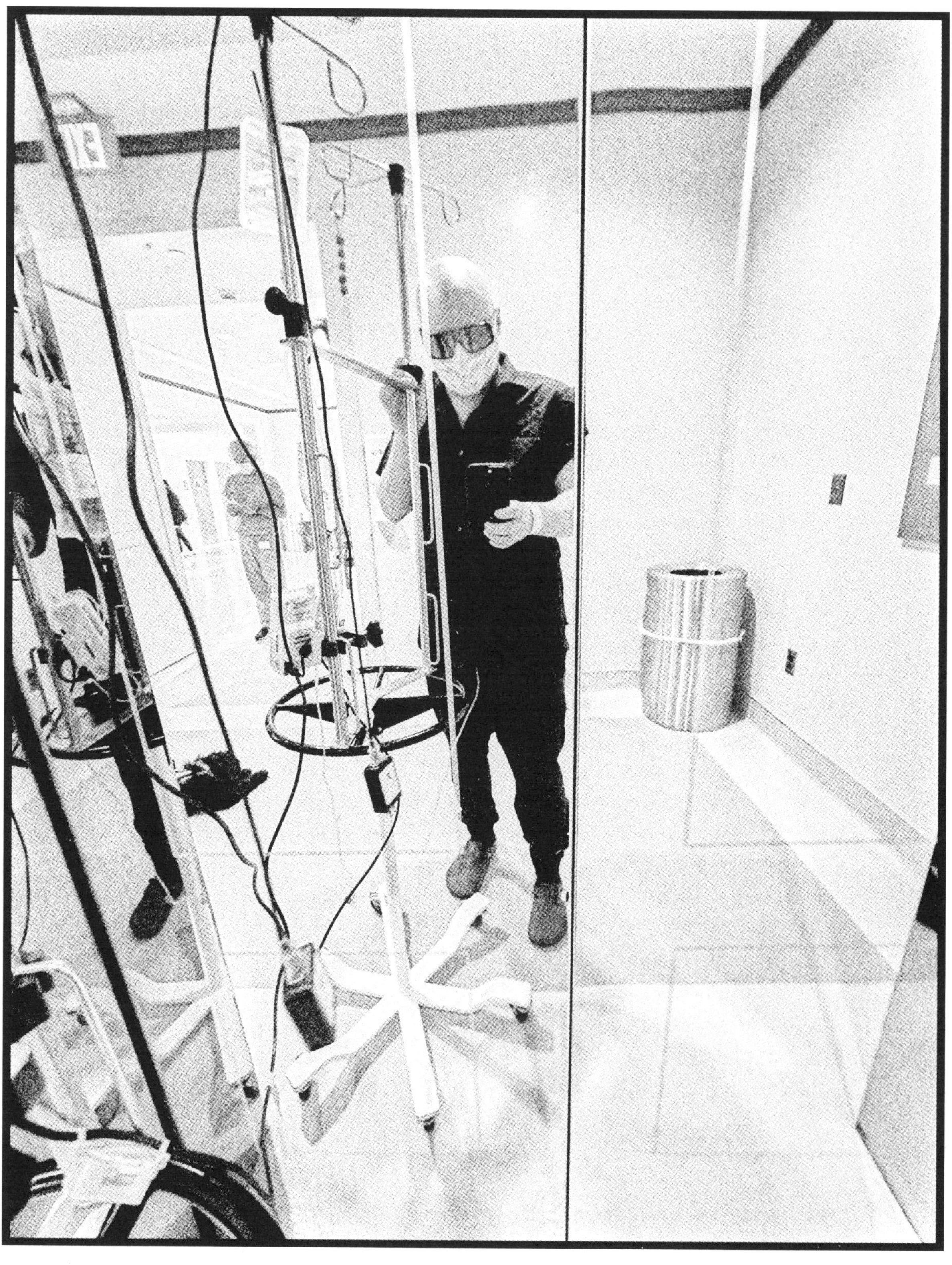

April 1, 2023

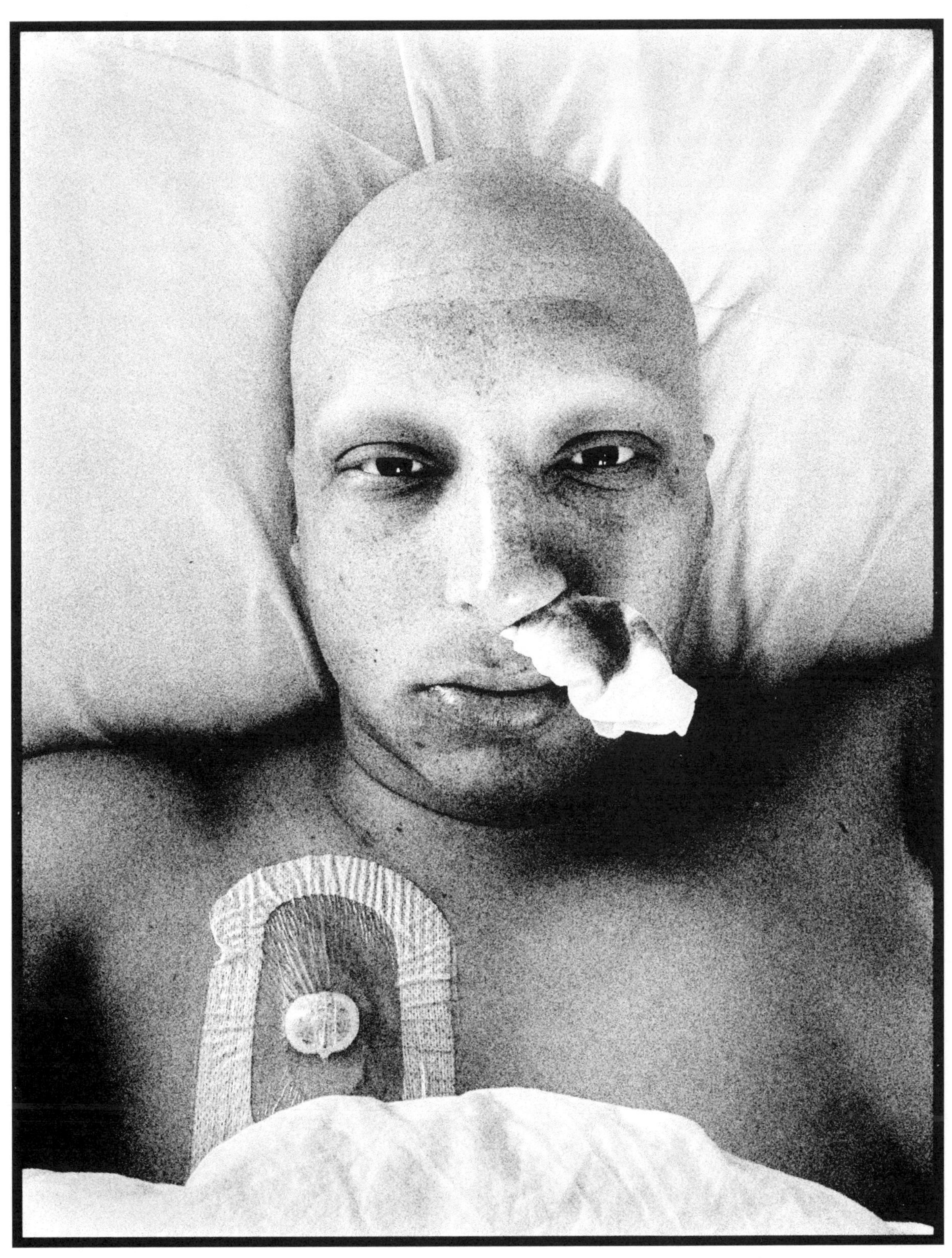

April 5, 2023

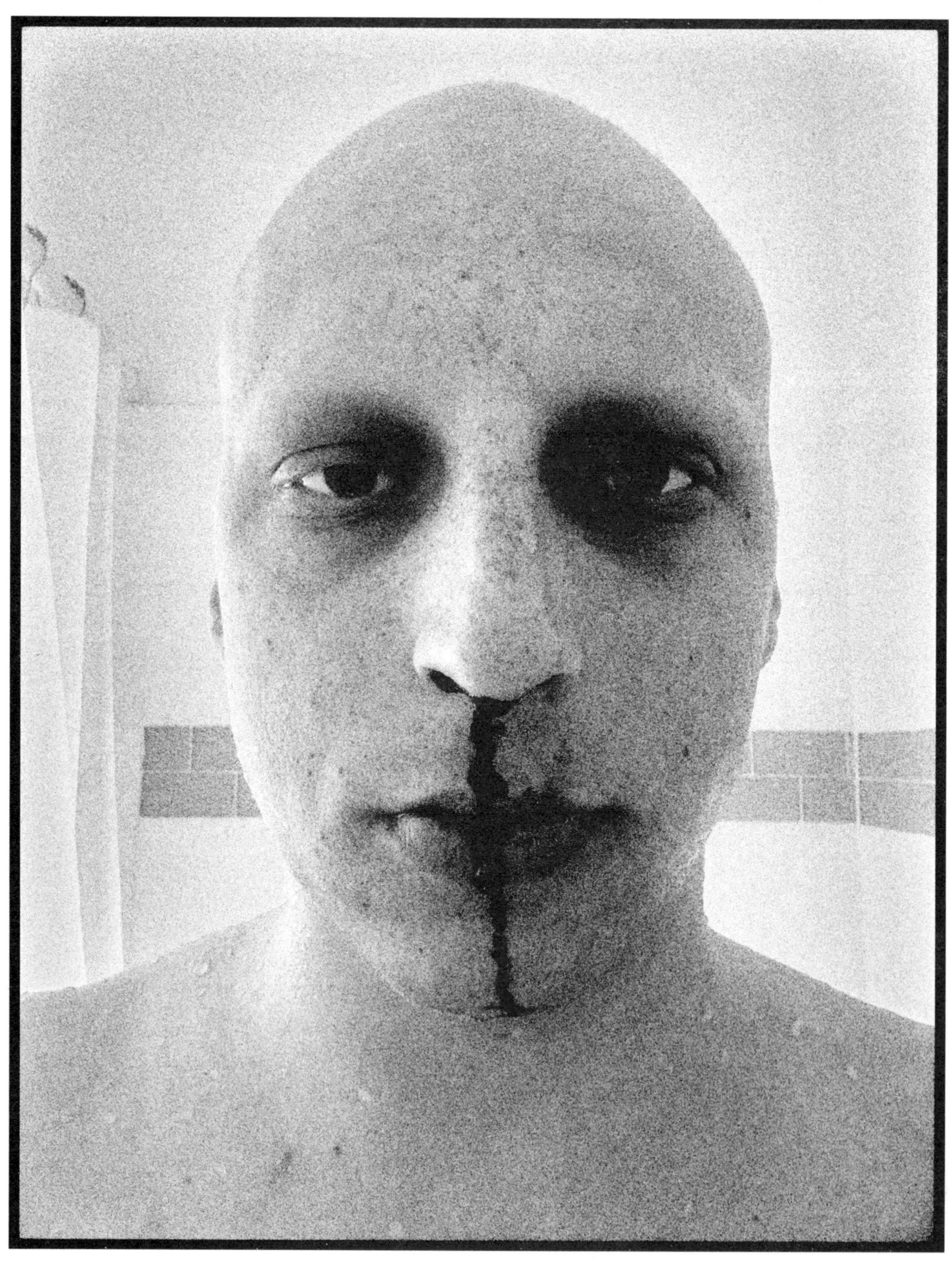

April 8, 2023

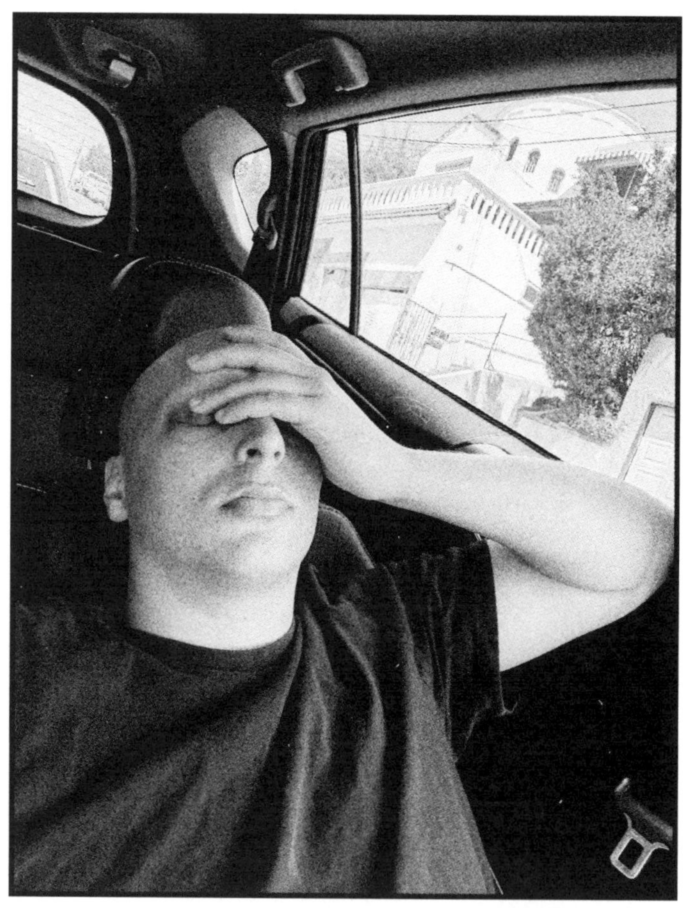

On set. Mind won't calm.

April 9, 2023

Blood is everywhere. Dripping out of my nose. In my stool. It hasn't stopped for weeks. It's just pouring out of me. In the middle of the night when I sleep. When I take a shower. It drips and hits the bathroom floor. Drop after drop. It pours all over. Everything's red like the Red Sea. This recent methotrexate was terrible. I was in the hospital for five days. Nausea and anxiety came over like never before. They had to do two blood transfusions. It's one of the most traumatizing things to see a bag of somebody else's blood sitting on an IV pole next to you, hearing it just drip into your body. I experienced that twice this time. Three all together. Something took over my whole mouth. Sores for about eight days now. It's impossible to open my mouth, eat anything. I can't drink many things because of all the acid. It burns from tomatoes, oranges, and vinegar. I've been basically eating apple sauce now for two weeks. The symptoms are so overwhelming. For some reason I assumed that as I got closer to the end it would get easier, but it's really the complete opposite. It's just getting harder and harder, and my body is getting weaker and weaker. There's no mercy. I don't share this to complain, just to paint a portrait of the current environment. I know this will all pass very soon, but right now it's a big challenge, and I'm so motivated with my work that it's hard to find time to rest, which is making me more nauseous. I've had this reflection recently from all the people reaching out. After my post, everyone is sharing celebration toward me just for enduring what I've been going through. It's such an opposition to my life's work. Typically I work hard, to be creative and share my work with those that celebrate it, but in this journey I have nothing to put out. Just something to get through. It reminds me of Holocaust survivors. Those who endured something and have been acknowledged for what they endured. They didn't choose that path by any means. It chose them. And they're honored and acknowledged for getting through. It's been a new psychology for me to realize that people are looking at me now for getting through something. My luck still feels very high. I feel tremendously lucky. I feel eternally grateful. I still look at the mirror everyday with great pain. Shocked by my portrait. It's been nice to get back to work this week. The dancers are happy. I'm happy and distracted. It's a nice reminder to remember where my mind was at prior to this diagnosis. Where my life was and my identity was prior to all this happening.

The last thing I'll share for now is that it caused me great pain to celebrate Jill's birthday in the hospital. We all gathered in the courtyard. I barely had any endurance to come down. I hadn't been outside in three days. Or even out of my room. So to be around so many people was so overwhelming. And also have so much attention on me when the attention should've been on her. And she shouldn't have had to face her birthday on that campus, but I'll make it up to her. And all this will be done soon. Thanks for writing, my love.

April 17, 2023

Day 1 of my last chemotherapy treatment.

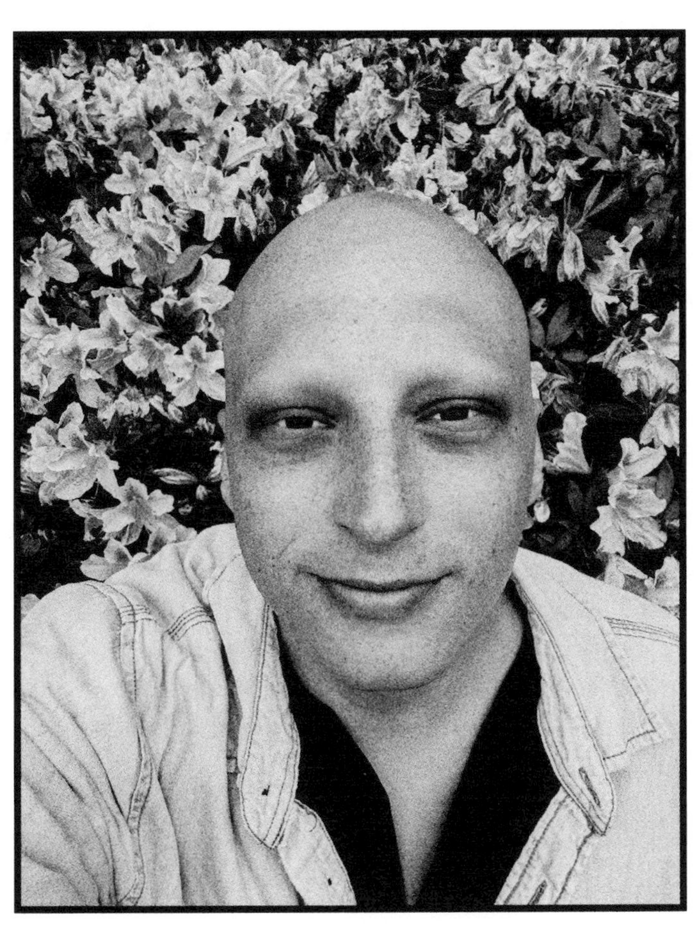

April 20, 2023

I just got my last bag plugged in at the clinic. I have 24 more hours until I'm not receiving chemo anymore. I'm so overwhelmed. This whole week has been so overwhelming.

It's so much to process, but it's all been going by so fast. Walking in on Monday, thinking this is the last week, and every day experiencing nausea, being plugged in, connected to this thing, hearing the pulse, getting my labs and fluids – all of it. It's crazy to think it's all coming to an end. There's a continuous wave of gratitude. I've made myself so busy with work – I think I've done it intentionally. I want everyone around me to be away from me so I can just process this myself. But I can't feel the next steps just yet. I still feel like I see the finish line. But the sun is shining, and I just feel very emotional. It feels so far behind me but still so far in front of me too. Very very lucky. I still look in the mirror with great question. And I continue to make my work. Thanks so much for writing. Love you.

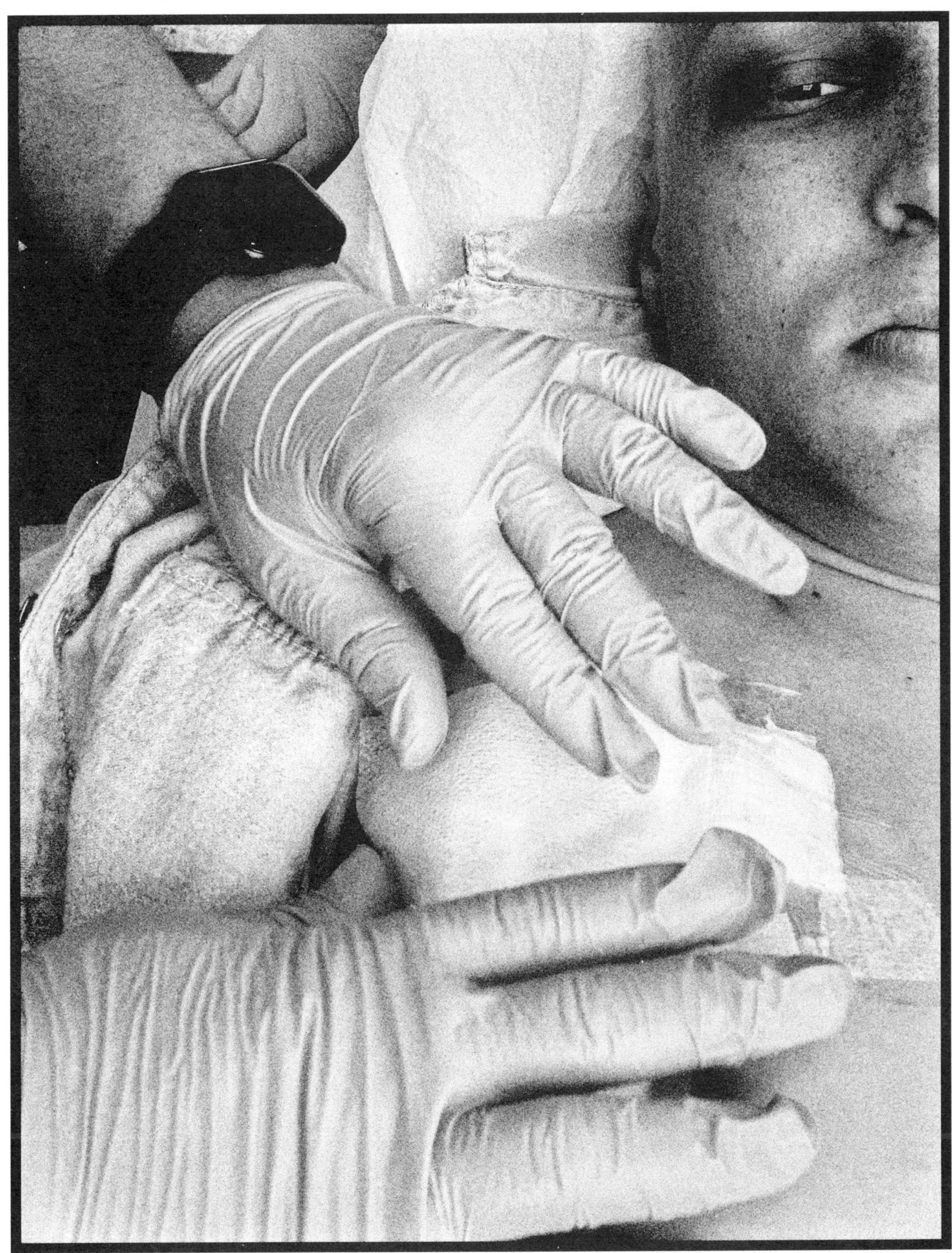

April 21, 2023

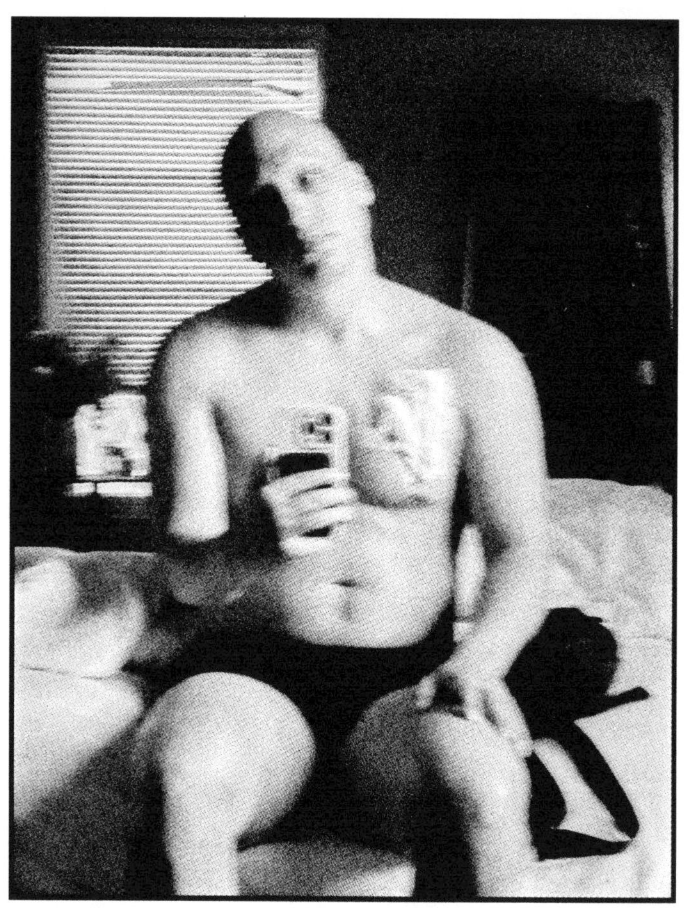

Last day of chemo.

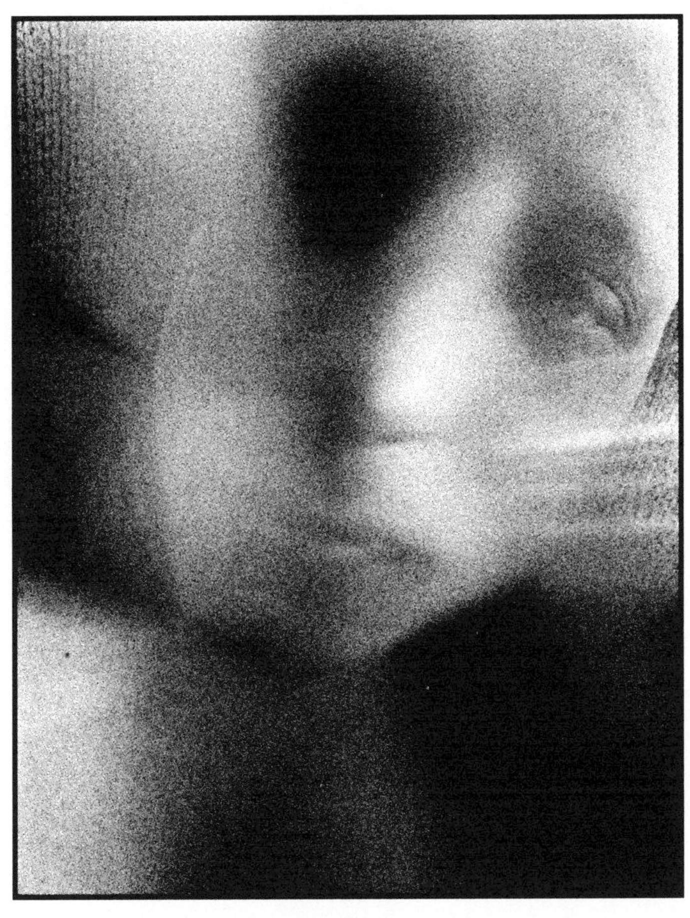

Last day connected to this tube.

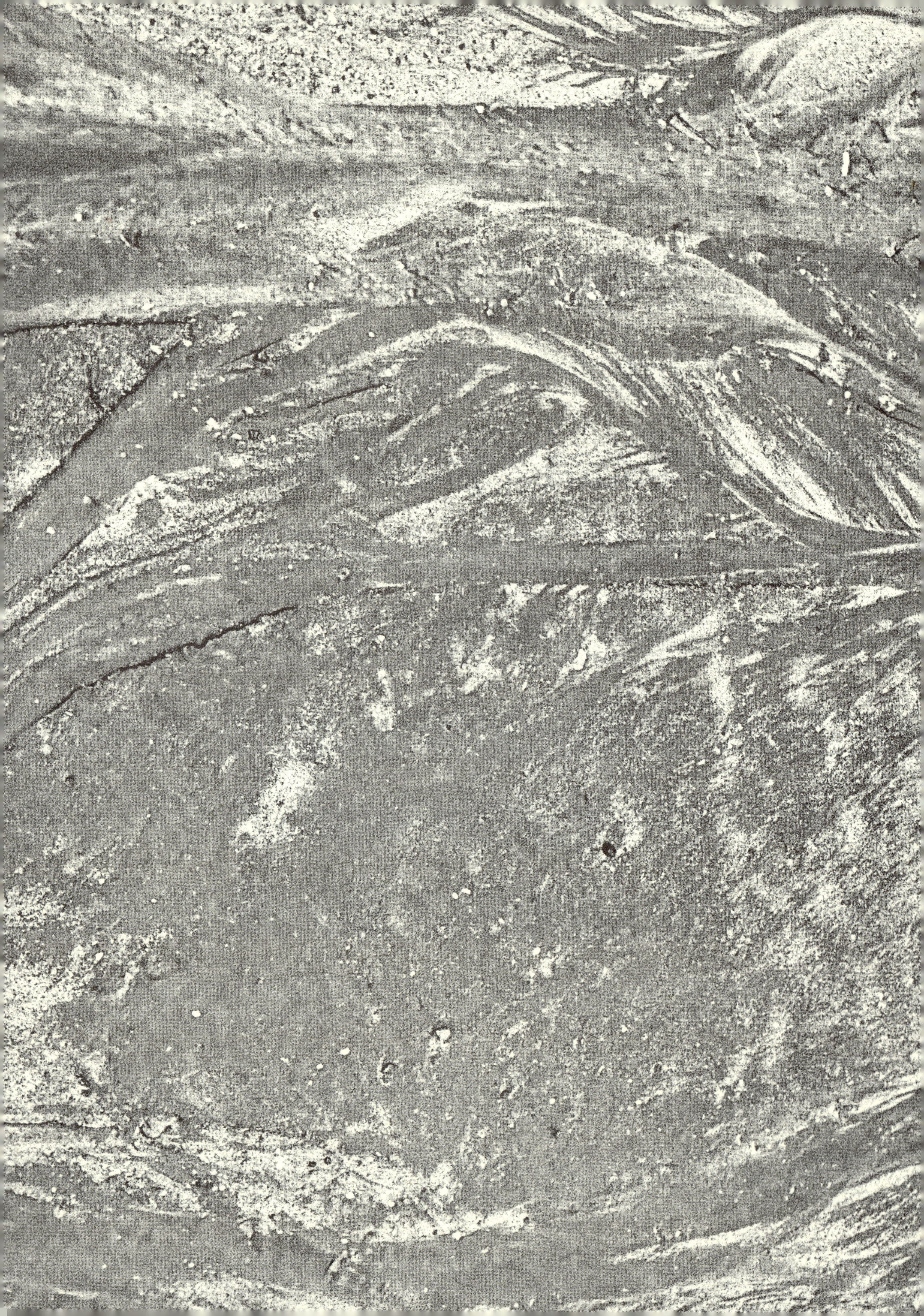

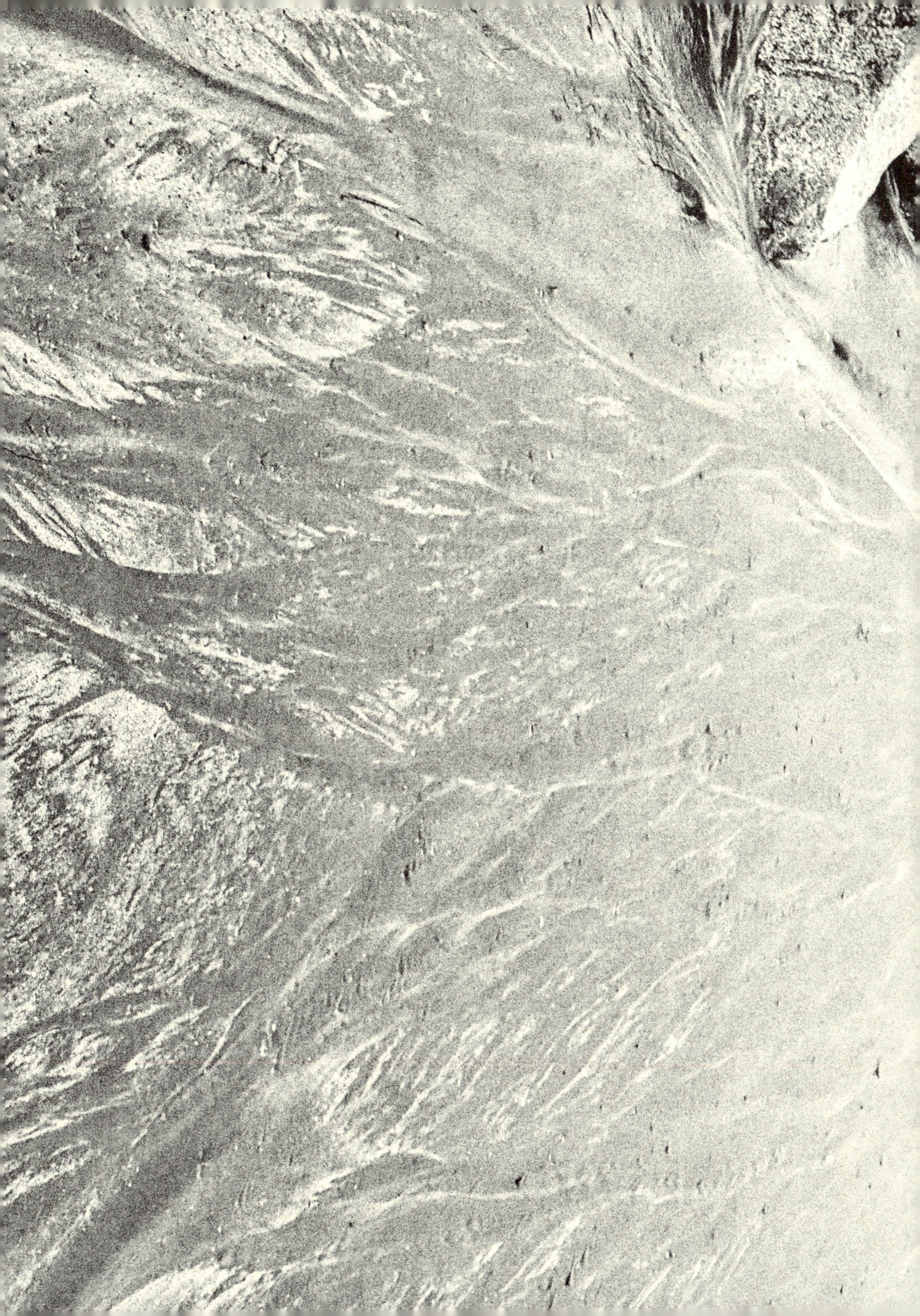

May 3, 2023

Beach walk with Mom.

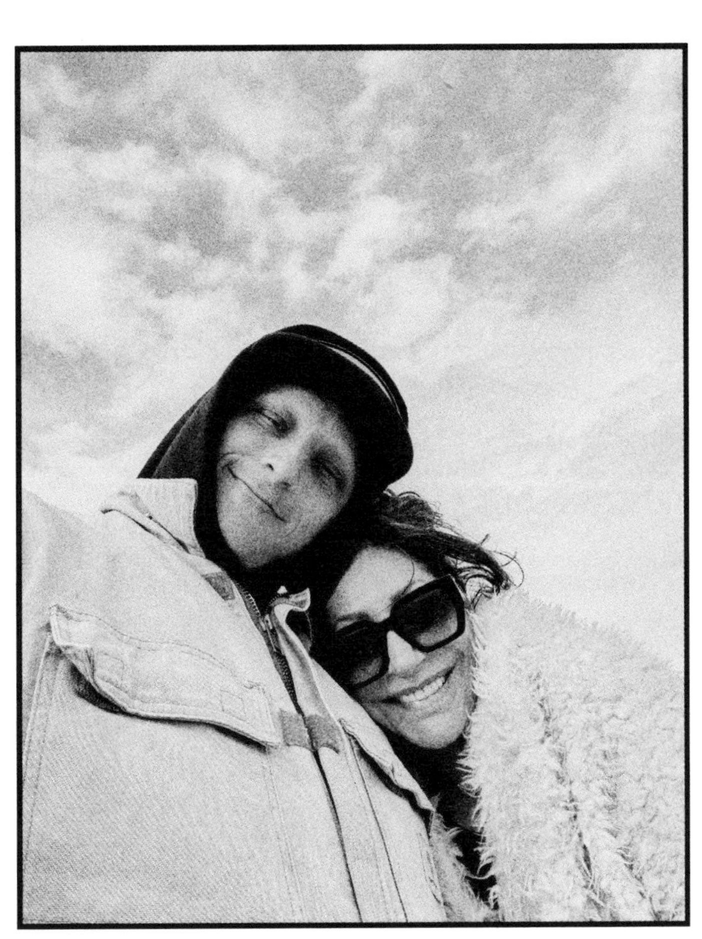

May 11, 2023

Our bodies should soak in water. The sun should shine. We're all created through an egg. The yolk represents that sun. Our breath continues. In oxygen, out carbon dioxide. The reverse for plants. No matter how far technology progresses, we will always need the natural elements and depend on these resources.

It's so easy to get caught up in our ego, but it's completely ignored when you look at the stars.

Our significance fades away. It's been a few weeks now since I've finished chemo. The bell rang. People cheered. I felt a deep accomplishment. A pause of celebration. A drop of salt water down my face, as the last IV sounds. But the journey continues – emotionally and spiritually. It hits hardest in the small moments. As I try to reacclimate back into social life, it's hard not to help but have everyone's voice muted. People complaining about their logistics. Their poorly strategized wealth and their cookie cutter lives. Everyone's wedding dress looks the same. There's a universal stress and loneliness that everyone is feeling. If only they could grasp their gift of being alive. There's an imitation of culture. Of popularity. A chase into darkness. My richness is transparent now. I want to be around good people, love my work, and be in nature. It's easy to forget my importance as time goes on, but I'm reminded in the stillness. I fear the recurrence. They say it's 30 percent. They say it will take six to 12 months for the fatigue to go away. I worked so hard during this whole process as a means of distraction for the pain. I worked so hard the whole time to be graceful and calm. It's shocking to have conversations with people now and see how distraught and hurt they can be by the smallest things. I think I need a break now. It's easy to create artificial busyness, but I think I need a pause until the universe tells me what to do next. There's too much output these days. Who knows the importance of writing this all down. Will it be read by one or many? Will it make an impact at all? There's a subtle fear, and excellent optimism for the future, and for however long that will be I will be grateful. Thank you both for listening.

May 19, 2023

Walks with Kanye on the beach.

An introduction to mental health.

May 22, 2023

Feet in the sand. The waves crash continuously. The cold water along my ankles. At its furthest expansion. Then it contracts by the moon, back to the sea. This process repeats. Life continues. A recent PET scan, labs, a visit with Dr Oliai today. Congrats you're in remission. It's all over for now. The focus now is healing. In a professional circumstance, in a personal one. With those around me, but also alone. My intentions have to be good. With all this information over the past six months I've needed a vehicle to get it out. The universe has reconnected me with Kanye. It's crazy because I've thought about him so much at the beginning of this journey. These waves are symbolic of the days ahead. They'll continue. They'll never stop. Some bigger than others. Some with more force and vibration and energy. Others with more calmness. But there's a humility in the continuation of them. Cancer may no longer be detected in my body, but there's an inner trauma from my life and what I've been exposed to in order to sustain health moving forward. At the end of the day, all people are good, just their circumstances and surroundings might be wrong. It's important to surround yourself with the right people, the right energy. Grateful for today that there's an official crossing of the finish line. That we've moved out of the Water Garden. And that I'm getting on a flight soon to start this next chapter.

I hope moving forward everything around me stays honest and pure. The house and car will come soon. But for now I want it to be led by honesty and nothing more.

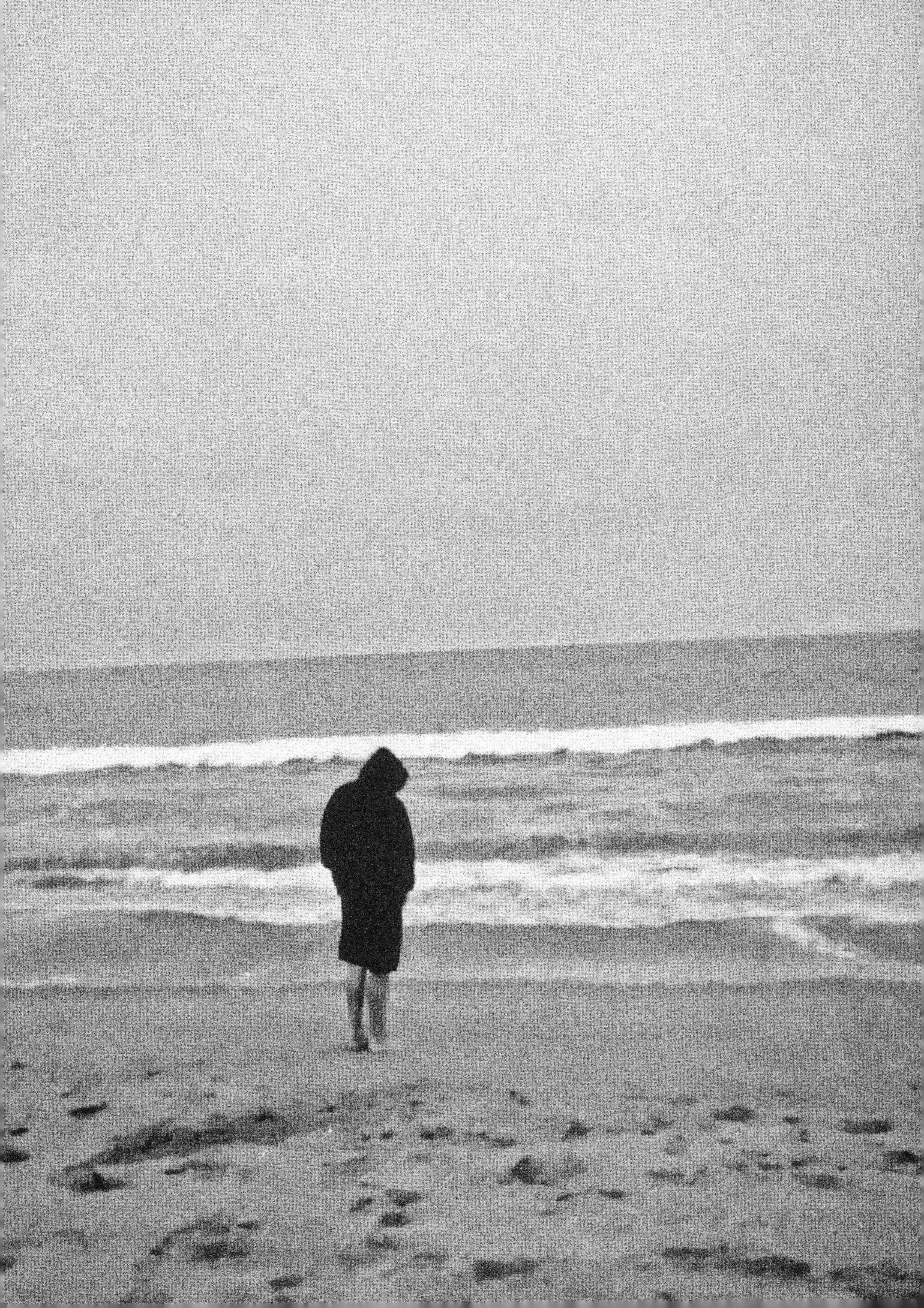

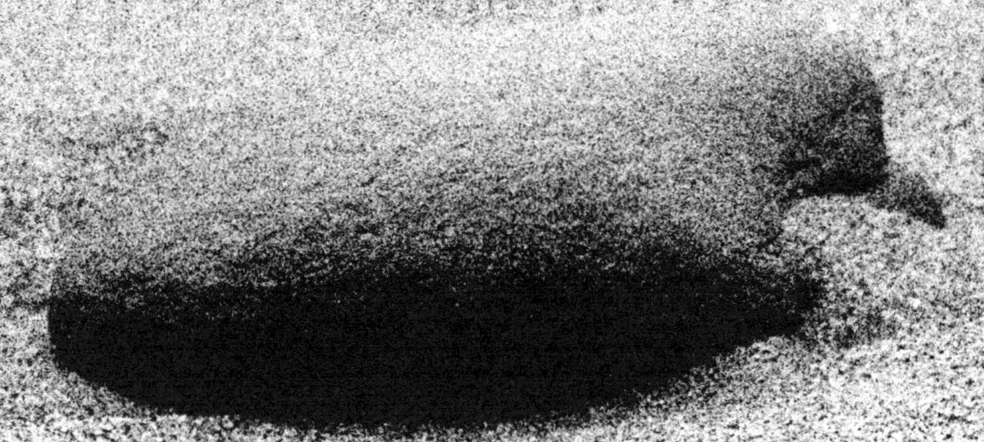

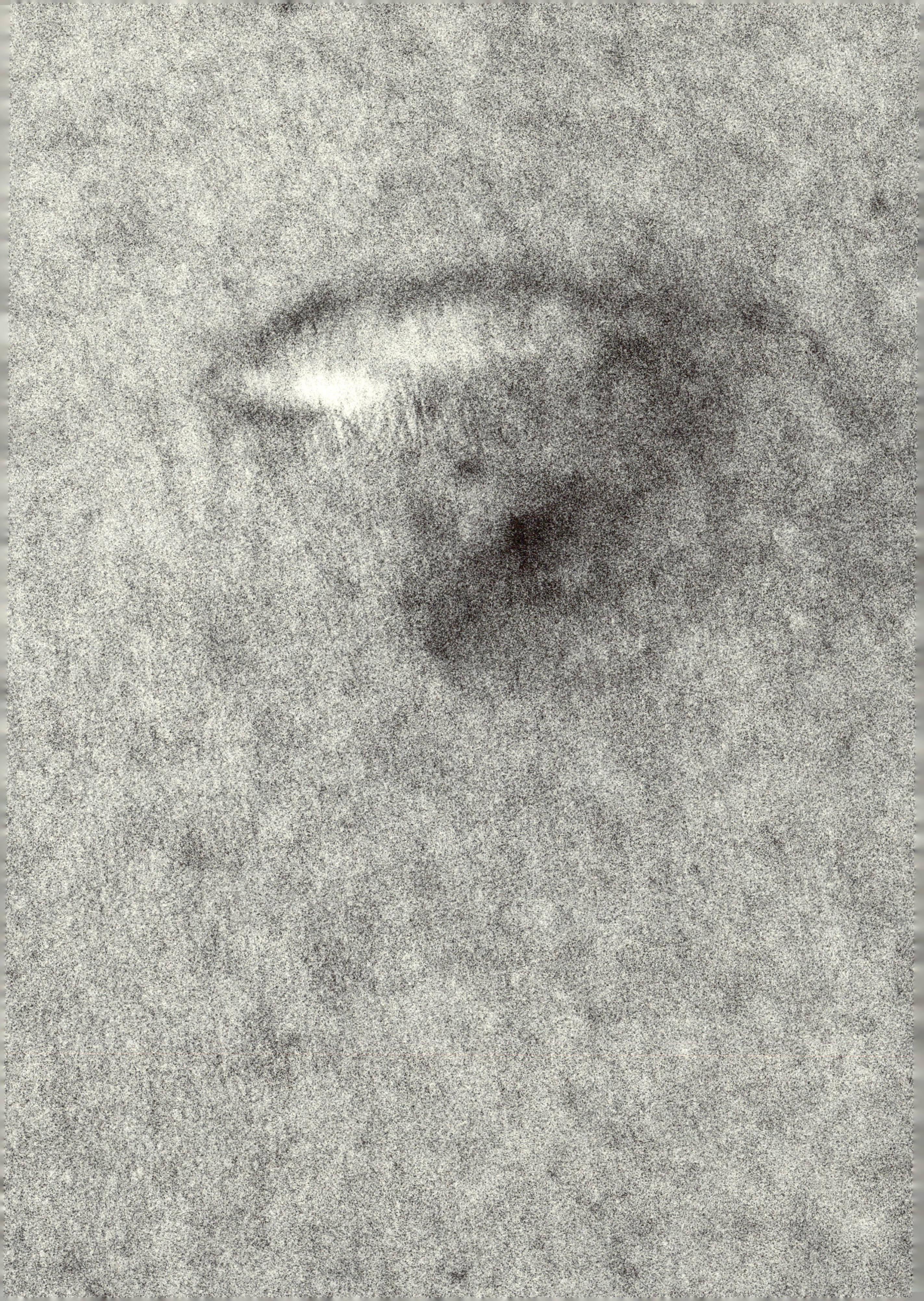

May 23, 2023

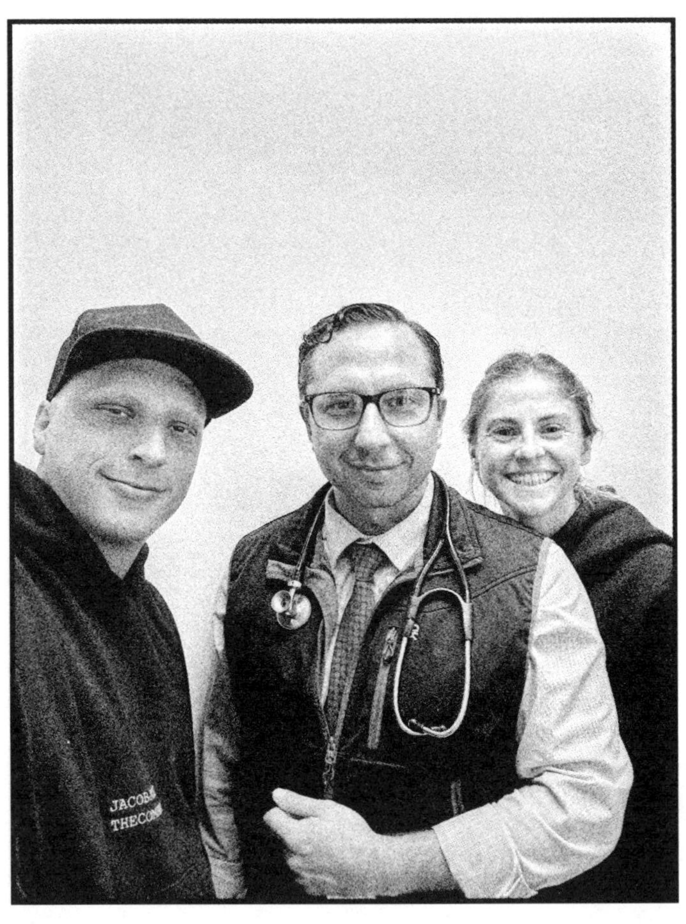

In remission.
With Dr Oliai. Port removal.

May 28, 2023

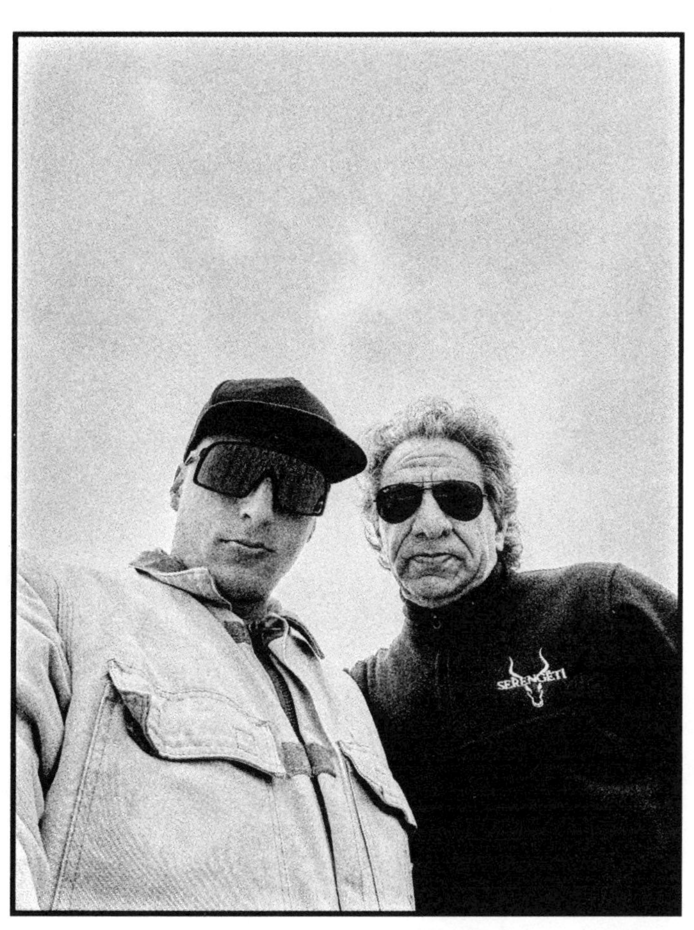

Beach walk with Dad.
Last moments in Los Angeles.

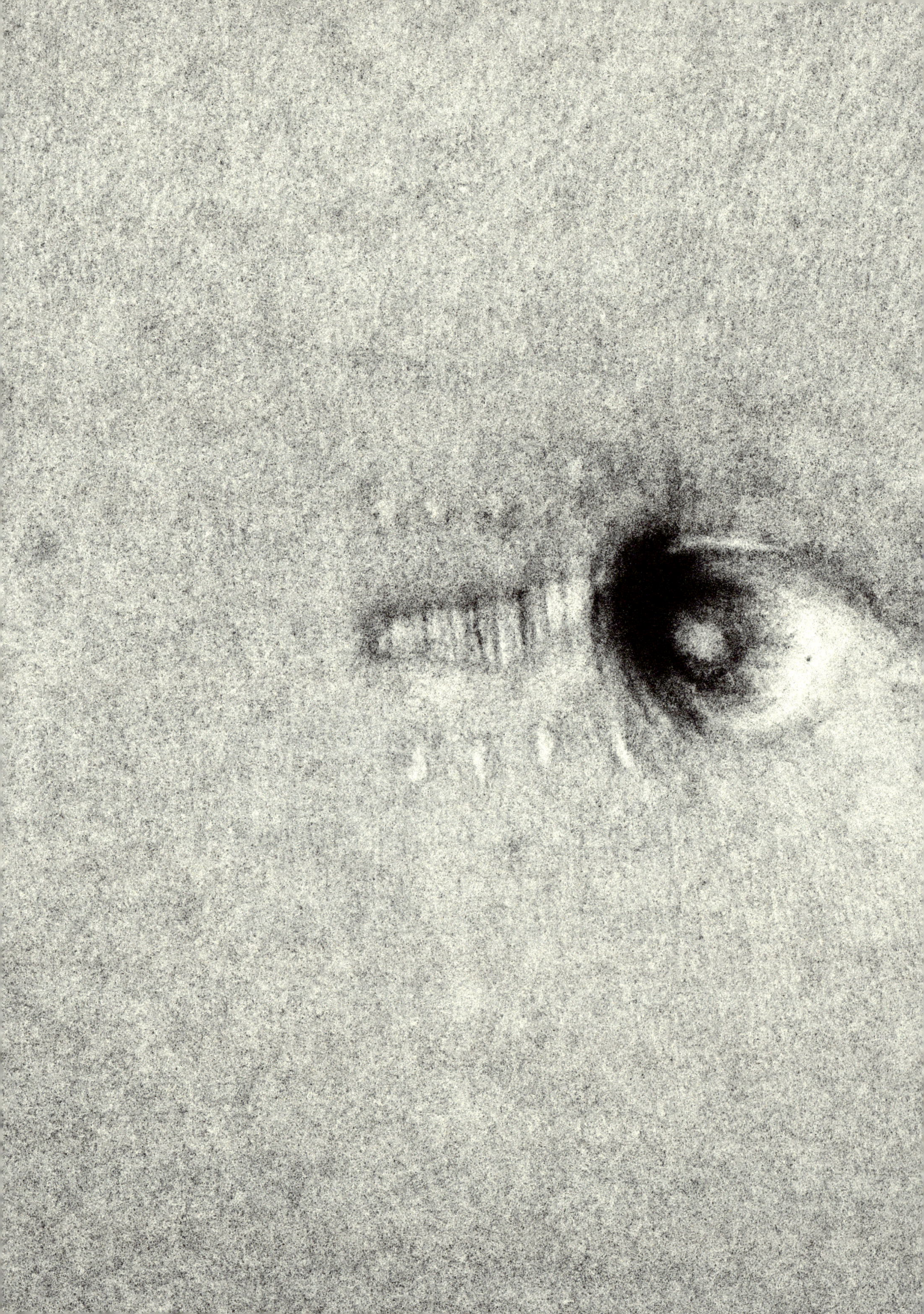

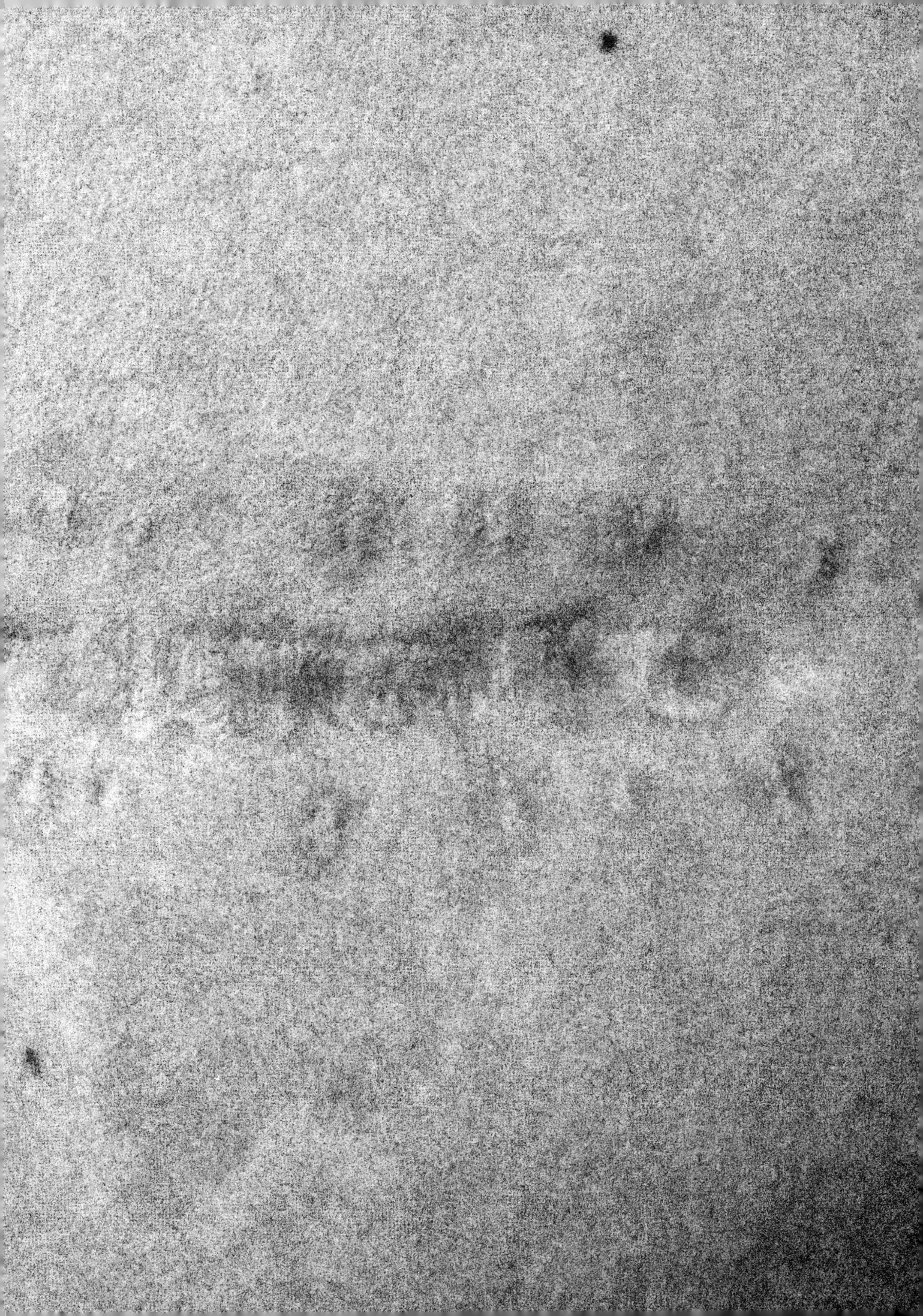

June 2, 2023

Malfunction. Shut down. There's a virus in my mind. It's trying to get me to shut off. Suicidal thoughts. Visualized actions. Jumping off a boat into a sea of darkness. Hand on the trigger. Pop too many pills. Put pressure on me. Choke me. Where's this coming from? The plane took off and I felt trapped. I can't sit that long. I need to lay down. Make sure your seatbelts are fastened. In case of an emergency, oxygen will come down from overhead. Pretend comfort. Are corporations' profits that important to sacrifice people's health? I said I need to lay the fuck down. They placed me in the galley between the two bathrooms. Twelve inches in between. Maybe 18. The doors on either side of me open and close. A loud sound of a shotgun. From vacant to occupied. Each time someone went in, the door would crack open, the light would hit, a slow motion disco the whole flight. I landed. My mind started taking over. Hyperventilating. Throwing up until there was nothing left. The paramedics showed up while I lay against the marble floor in the airport. I thought this journey was over when I went into remission. But this trauma after is a whole new disease. It's been three days since. And my mind keeps going. Every second. Every minute feels impossible to get through. I look at her and tell her I love her. That I'm sorry. Why are you with me? You could have anyone. Drugs are the only thing that took me out last night. Forced rest. The wind calms down. Before that, artificial meditation soundtracks. Four counts to inhale. Seven counts to hold. Eight to release. A call with Danny. He walked me off the ledge. Literally. I really wanted to die. It seems like there's nothing to look forward to anymore. Nothing to learn. I don't get how people die of old age. How do they make it so goddamn long? I forgive myself for judging myself. Maybe the resort on the beach wasn't supposed to be perfect. A permanent panic. A fear of recurrence. I woke up. It was 8:23 p.m. I thought it was the morning. I can't believe I slept through the whole day. I feel calm. Jacob, go walk outside. Put one foot in front of the other. Step on the grass. I want to be in Santa Monica. I did my best to show up at my cousin's wedding. I'm sorry if I ruined it. I'll try my best to carry on for now. It's hard to pretend significance. When you look at the sun each day and see the moon and know how really insignificant we really are.

Being told you have cancer, you can really visualize death. I'm not scared of dying anymore. I'm scared of living. I love you more than you know. You're much stronger than I am. And deserve much better. I might have dug myself too deep. My whole life flashed in front of me in a matter of seconds. Holding her hand in Vegas, playing trumpet, my fourth-grade teacher Ms Lightner, SeaWorld with my mom, drives out in my dad's Yukon XL, skating down San Vicente. Then my breaths get faster and I start counting them. Within seconds I'm at 89. I wish I was in the ER room in Santa Monica. Or in a hospital where my comfort lies. How did I get stuck here in Athens? This little room feels like a hospital. Sprained brain. Go away. Please don't come back. I love you with all my heart.

If I get too far trapped, find freedom.

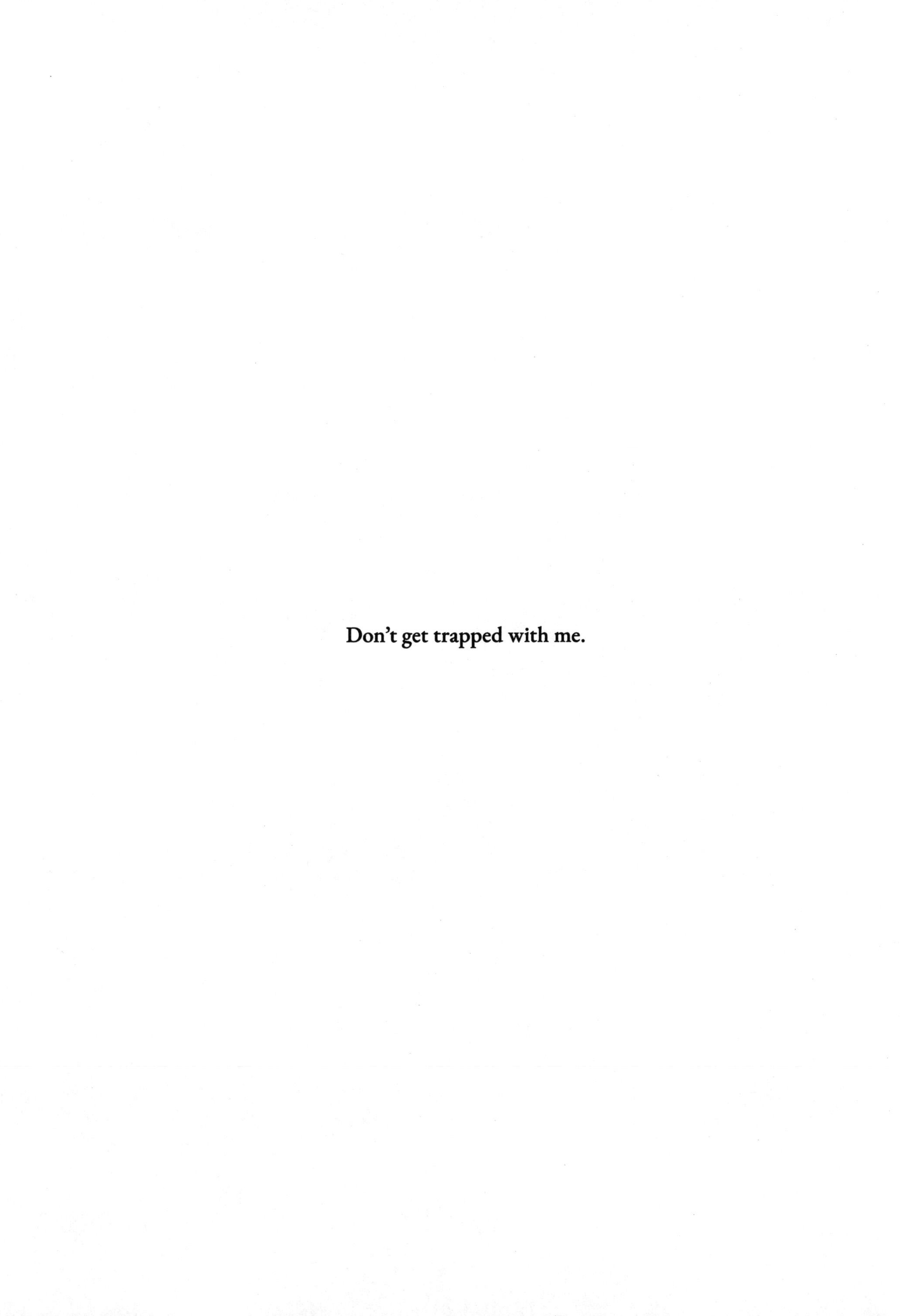

Don’t get trapped with me.

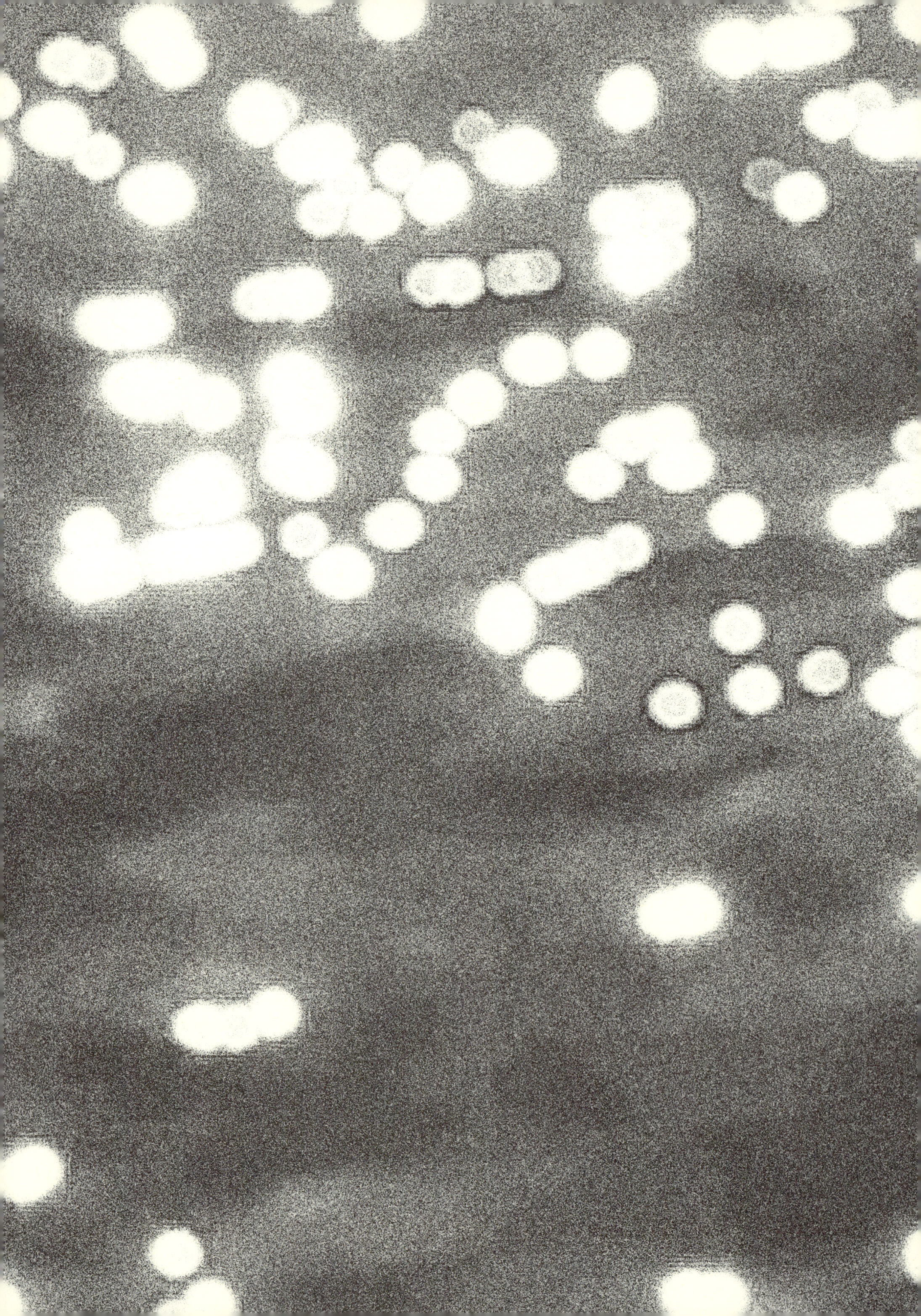

June 4, 2023

Everybody is doing the same thing, but there's this inner feeling that they're all trying to be different. They think that they're being different – in how they dress, the car that they drive, their outward taste or sense of creativity. But, in truth, everyone's doing the same thing. Elon Musk recently said at a press conference that his hope with Tesla is that everybody drives the same car. The same way that people use what Steve Jobs created. That there are hundreds of different kinds of cars around the world, and that his goal is to have everybody drive the same one. The same way there used to be hundreds of flip phones and mobile devices but now most people only use an iPhone. I'm not sure if it was from my recent battle with cancer, thoughts of suicide, or questions of mortality, but I'm finding I have a much smaller sense of patience to accomplish a lot. And a lot of big ideas. It's hard to watch the behind the scenes of Pixar. Andrew Stanton leading a team to create *Finding Nemo.* To hear the Q&A with Elon Musk and his senior leadership team. Realize these are the people who are changing the world. It doesn't seem hard to do. I just need to put my mind in the right place and make sure that whoever is surrounding me is wanting me to achieve my vision. Because I know my ideas will change the world. Having traveled, you go to every big city, and it all looks the fucking same. The same buildings. People live the same. The architecture is the same. It's the same populated downtown area with the same stores and the same food. The only thing that's different when you travel is the natural environment. The lakes, the oceans, the caves, the vegetation. But the birds still fly, insects all around. Everyone's a predator looking for their next meal. Although we think we are trying to be different, with our outward expression, are we really ever going to be? Can someone's cells really be different? Can human nature – or even nature in general – be different? Or is everything really just the same? Oxygen is the same. Carbon dioxide is the same. Water is the same. But until I can't anymore, my attempt will be to create vibrations and frequencies that affect something new. It's impossible to look people in the face anymore and not imagine them having sex, what they will be like when they're old, how they sleep, how they sit on the couch and do nothing. The complexity of how I see human life is evolving. My mind is rapidly going.

June 5, 2023

Hair regrowth. Introductions to trauma.

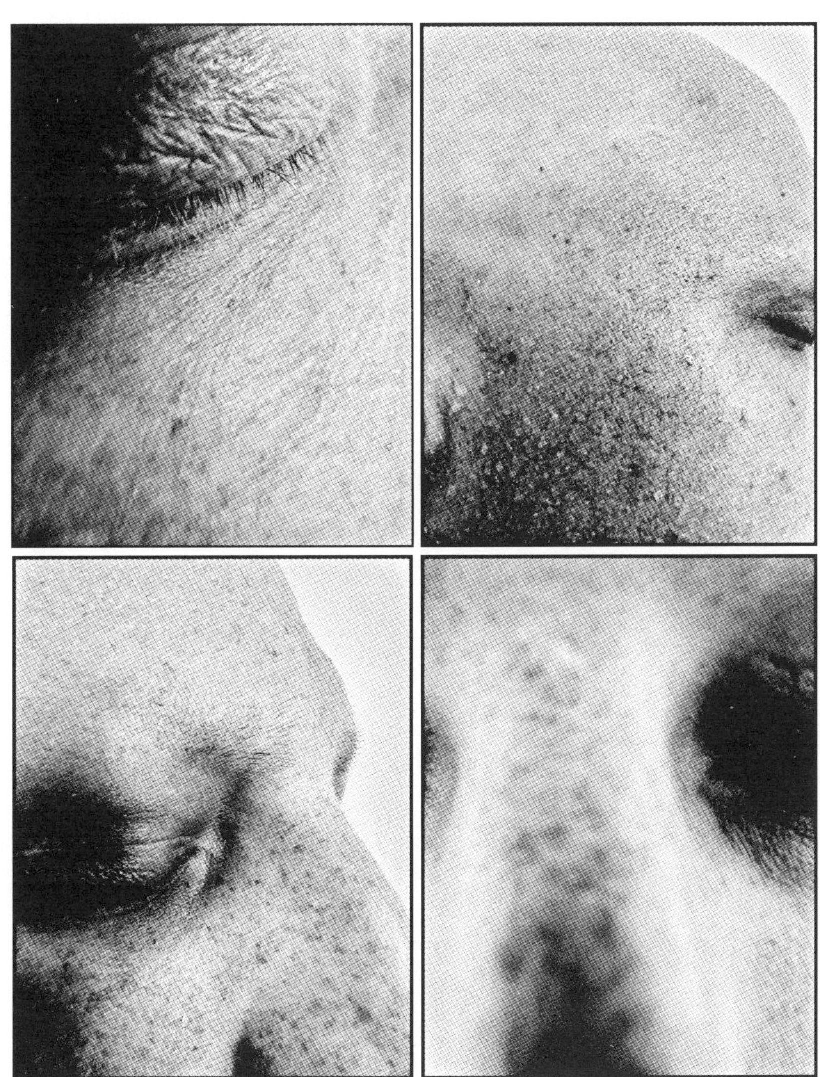

June 15, 2023

Something has taken over my mind again. For a second time it shows it's not an isolated thing. Difficulty breathing. Difficulty thinking. Maybe the best thing for me to do right now is do nothing. But what does nothing look like? Is it not working? Is it not being distracted? That might actually hurt my mind more than help it. I'm finding that the places that appear to be the most beautiful are really the ugliest. It's too challenging to coexist with the beauty. I keep moving from place to place. An absence of grounding. I miss my dog. Everyone says I need therapy. To talk through my problems, get different perspectives. I'm open. I still don't understand how people get to an old age. How do they live so long? The whole time I was fine battling cancer. Until now. Now I really feel "why me?" These thoughts are too strong. They won't calm down. Is death a bad option? I have a lot more empathy for people who have done it. I think my weight is too much to bear for those around me. My love, she's so strong. She's not that strong. This has been too long of a journey for her. She told me I'm like lifting a boulder up a hill. And that when she finally gets to the top there's no celebration. She needs to rest. I feel like I haven't let her rest in a long time. There's so much work ahead of me right now, and all I want to do is go home. But part of me is curious about the challenge of navigating through the work. But I fear the relocation. The new bed. How to get there? The fear of sitting. Sitting for long periods of time. I dream about the place that I'm in right now. Surrounded in nature, the sunlight hitting my face, water, good food, good people. I just can't enjoy it. Why is it that the most beautiful is the most ugly? I think Kanye coming back into my life was the world's way of telling me that I'm going to now be dealing with mental health. He says in one of his songs: maybe it's not a disability, maybe I'm a superhero. I like that. I feel I have a conscious mind right now, but it's scary when I don't. I guess I just need some peace. I love you more than you know. I really do. You're such a gift to me. Thank you.

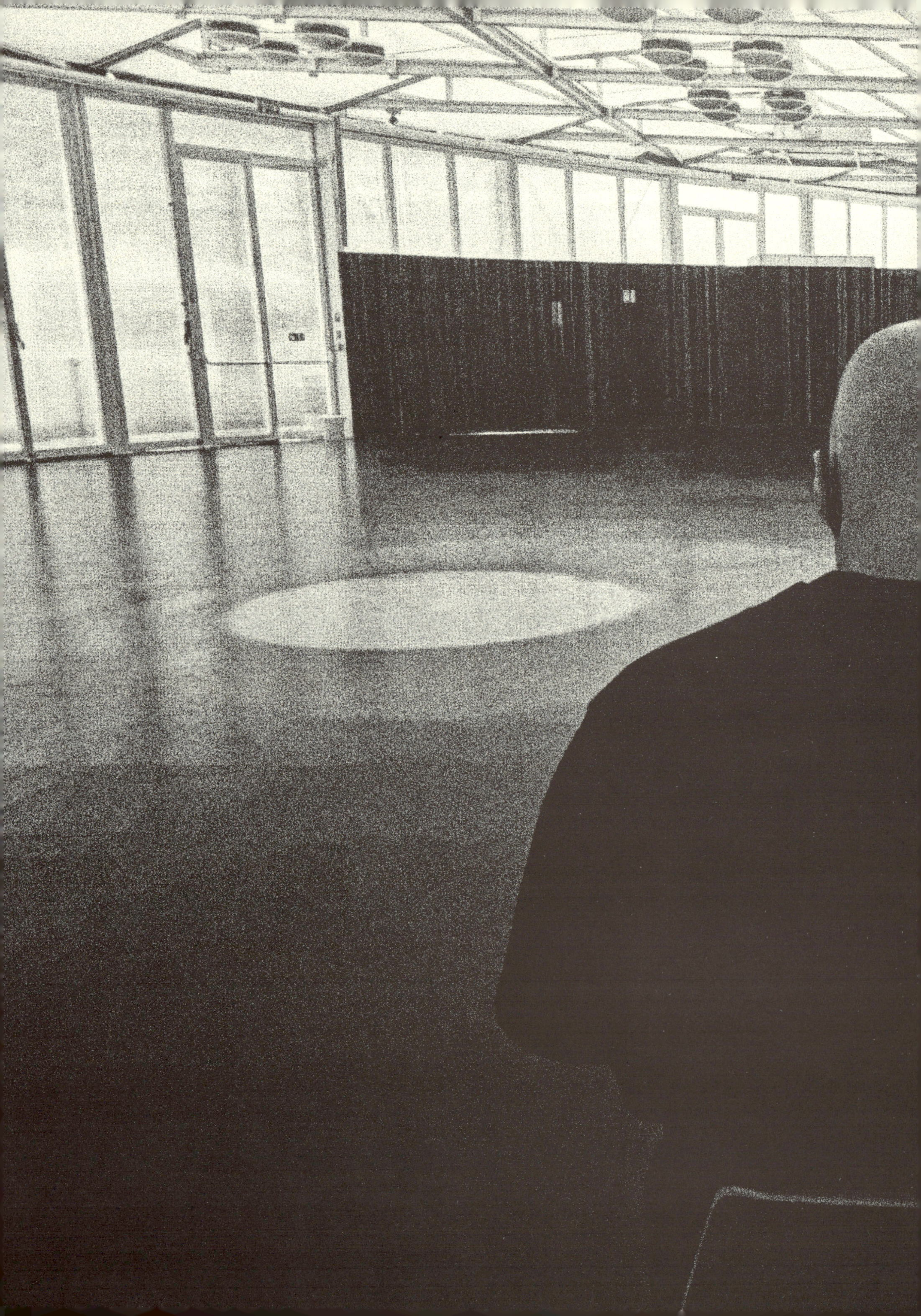

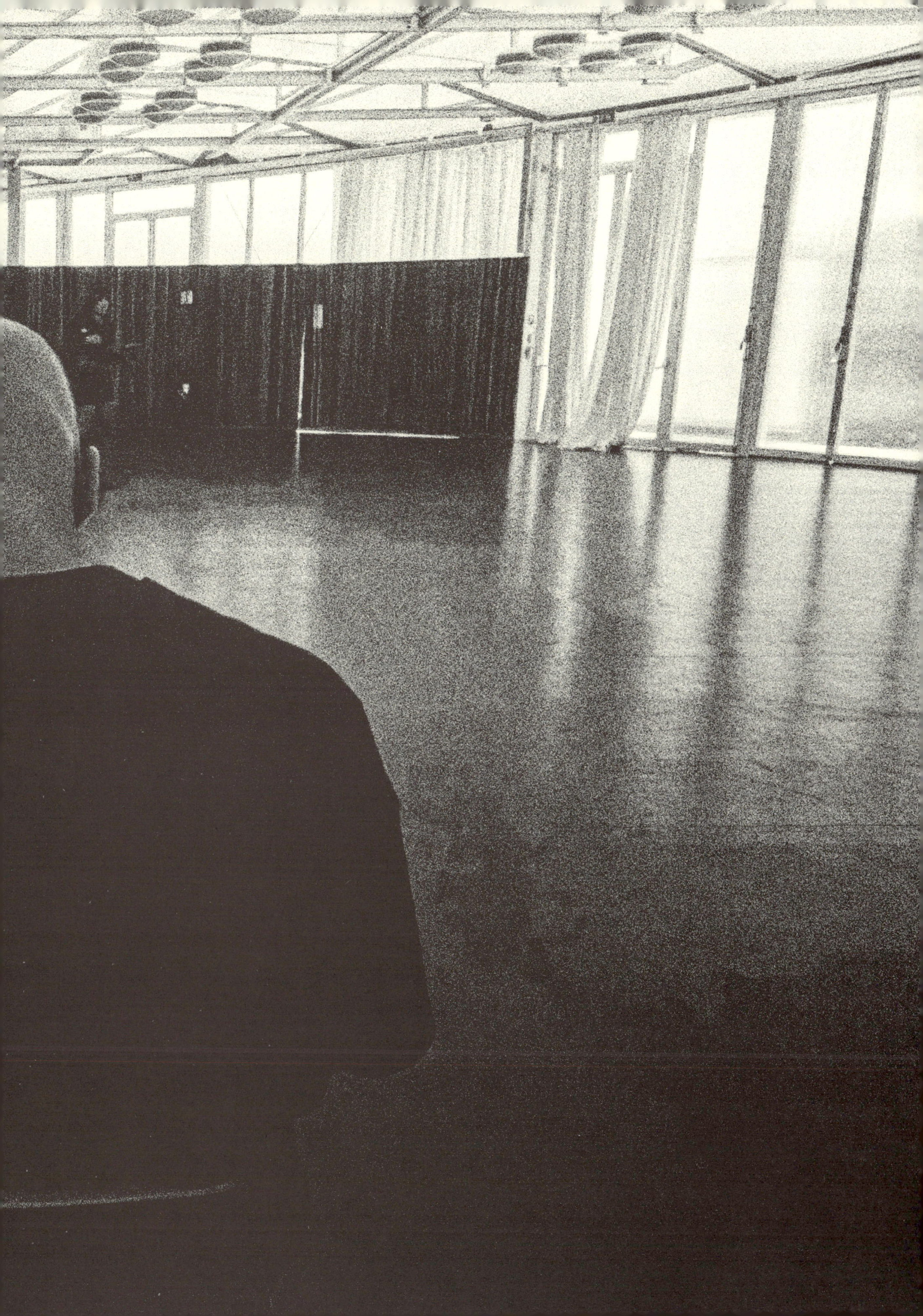

June 16, 2023

An attempt to work again.
The mind is trapped, but the body is moving.

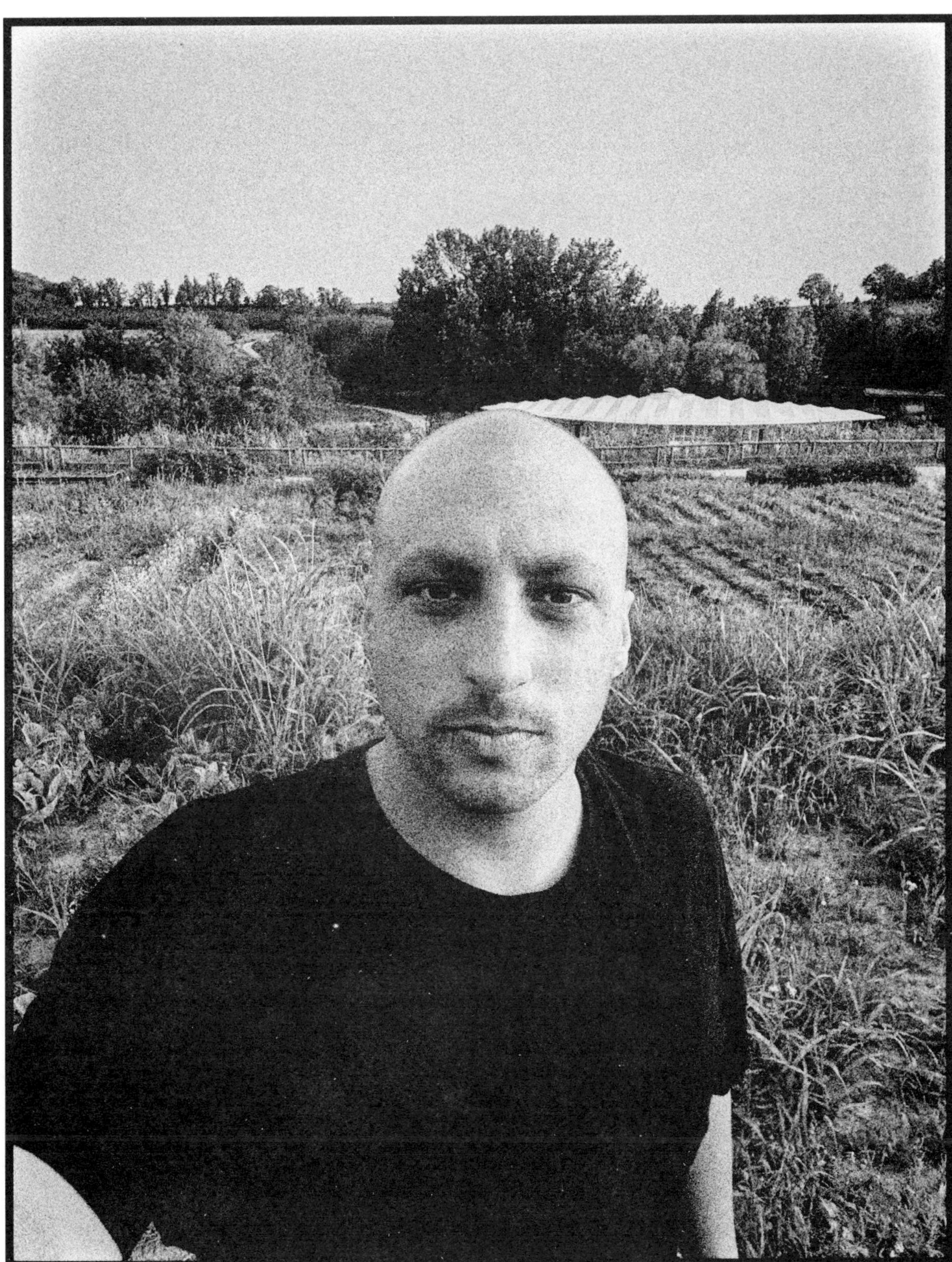

June 27, 2023

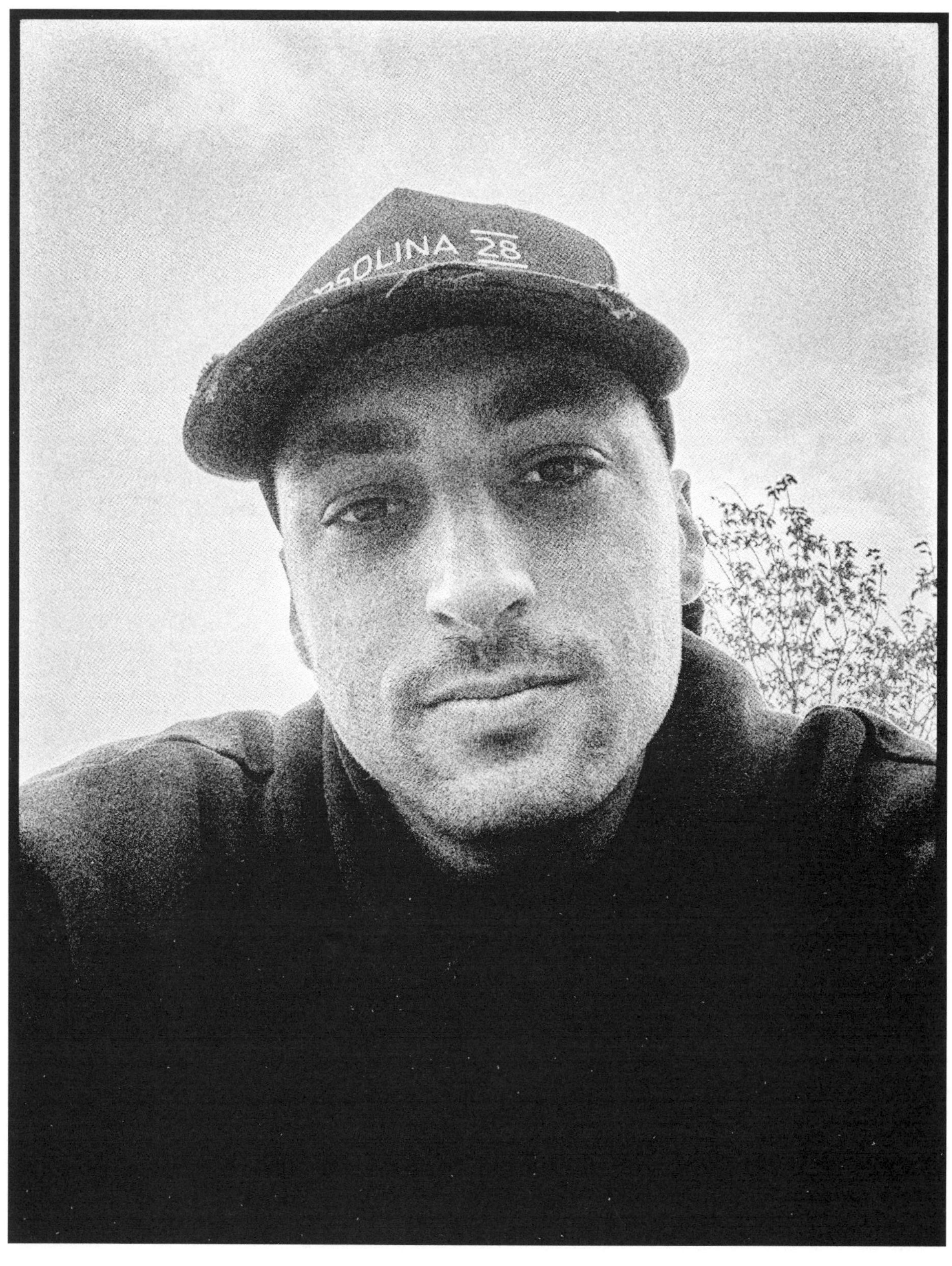

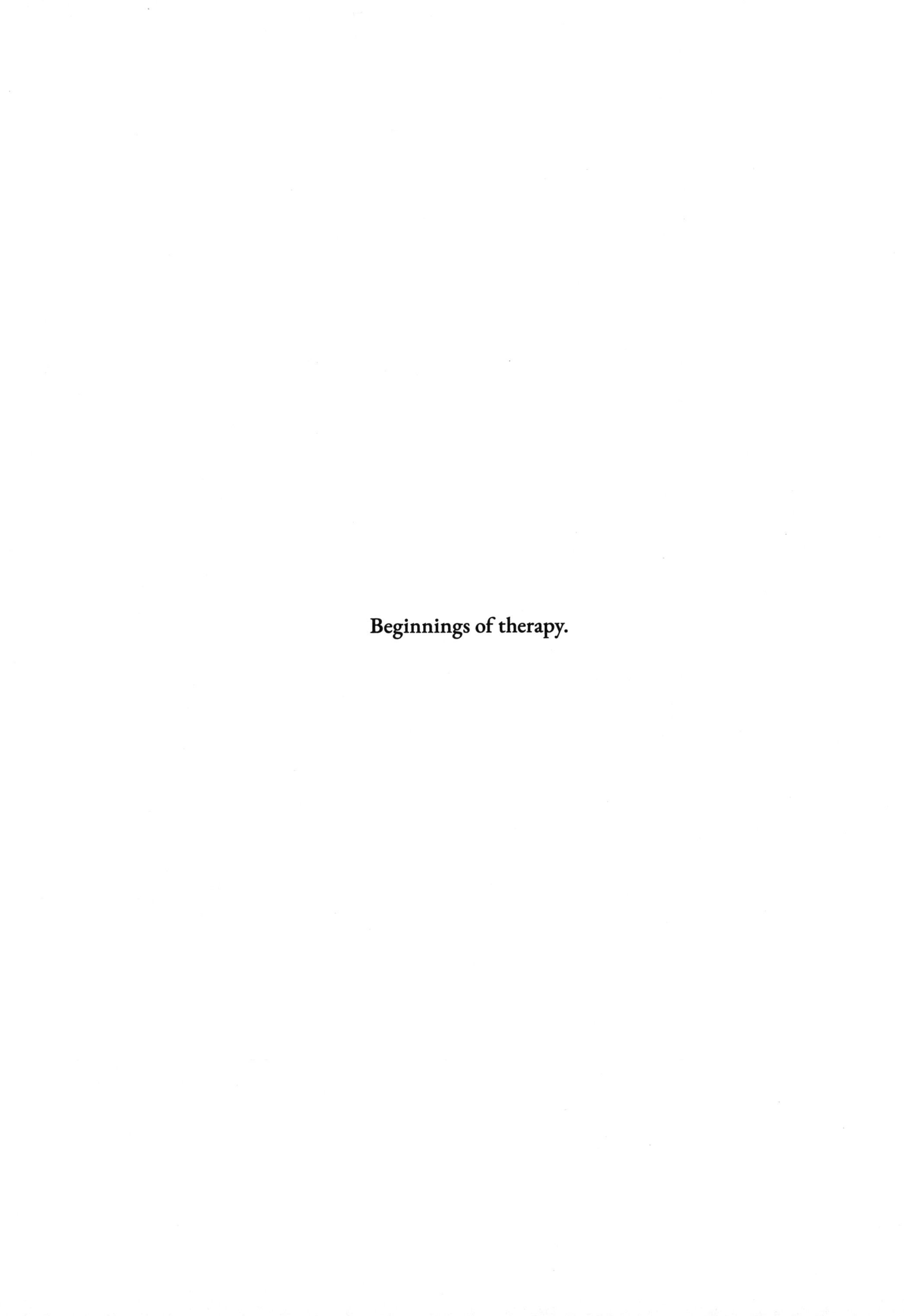

Beginnings of therapy.

July 5, 2023

Back in LA. Post therapy. An understanding of trauma.

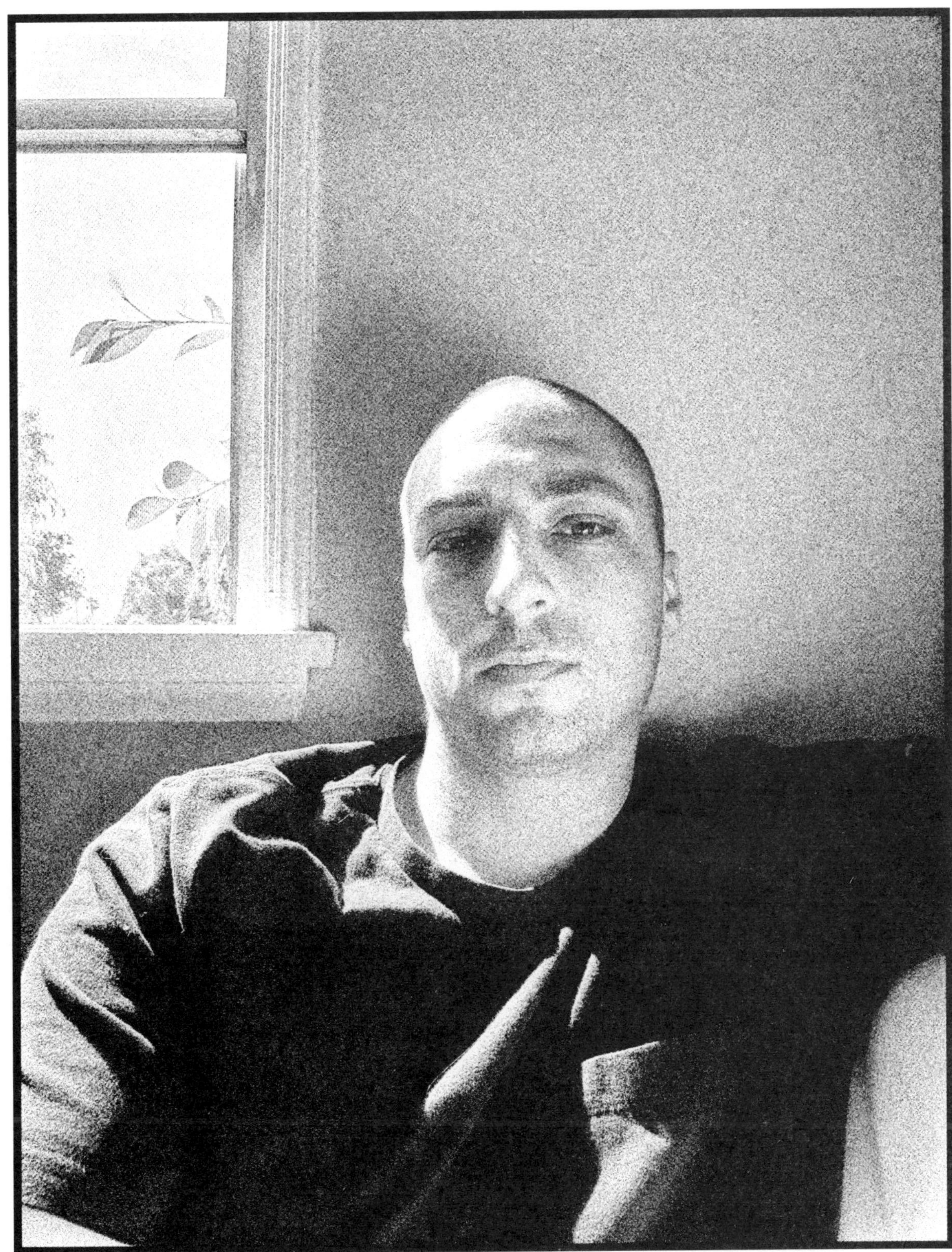

July 6, 2023

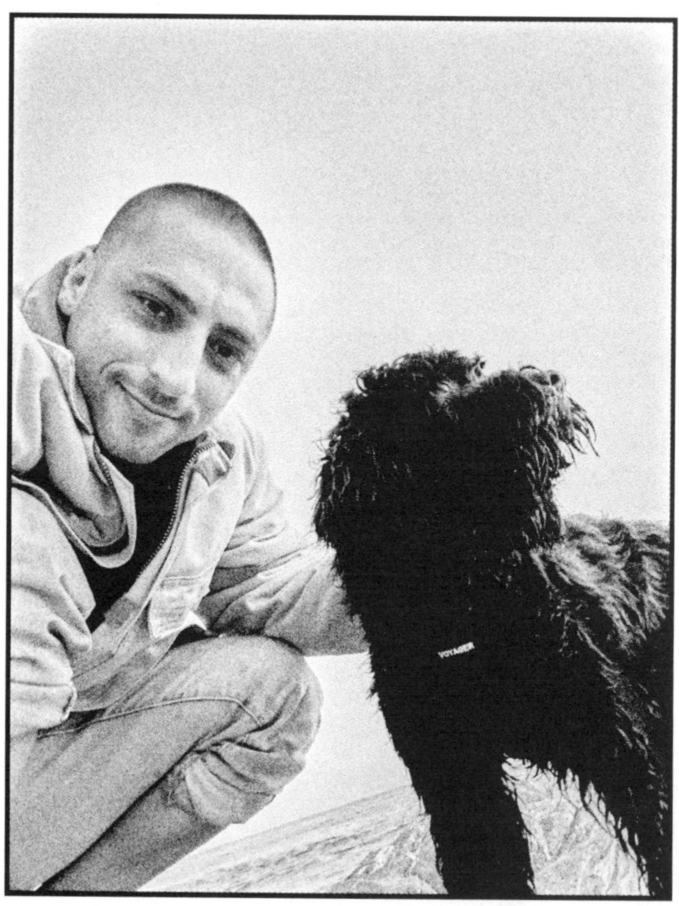

The wound is slowly healing. Sam and salt water.

July 7, 2023

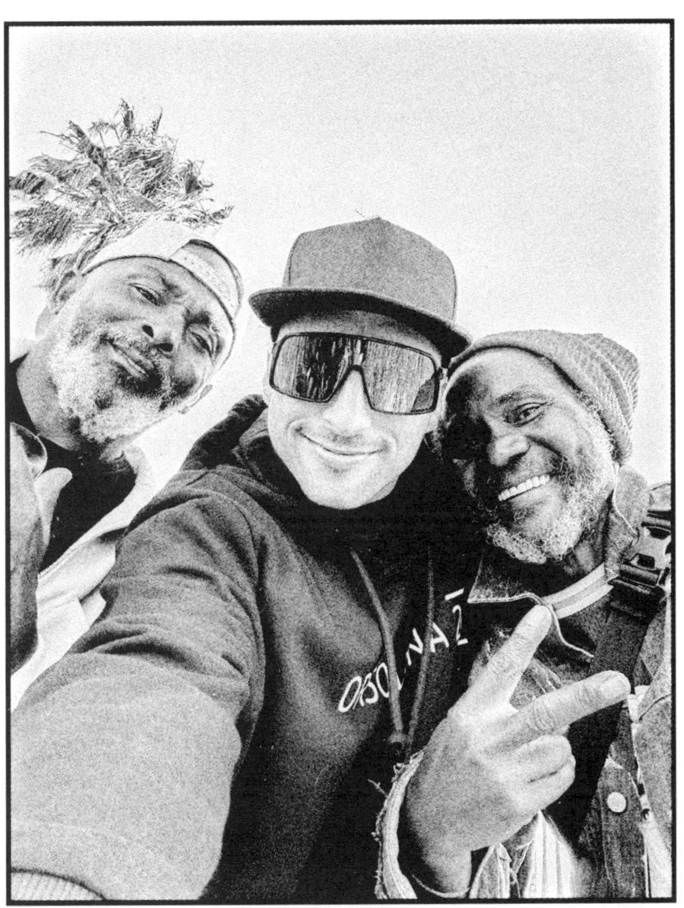

With my mentors. Revisiting where it all started.

July 14, 2023

Meeting my nephew for the first time.
Overwhelmed by the circle of life.
Troubled by how I wanted to end mine.

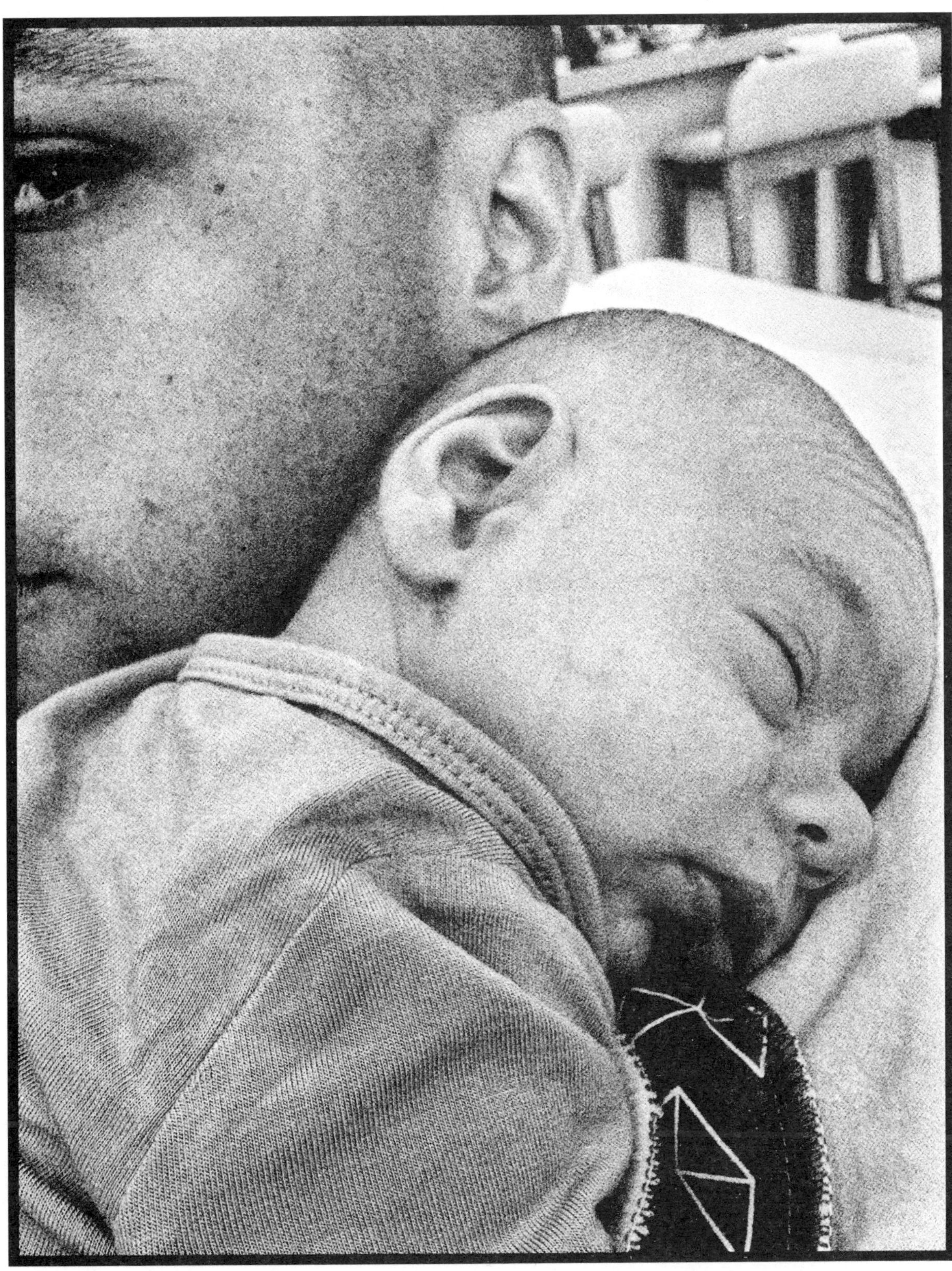

They don’t say how difficult

life is after cancer.

July 27, 2023

7.27.23

They dont say how difficult life is after cancer. Deep trauma exposes a heightened fragility. Its no wonder so many songs are about coming home. Unable to work. I needed this return to something familiar. The body's been overworking itself for so long now. The mind's just starting to catch up. Deep considerations on suicide. Time keeps slowing down. Are these mental games and visitors about my cancer? or Is it from childhood? They say the body's keeping score to your pain. Is that why I had crohn's? Is that why I got cancer? Is it all from what I was exposed to in my childhood? Does everyone have trauma and pain? I was good for a few weeks there but then it all came back. I love everyone so much. The last thing I want to do is hurt them. But the thought of finishing seems so right. 988. Its ok you're gonna get through this. Thanks for calling. She left for the first time to Tinsley last weekend. It was the first time we disconnected since my diagnosis. If I cant get through these things how am I going to make it through in the future? Too much is gonna come up. All these musicians are writing songs about pain. They're all taking mental health breaks. Deep breaths and cracked knuckles. Its time to finish it. All to start again tomorrow morning. I've got a lot of work to do if I want to get through this. I'm sorry if I ever go. Because I love you so much. Thanks for writing my love.

Deep trauma exposes a heightened fragility. It's no wonder so many songs are about coming home. Unable to work. I needed this return to something familiar. The body's been overworking itself for so long now. The mind's just starting to catch up. Deep considerations on suicide. Time keeps slowing down. Are these mental games and visitors about my cancer? Or is it from childhood? They say the body's keeping score to your pain. Is that why I had Crohn's? Is that why I got cancer? Is it all from what I was exposed to in my childhood? Does everyone have trauma and pain? I was good for a few weeks there, but then it all came back. I love everyone so much. The last thing I want to do is hurt them. But the thought of finishing seems so right. Call 988. It's OK, you're gonna get through this. Thanks for calling. She left for the first time to go on a trip last weekend. It was the first time we disconnected since my diagnosis. If I can't get through these things, how am I going to make it in the future? Too much is gonna come up. All these musicians are writing songs about pain. They're all taking mental health breaks. Deep breaths and cracked knuckles. It's time to finish it. All to start again tomorrow morning. I've got a lot of work to do if I want to get through this. I'm sorry if I ever go. Because I love you so much. Thanks for writing, my love.

August 16, 2023

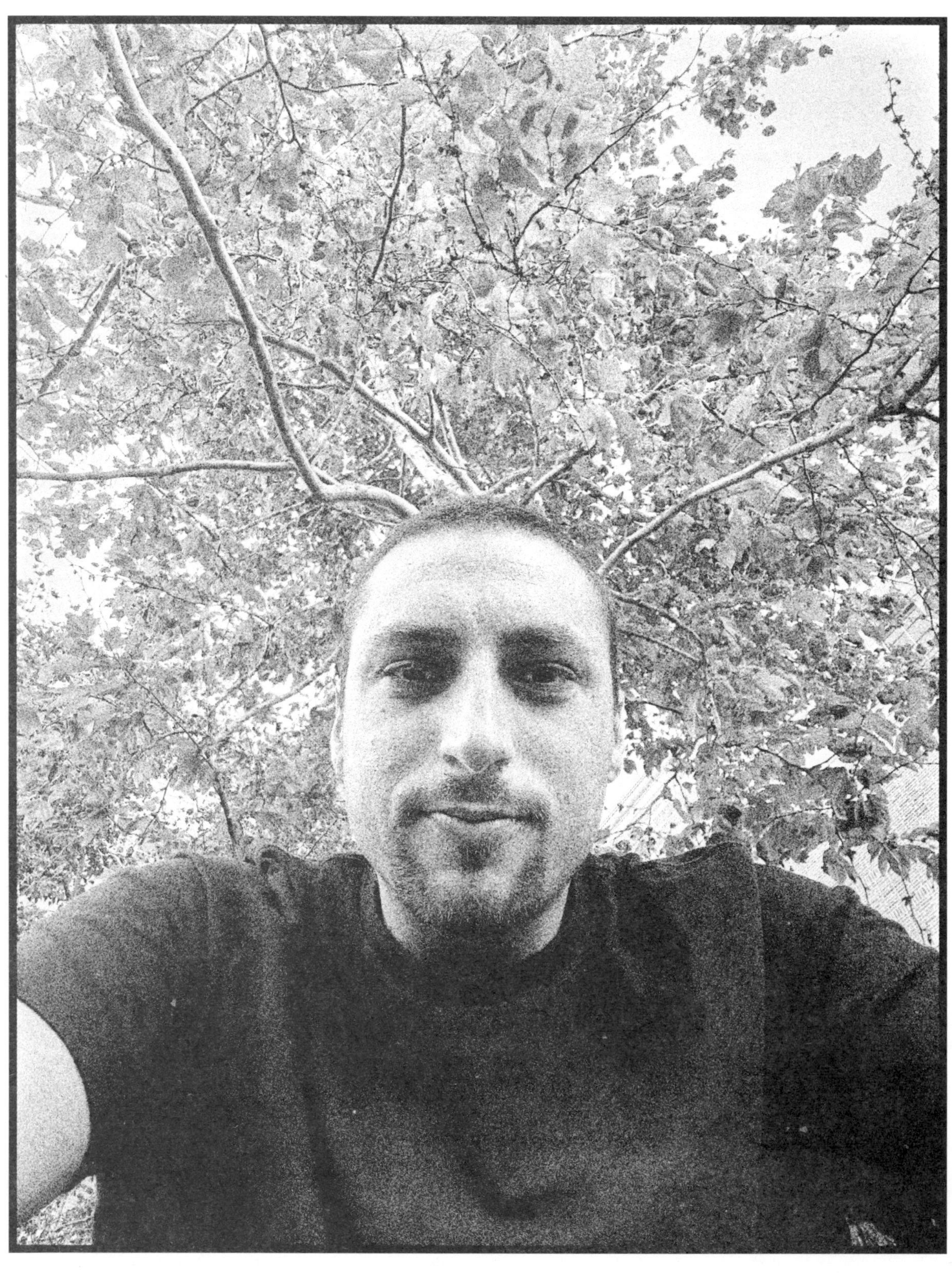

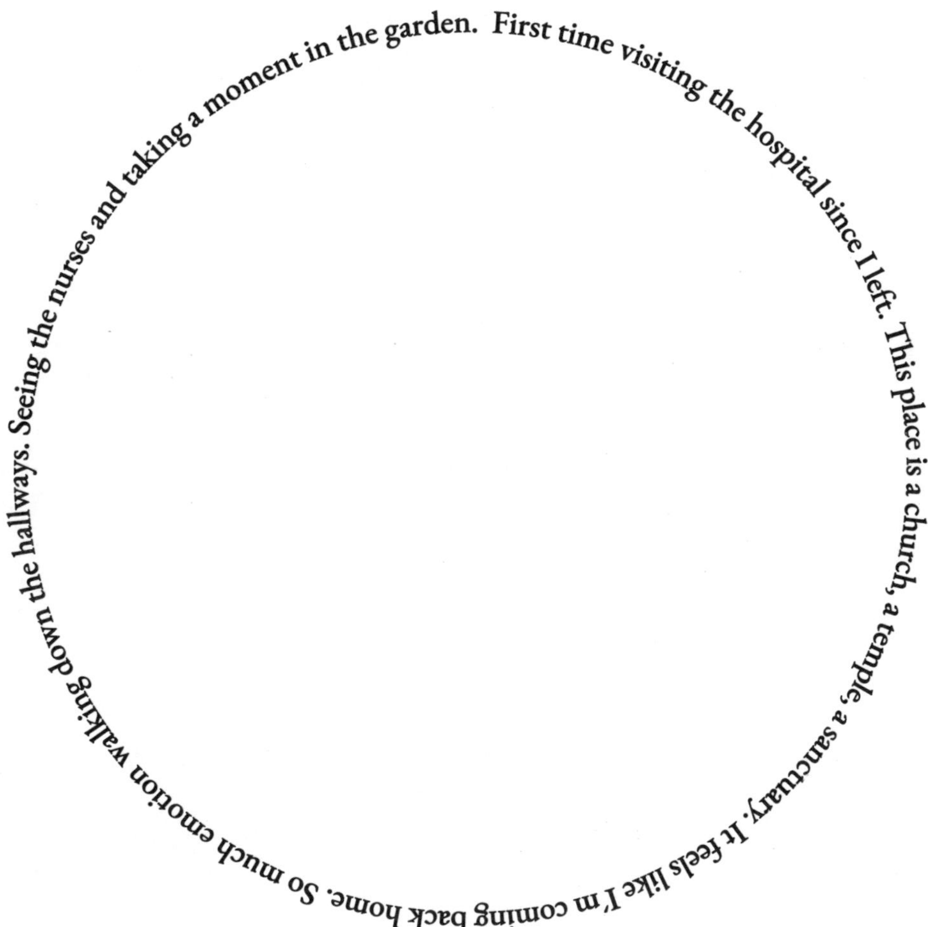
First time visiting the hospital since I left. This place is a church, a temple, a sanctuary. It feels like I'm coming back home. So much emotion walking down the hallways. Seeing the nurses and taking a moment in the garden.

August 22, 2023

PET scan.

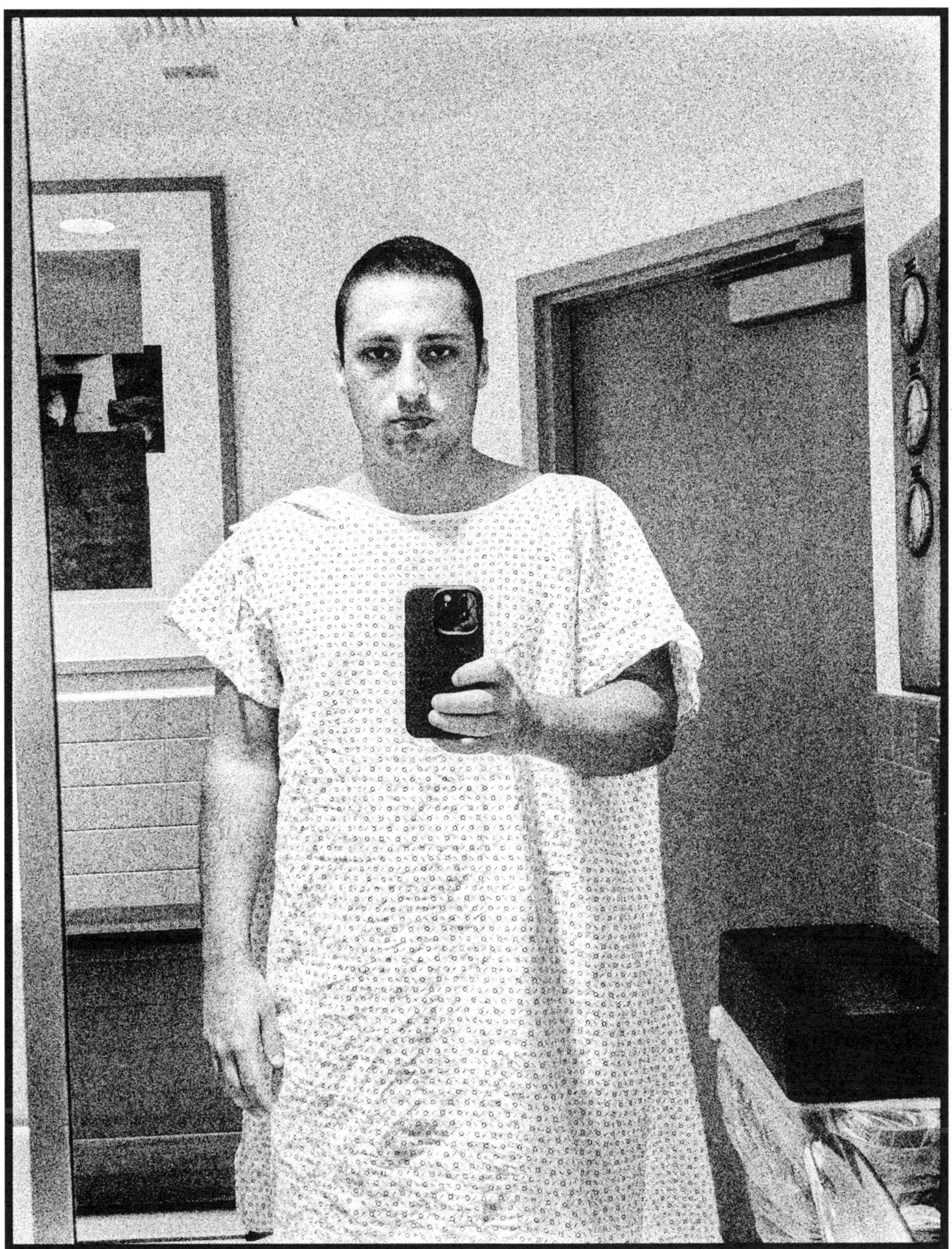

August 28, 2023

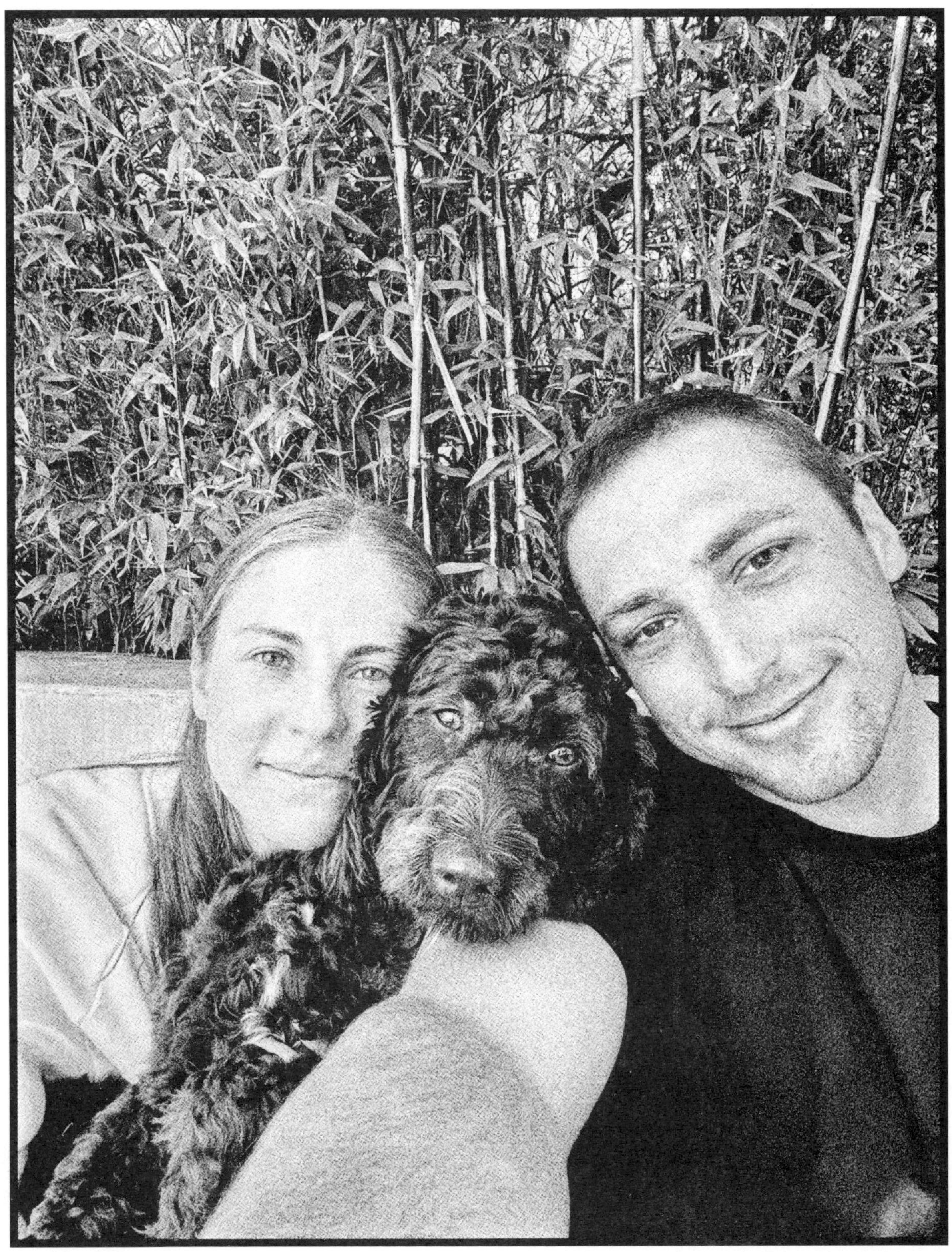

Dr Oliai visit. PET results. Gratitude.

Leaving Dr Oliai's office. First check-up since put in remission. Three months out. The results of my PET scan this week are that I'm still in remission, which is great news. It's been really interesting to experience such deep psychological effects from this illness, and in talking to him just now, understanding and learning more about the gravity of mental health and trauma that comes from going through such a severe cancer. It is a very difficult road getting diagnosed and going through treatment, but your head is down and you're so focused because everything is so immediate in the future to get through. It's not really until you finish that you realize the severity of what your body endured and also your mind. Another thing I found interesting was the discussion about profit within a capitalist country and medical world. That although some of these drugs are helping to heal us, there's someone at the back end making a significant amount of money through our illness. It's scary to think about and conceive that there is so much money involved in this system. And that even if they did find a cure for a specific cancer like lymphoma or colon cancer or liver cancer or breast cancer, it would likely not be distributed because these big corporations would make more money from us taking these medications. Or that if it was discovered (which it's likely to be in the coming years because of AI and other developments in technology) that the price point would be so unattainable, prioritizing you to use more harmful drugs with deeper side effects. So it's one thing to go through treatments, but it's another thing to step out and realize this is the system that we're in. We also talked about prevention and the availability to be sick in our society. The fact that so many products have warning labels for cancer, and people still buy them. That there's a knowledge of how much sugar and corn syrup are damaging to the body, and yet they are so available. That cigarettes and alcohol are still so used, knowing the potential for illness. And how many pesticides exist on non-organic produce and how those cause so many damaging effects chemically to the body.

When I asked Dr Oliai what would happen if he were in my shoes, from a diagnosis standpoint, he said he'd have to stop working and that it would cause him great mental health issues as well, which gave me a lot of peace and calmness. I think it's weird to live in a society – and I would say this even without having cancer – where there's such a desire for stress and productivity today and how we know how much stress damages the gut biome and our health. In addition to that, there's such a falsity that we need to be so professionally productive. But when you're going through a situation like mine for six months and then the after-effects mentally for three to six months, it's nearly impossible to have a professional identity. You really need to stop – if you have the ability to. Dr Oliai talked about single parents who have multiple kids and how it's impossible to stop, which gives me much greater empathy for different situations. The use of technology and social media and the mental health effects with kids. All this stuff is only going to accelerate and raise stress levels, and the way that diet and nutrition are evolving with seed oils, sugar, and corn syrup.

I just feel like we are going to become more and more susceptible to cancer in our society, and it just causes great fear. But with all that being said, I am so grateful to be supervised by a doctor who really cares so much and is so great at what he does, both academically with his intelligence and also emotionally and through his communication and availability. I think it's rare and also really powerful. Feeling overwhelmed with information, but emotionally optimistic as time goes on.

September 12, 2023

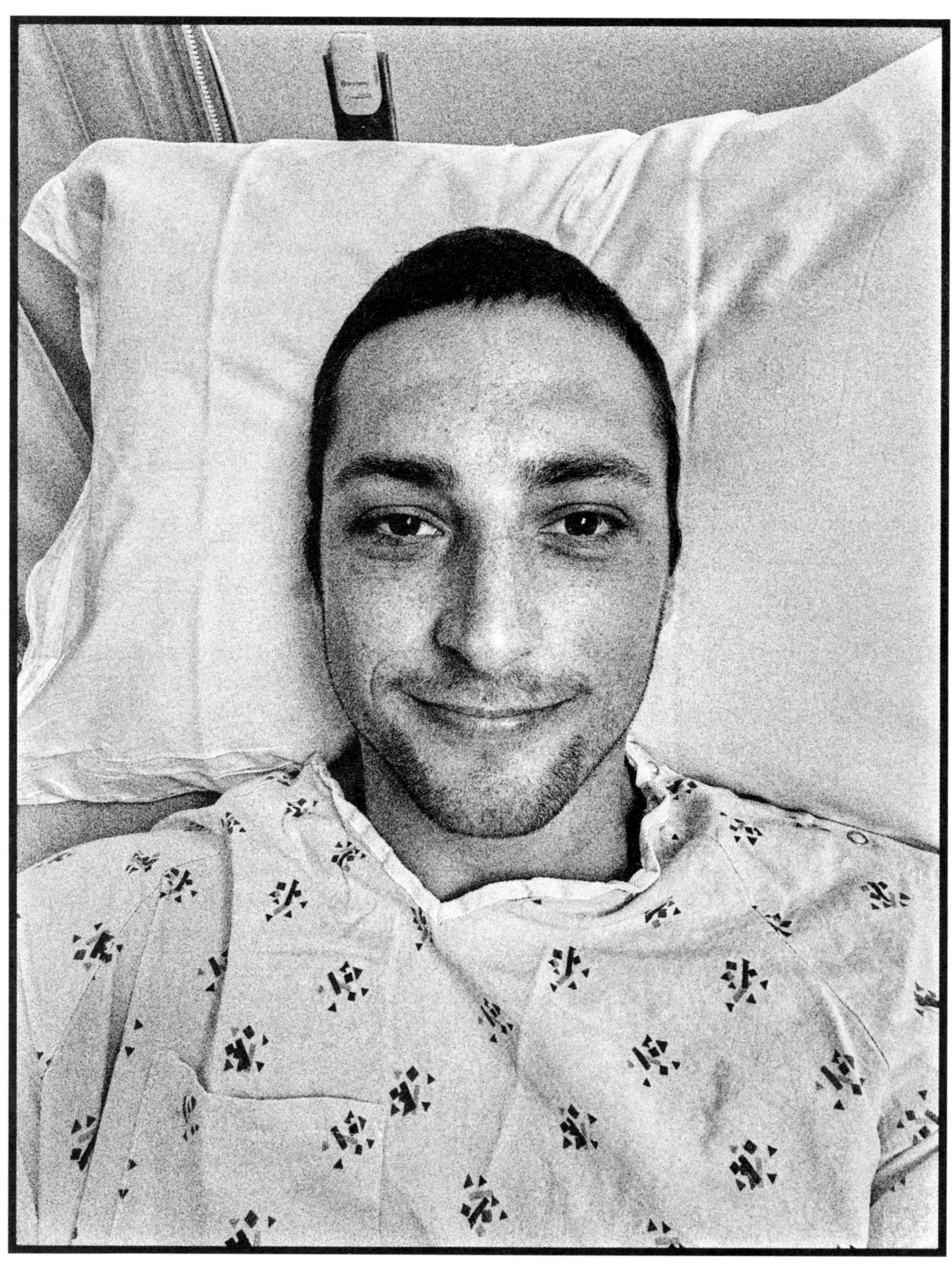

Done with cancer. Still have Crohn's. Colonoscopy.

September 19, 2023

My happy place.

As time goes on and I slowly reacclimate back into my real life, I'm reminded of the stressful patterns that I would create chasing my ambitions. That led me to stress and unhealthy habits. As the mind games slow down and the intruders leave, I'm left with my professional identity, but I'm not sure if I want to keep going back to that space. Thinking about all the people trying to find their own professional identity, constantly chasing a dollar or a purpose. These inner stresses are unproductive. But I'm so happy I got this dog. I see him lying on the floor while I work in the house, constantly staring at me to go outside. He's so happy being in nature, chasing the ball when the waves crash on the sand. Seeing the sunlight. He wakes me up in the morning, kissing my face, so I know to wake up and get out of bed. Not sit too long with depression. He barks when he's cranky from being inside all day. A reminder to me to get outside. I've been watching this show about how to live to 100 on Netflix. It's so powerful to really shut down and think about health. To think about community and physical activity and diet. I wonder if I just forcefully stress myself out too much on purpose. I think I need to stop chasing, and trust the universe is going to do its job for me. There's only so much strategy that can make you move along. I think the truth is in the work. It's in doing the work. But I'm here at the beach. A beautiful day in September. The sun hasn't set yet. The birds are flying in the sky. The water's warm along my ankles. Sam's so happy and curious about everyone and everything. So beautiful. I think that's the definition of true health: seeing the beauty. Just experiencing it. Thank you, Sam.

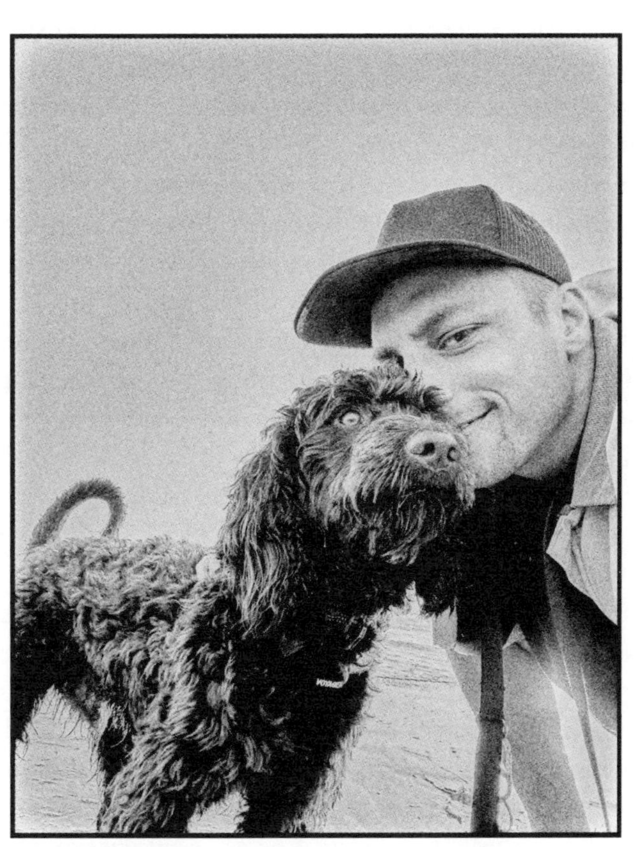

October 18, 2023

Just left therapy. Sitting in my car with the sunlight on me. So much came up this week. So much has been happening the past few weeks. I finally got back to work with my dancers with a goal to bring happiness and positivity to the process. Something that's been absent for a long time. I communicated that I had so much fear in me right now and I wasn't sure why. I was asked to hold on to that and feel what it's like in my body. All I could think about were the beautiful things in life, the natural things like water and fire and sunlight. I'm having a really hard time with time right now. It just doesn't seem to stop, and I feel so uncomfortable in the moments that aren't planned or scheduled, and I have such high expectations to become something more than what I am right now. To make more money or to have more opportunities or to accomplish something more. It seems like this endless chase that won't stop. But I felt the friction and vibrancy of this prior to my diagnosis, and maybe that stress helped contribute to my sickness. Maybe the stress now might equate to a recurrence. Having shows this past weekend was so invigorating. Having audiences come and value and celebrate my work gave me so much inner value. Having the dancers feel so much pride from performing. Everything just felt right. Felt amazing to be with family – both blood and not blood. People that I look up to. People who are supporting us. One of the things I've talked about with my therapist was my fear of discomfort. How I keep thinking about my body being in comfortable positions. How being still is so hard. And she reflected on the fact that maybe stillness is difficult because growing up I was around so much aggression and pain. Hearing my parents fight and argue all the time. Or waiting while I was receiving chemo. That being in moments of stillness is actually really scary for me. That I need to constantly be active or productive. It brought back these weird triggers and memories of a kid. How I used to wait for my mom to pick me up from school all the time, or my dad and stepmom yelling and fighting and me running out of the house. These vast feelings of concrete kept coming up. Just like lying on concrete. It's something that's just never going to be comfortable. And that maybe finding peace is just relaxing. I feel the sunlight. So beautiful.

November 2, 2023

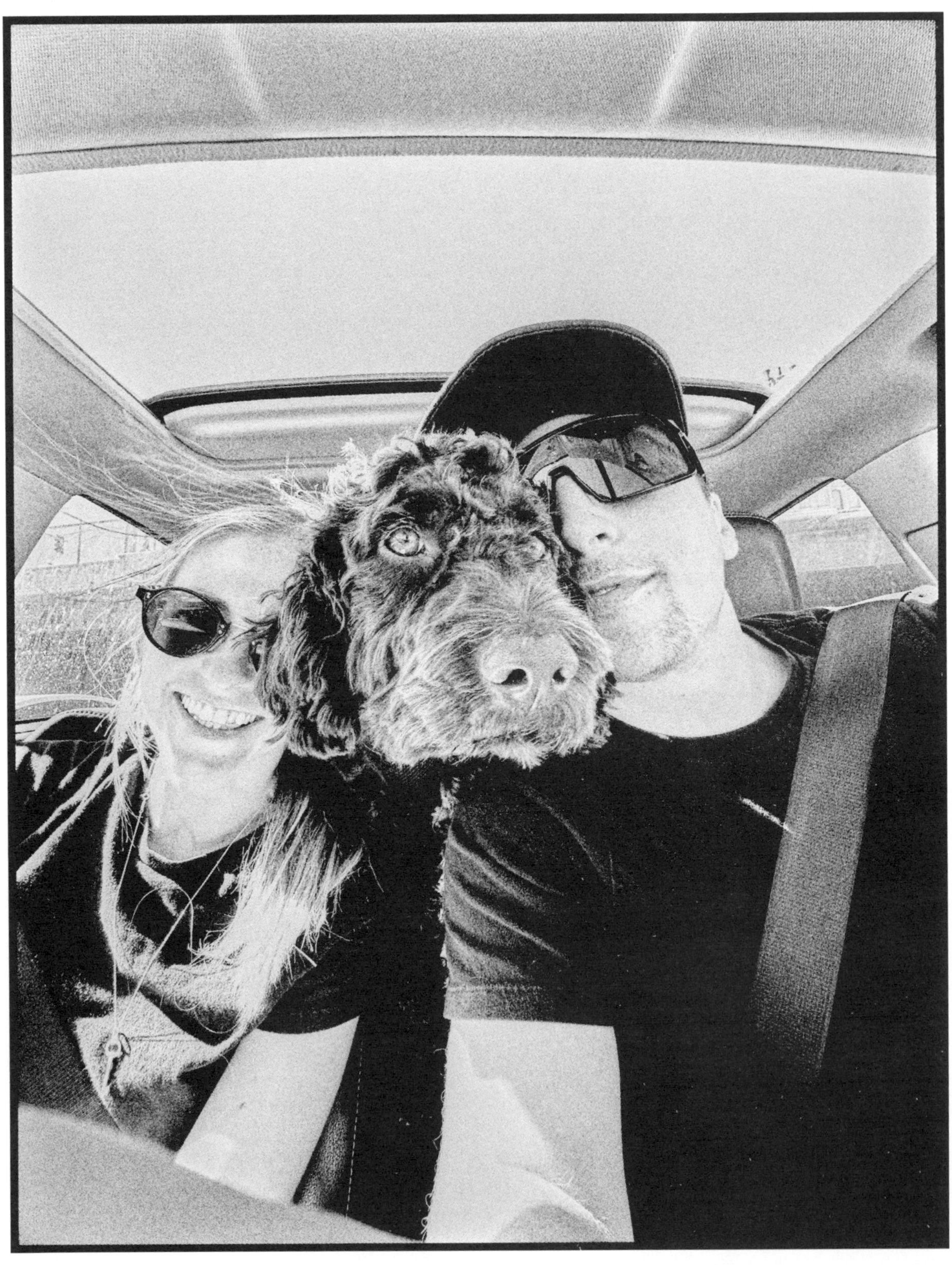

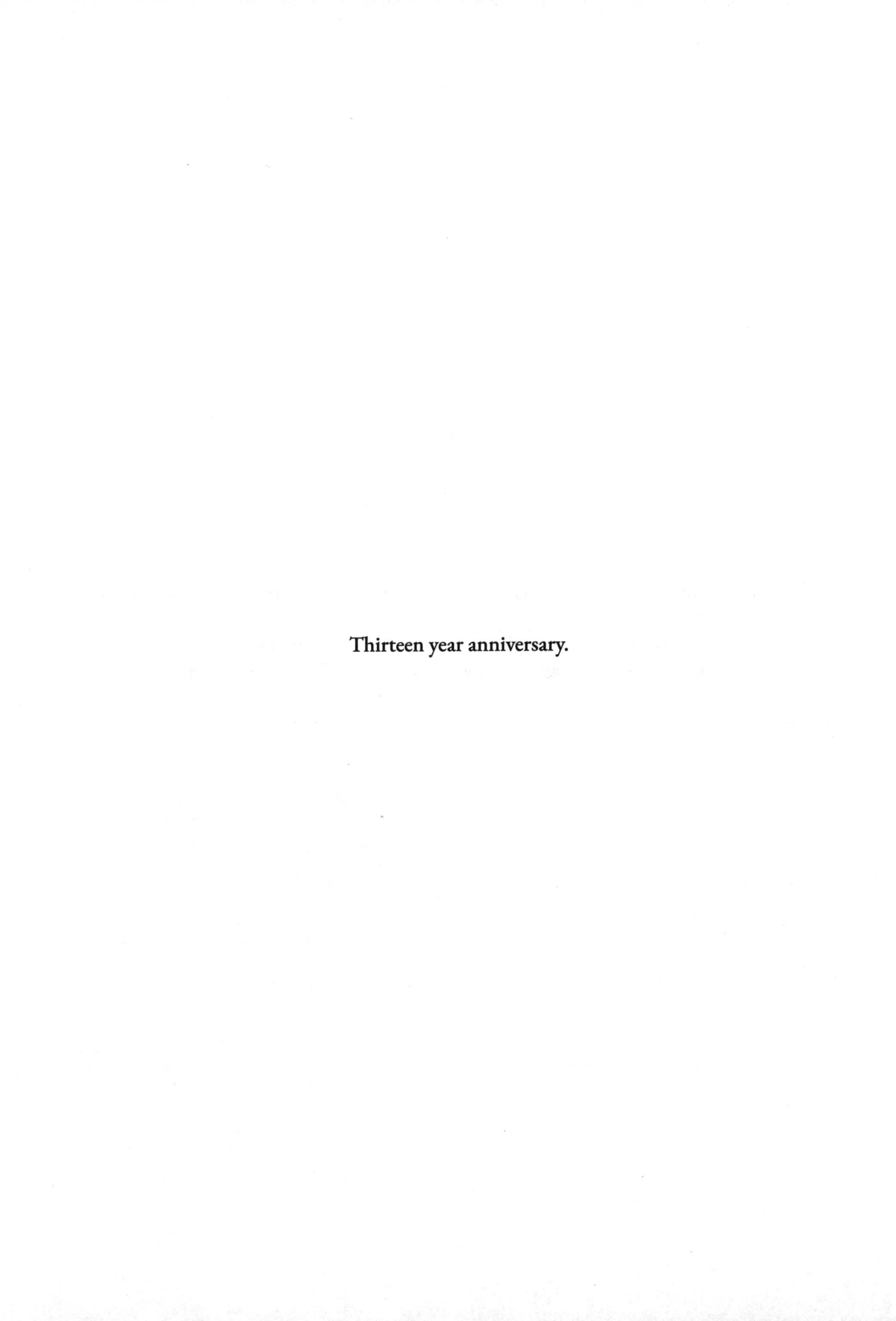

Thirteen year anniversary.

November 17, 2023

One year anniversary from my diagnosis.

We performed tonight in Scottsdale, Arizona.
Exactly one year ago we were performing as well.

Felt full circle. Finding joy.

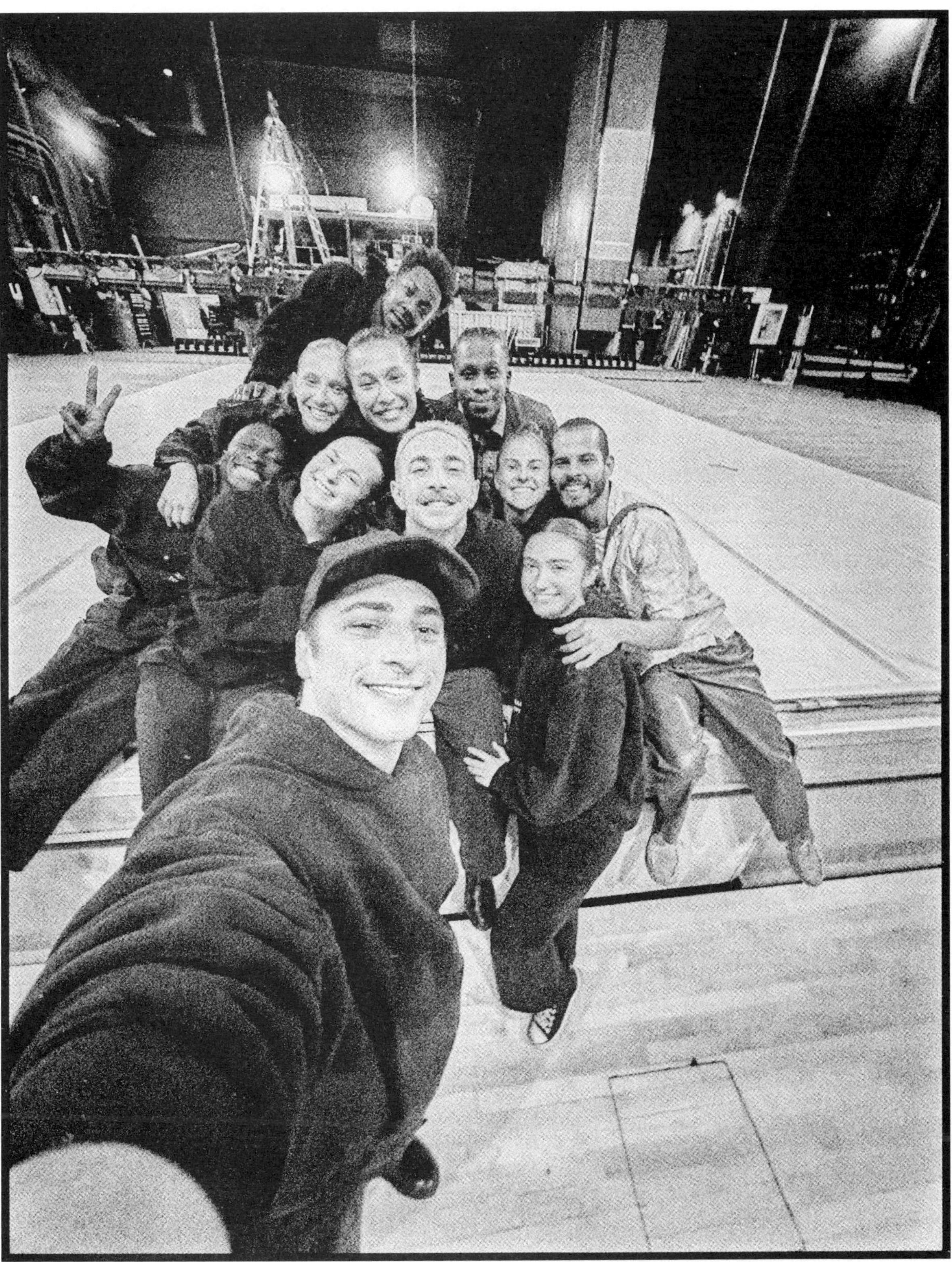

November 23, 2023

A morning ocean dip for Thanksgiving. This time last year I shaved my head and it was my last day before starting chemo. With the two rocks of my life.

A lot to be greateful for.

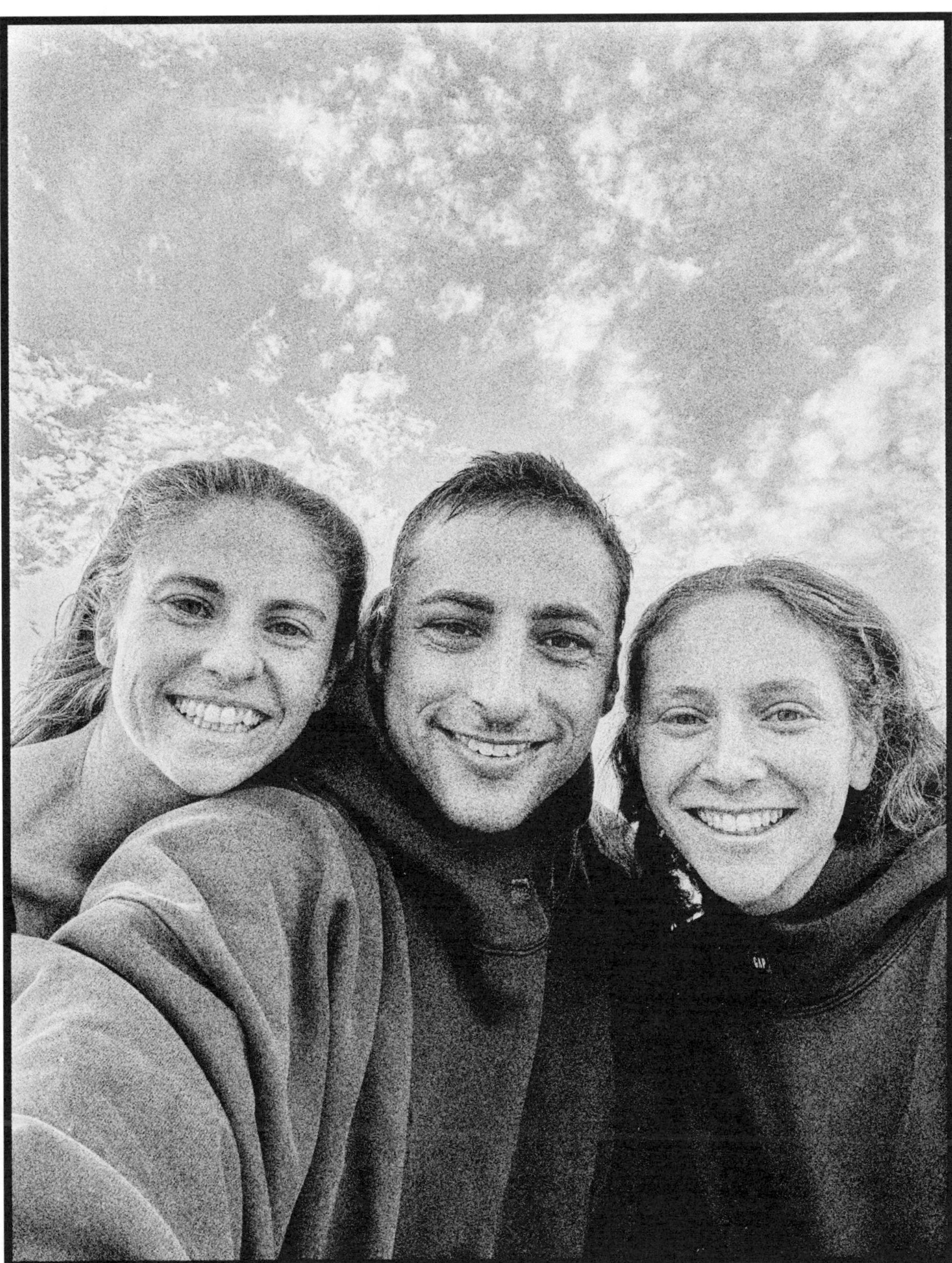
GAP

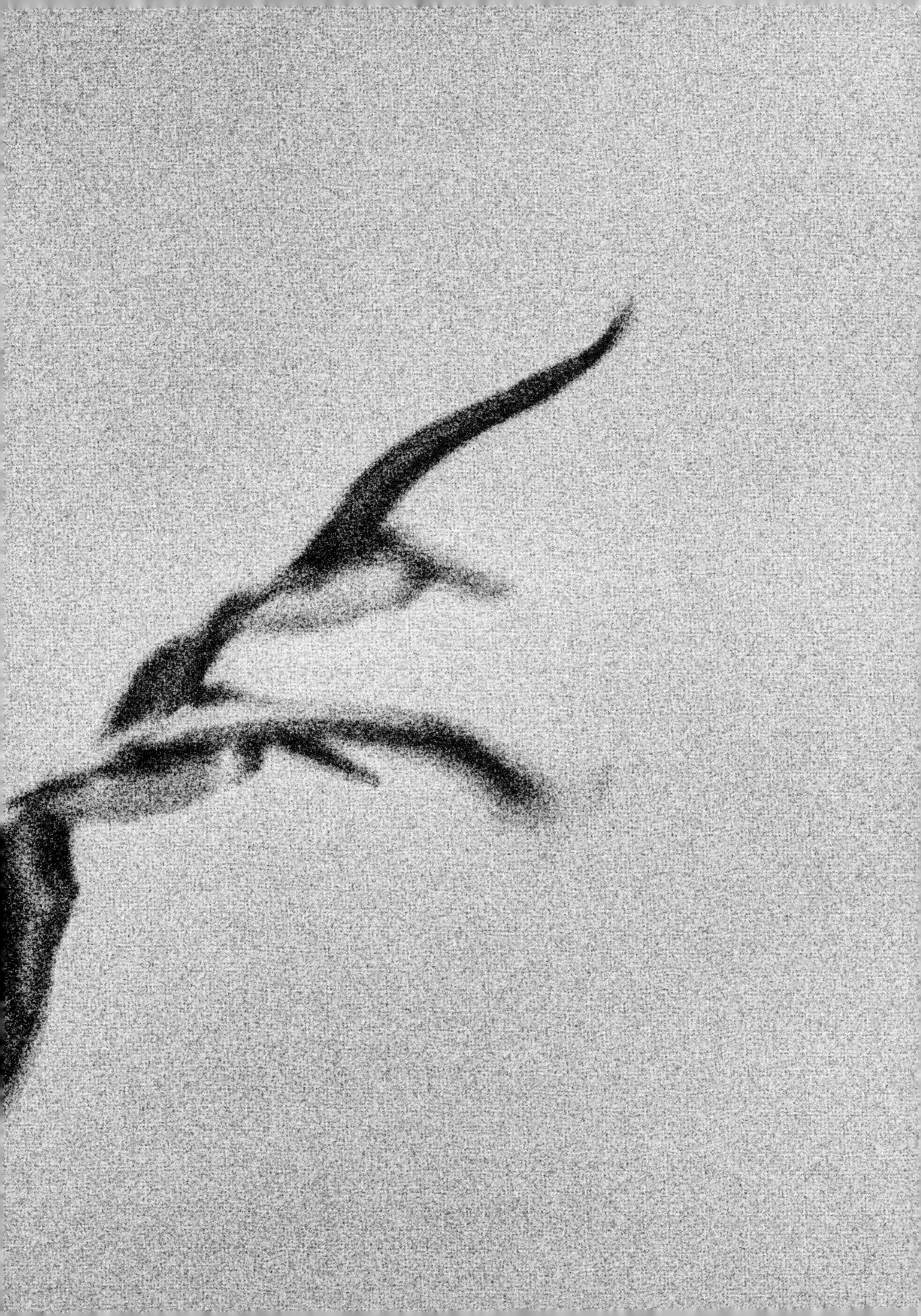

November 26, 2023

My mind has been speaking so loudly recently. But only during the inactivity. When everything stops, the phone is down and I am peaceful with my stillness. There is so much dialogue rushing through me. So many questions. Where am I going? Am I alone? Who is with me? Thoughts about the longevity of my life. How long will it last? Will the cancer come back? Will the suicidal thoughts return? If they return, will I beat them or will they beat me? Comfort and the constant chase for it. Financial stability. Growing my company. Growing our company. Dancers leaving, starting to make their work. Everyone is leaving. Did I do everyone wrong? Is my absence more powerful than my presence? Should I leave? When is the last time I have actually been alone? Thoughts about marriage, about forever. Not knowing what's happening now. Having kids. The responsibility. The hate of exclusivity. We are never really exclusive. But for me, sexually. The desire to continue to be curious. Having kids. Caring for them more than myself. Providing for. Commitment. What if this all stops? What if I need to get a job? What if my job stops working? What if I need to provide for myself and for her and for kids? What if she leaves? How do I support so many? Where is my business? Is it just a hobby?

So I get in the car with Sam. Head south to Mexico. First time with my own thoughts in so long. A conversation the night before about the work. Whose responsibility is it to make the work, then get the income, to come up with the ideas, to grow? Then I wake up to the fact that I am not supportive, that I am not present. Maybe my presence will never make her happy. Self-fulfilled. Powerful. Why can't she take over the world the way I see her taking over it? Why can't she see in herself what I see in her? Why can't she run the business? Why can't she believe in herself? Why does she have so much fear?

I finally arrive in Mexico. I can't remember the last time I have been alone. I can't remember the last time I have been alone. I can't remember the last time I have been alone. Why am I so scared to be alone? How do so many people live alone? Why have I needed to have people next to me constantly? Co-dependent. Coexist. Cohabitate. Judgment. Self-judgment. Separate. Need. A hospital. Nurses. Call button. No visitors. Me and my thoughts. Panic attack. Waves crashing. Too beautiful. Is it too beautiful? Sam needs me. Repeat again. Where are the dancers? How do I make the dance? How do I make it again? Why is my aloneness causing others pain? Why are we all causing others pain? In our success, in our failure, in our presence, in our absence, in our health, in our growth and in our limits. In our togetherness. In time and in space. I noticed I have too much going on in my head. I wonder if I am doing it right? Or, rather, is anyone doing it right? And why is everyone leaving? Have I treated everyone poorly? Is my process bad? Am I too intense? What is intensity? What is doing it right? Or wrong? What is doing it? What is not doing it, and why is that doing too much? Why won't it all stop? Continued thoughts.

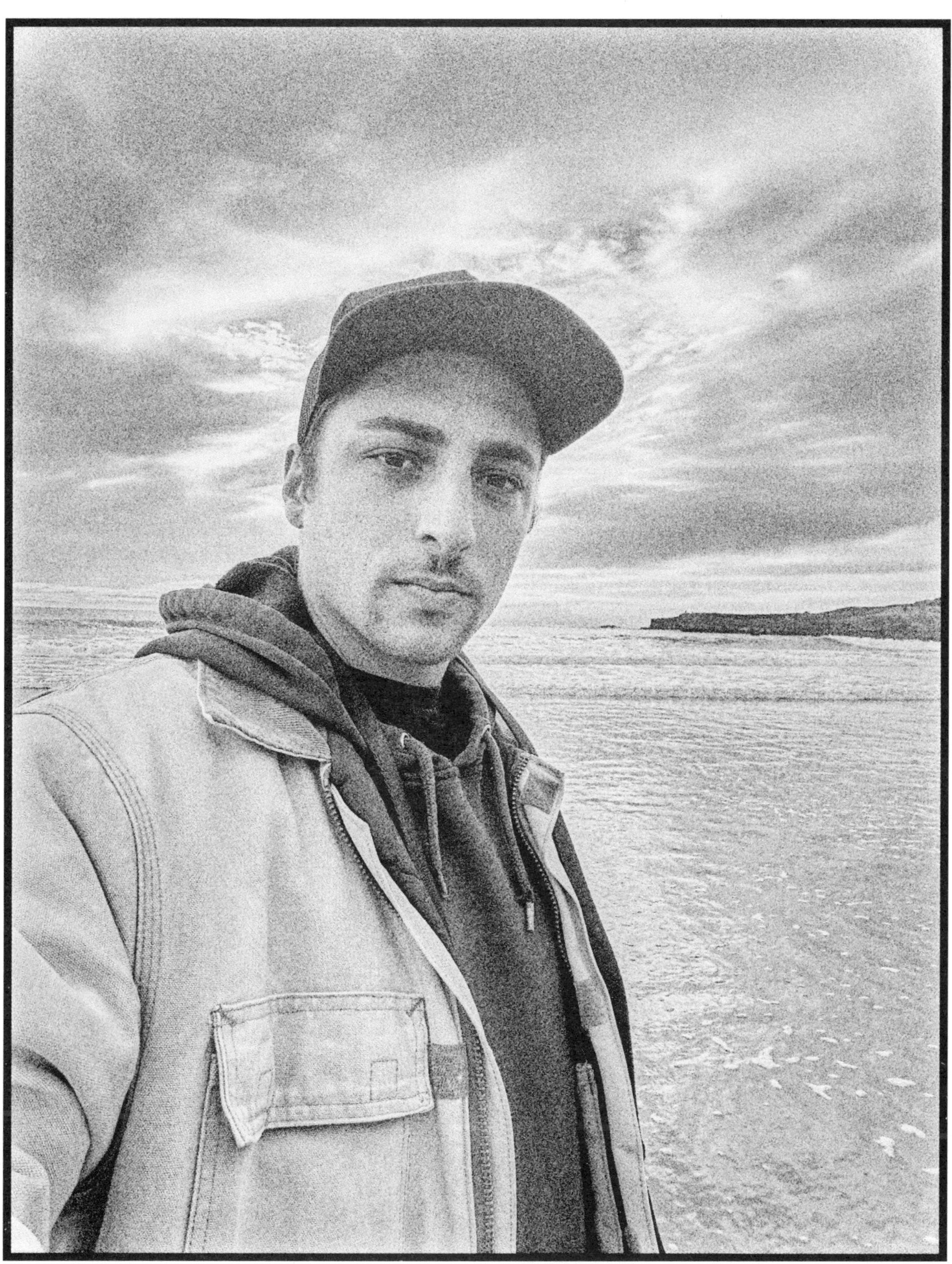

November 27, 2023

Alone in Mexico with Sam.

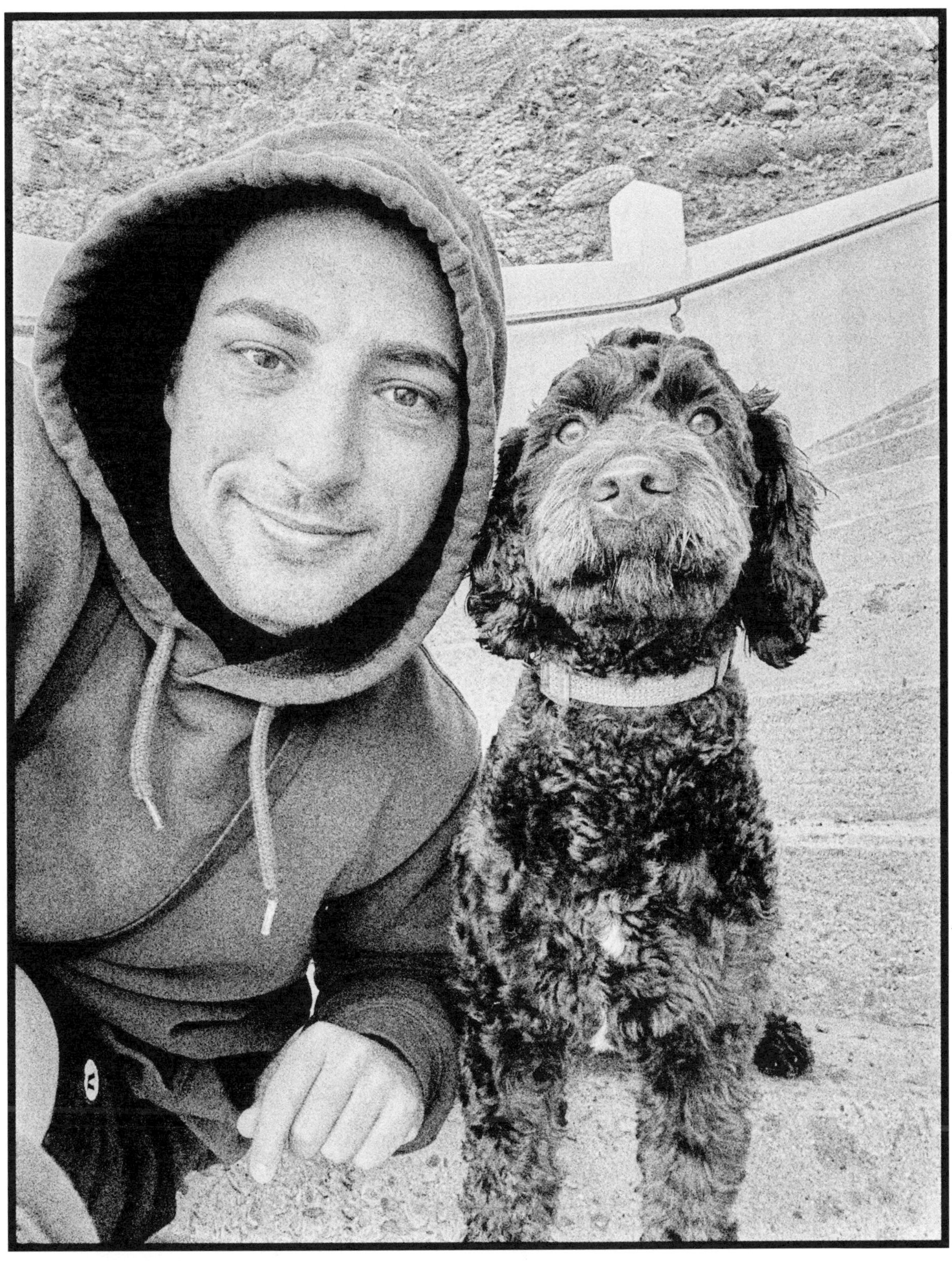

November 27, 2023

Maybe you are doing it all right but just with the wrong perspective. That is the last thing Anibal said to me before the call dropped from a low battery. I then jumped in the ocean. The salt against the body. The fear of drowning. Unsure of what's become of me. What is this constant chase? I want to change the world. I want to grow. I need help. I want to be more than I am. To have a larger vision. To work on bigger projects. I need help. To be the artist. But maybe I am doing it all. Maybe it's all happening the way it's supposed to. It's just my perspective of what's happening is all wrong. I look at the people on the internet with such distraction. How are they doing it? But so many are looking at me in the same way. I just don't want to worry. Inherited worry. Lonesome.

While teaching in Scottsdale, there was a self-conscious student too scared of herself. Too scared to come out and dance. I replied that it is selfish to have this belief because there are too many watching you who you can inspire. Who you can help. The circle of life.

Do I care too much for the people around me? And is that care selfish, for my own benefit? Do I need to be left alone more, in my own thoughts? Is it that I don't want someone else to be lonely so I give them company? "Or am I selfish to make them want to feel good, as it makes me feel better?" Or is it that I don't want to be alone?

Would this all work better if I weren't here? Being alone isn't working. I can't find peace. I can't reason. Or am I just looking at this all wrong?

I talked so often about identity. But I can't be alone. My identity isn't actually in myself, it's in others. It's in my work. It's in the sun. The waves crashing.

How can I actually be in a relationship with someone when I am so lost? So confused. But also so sure.

Sam gets so much joy being at the ocean. Chasing the ball into the water. When I lay around too much, he gets antsy. He wants to do things. I just find myself not being able to. I want to give up.

But maybe it's like a sickness. Like when Sam was sick. We all just waited for time to pass. He sat in complete despair. But time did go on. That's all we are striving for – to find ways for time to go on. To not stop, or rather to not stop time. But it will all continue. The waves crashing, the sun rotating. The dances will keep being made. It will all continue. Isn't that the point? For it all to continue?

Why do we all sit in pain from each other's absence
when we can just be together?
Why can't we all just be together?
Why aren't we together?
Why am I alone?

I'm alone.

November 28, 2023

Forced isolation. Recalibrate. It's learning how to be inactive before I can be active again. Learning how to stare out and do nothing with my thoughts. To focus on my breathing. To understand how to let time go by in peace. To not need anyone to constantly talk to or be around. To share ideas with or know how they are feeling. That's a luxury. But to be in stillness. To think about our ancestors. Watching the clouds for hours at a time as the earth slowly spins. Feel the presence of life. Notice the heartbeat. I need this time. I need to know how to let time go by. Without needing anything. To be anyone. I'm reminded why our society really is such a trap. The perception we have of ourselves when watching each other. The real gift is just being alone. All we really are is alone. There are so many in my life I can call. And I do. They all share their fulfillment in being alone too. That those moments are rare but they are so rewarding.

It has been about a year since my diagnosis. Since I was throwing up. Since I shaved my head. Since the hospital. It's been a year since everyone started to worry and show up. Since I got daily texts and calls asking if I was OK. Since the chemo started destroying my mind. Since I left the old me. The guy with the long hair. The guy constantly chasing for more. Always wanting to be bigger, to have more. To make more money. There was so much time in that hospital room where I was forced to sit with my thoughts. To allow time to pass. So much was entering my mind. I dreamed I was flying like a bird. Escaping this reality. I felt on top of the world. Like the ideas I had were more important than anything out there. Like the stories I wanted to tell and the visuals I saw needed to be created and told. But then time passes. You can't remember those ideas as clearly. The inspiration fades to make them come to life. People stop checking in on you, asking if you are OK. They are still there. But it's not as frequent. They stop checking in on the people that are taking care of you. What you shared about current pains or feelings don't seem as important to share anymore. Maybe it's best not to share anything. Constantly caught in a trap if I am sharing too much or not enough. Or not listening enough. As time goes on, I try to settle back to normal life. The life where everyone is busy. Where their phone is the addiction. The constant comparison to everyone else's perfect life and creative work. The one where people are still buying food that causes cancer. The one that's moving so fast that I am blind to my speed. Then I am running with no energy, no endurance, just to keep up. When I am still, no one is around teaching me how to be still. How to stop. I am just running out of breath.

This little moment away is peaceful. Full of fear but powerful. It's nice to be with Sam. A reminder to have routine. To eat. To get outside, walk on the beach. Play. Feel the sun. Observe. Not be on technology. He barks when he needs something. Food, time to go outside to use the bathroom. It's powerful when he barks just to have attention. Just to be seen and cuddled. As I crave this time of isolation, he never leaves my sight. I move through the space and he is always right next to me.

He doesn't want to be alone either.

Even going up and down the stairs, he is on the same step as me. Always looking at me.

The point of coming down here to Mexico was to conquer a fear. I got on a plane to conquer a fear. This whole time experiencing mental health and trauma, I have visualized with great pain anything I was scared of. But as time goes on, I get through it. It all gets easier. It all gets more comfortable, even the things I found uncomfortable. Sitting instead of lying down. Being alone. Being in stillness. Not knowing what to do. Therapy is to be credited. Talking to a therapist. Sharing the problems. Getting new insights. Getting new tools. Talking to friends. Knowing so many are going through what you are or have been through, just in different forms. In different accounts. Plant-based therapy. Psilocybin. It has removed the visitors, the bad thoughts. The thoughts that make me want to die. Alternative medicine. Western medicine is what got me sick in the first place. The FDA, the government, bureaucracy, they are the ones poisoning us. It's not to say that they aren't good people. That they do save lives. But we need to consider plant-based medicine too. Eastern and holistic philosophies. We need to talk about healing and health more openly. We need to force ourselves to be alone. To be in nature without technology. To be in company with others. With no agenda. Just to learn how to really coexist.

Learning inactivity is a tool. Learning how not to distract yourself with artificial busyness but to really sit in productivity with stillness is a talent I think few possess.

It's time to watch

the clouds move.

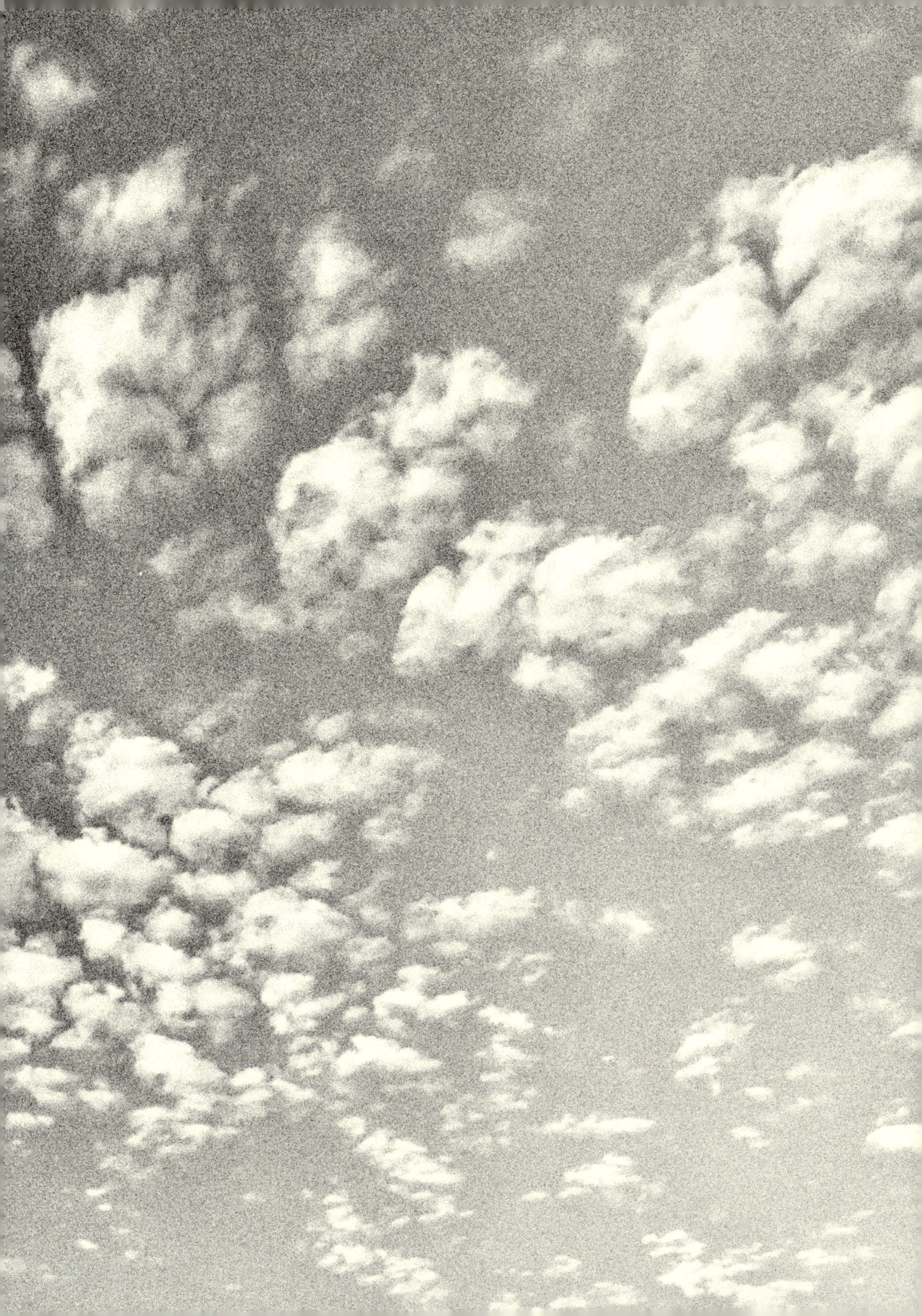

November 29, 2023

Salt water against the face. This journey stops here. Last entry for now. The sun rises. Time with Sam. Thank you for this opportunity, for listening.

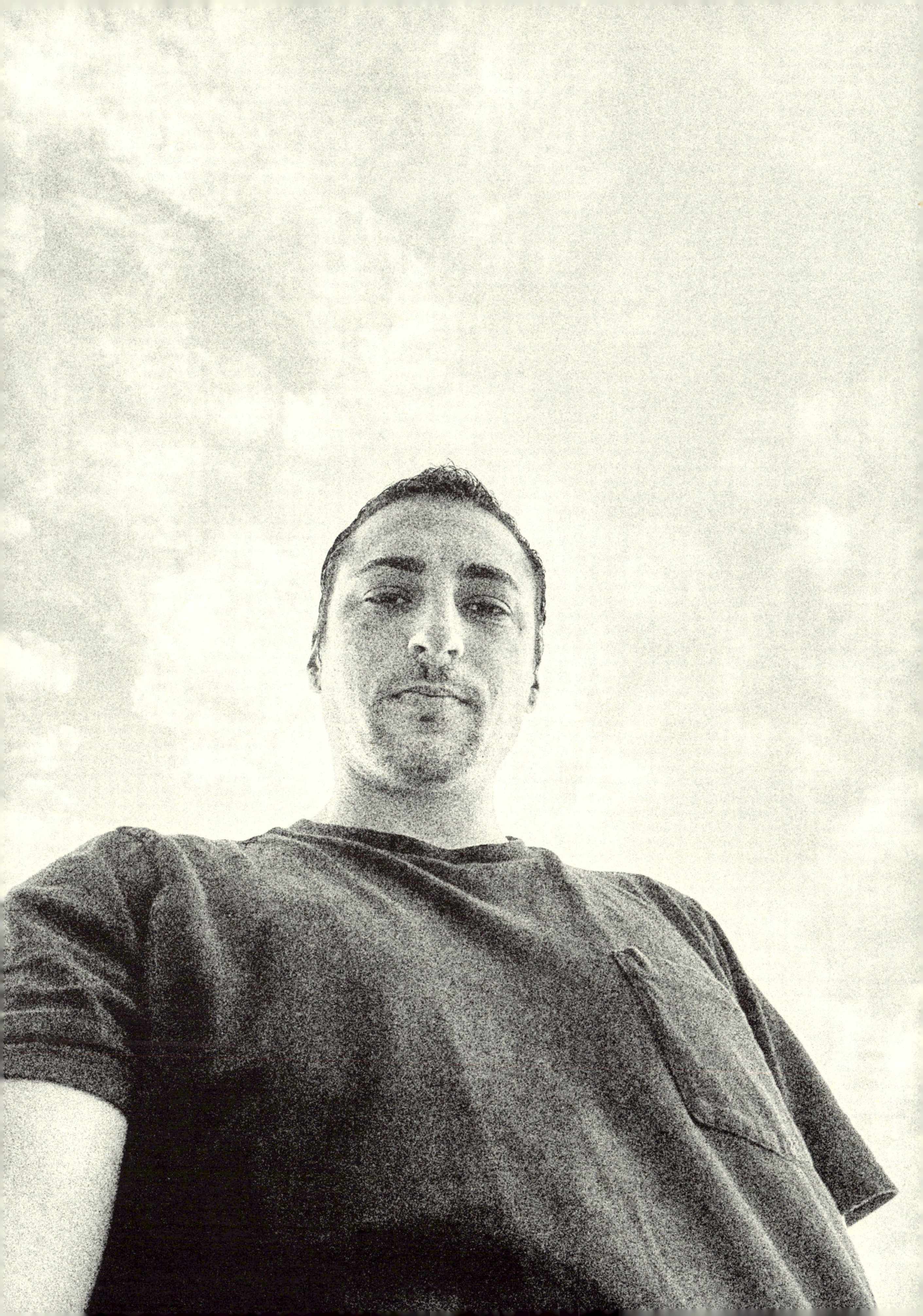

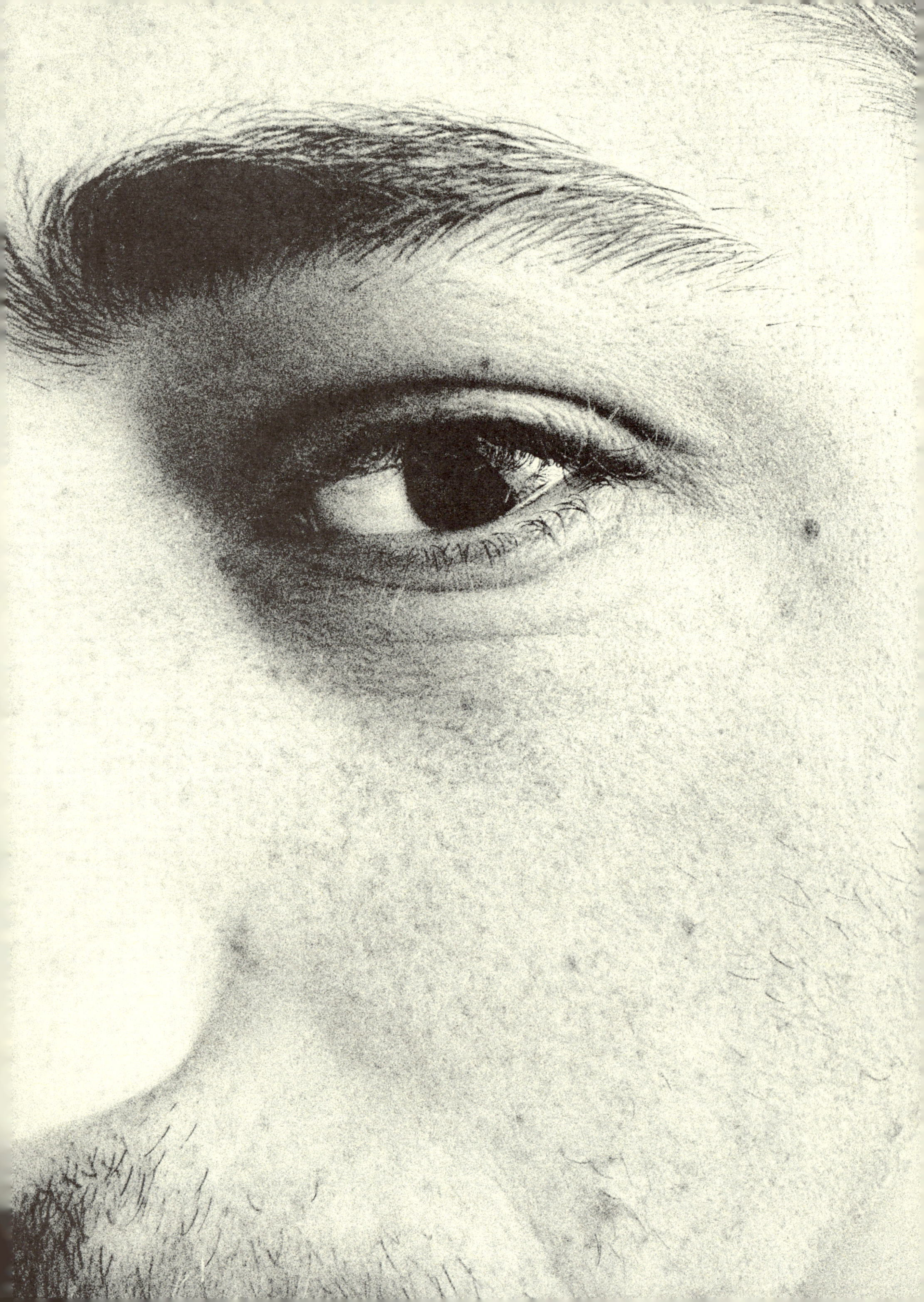

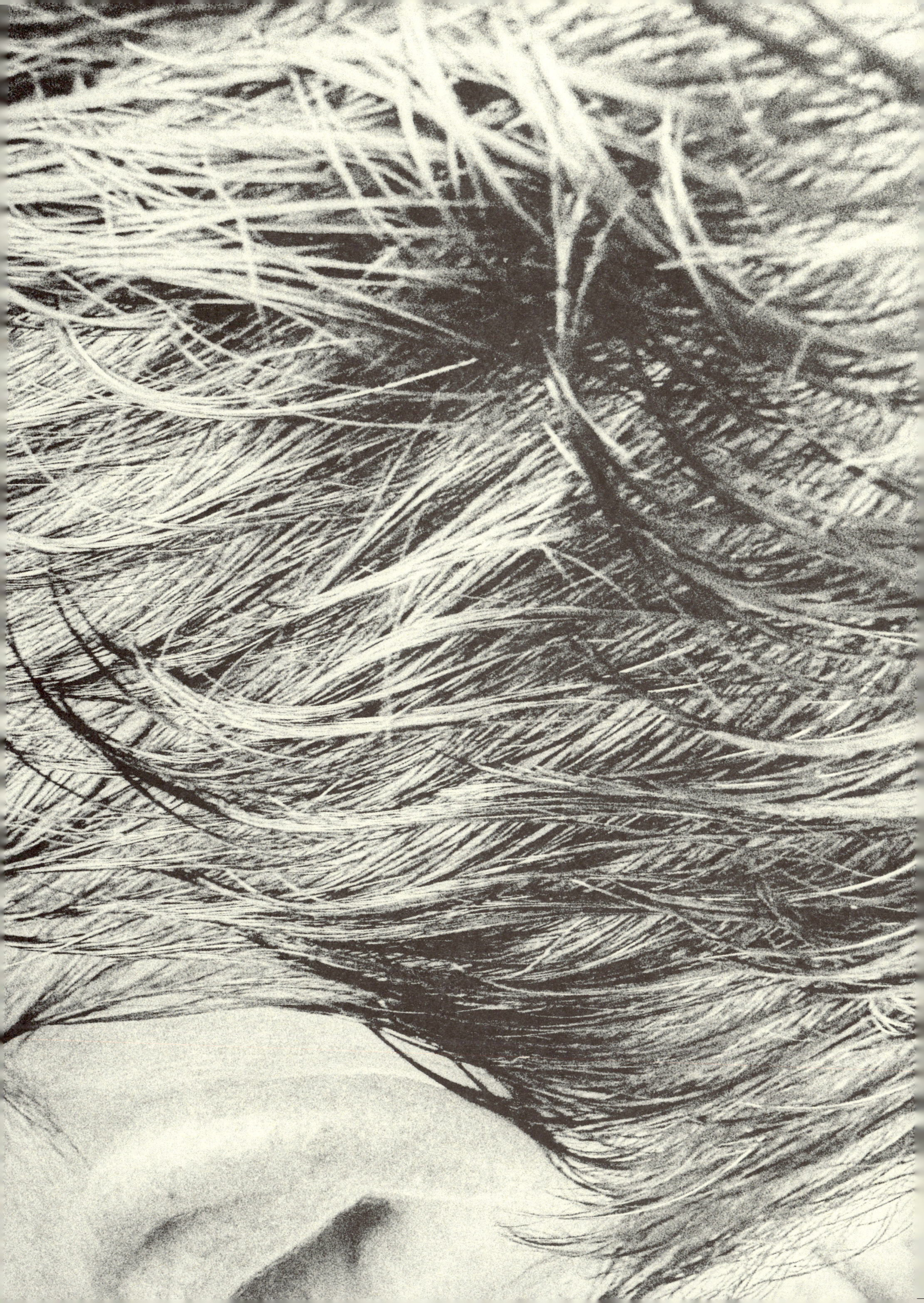

I look out to the sea of darkness.

The waves crash. The white caps continue to break toward the shore. There's no light around except for artificial ones and the boats far away. Sam stares out with curiosity, standing on the ledge. I've just spent the last few hours reading through this journal – every entry since my diagnosis. I feel so grateful that I've documented everything. I'm not sure who will read this or if it will ever be shared, but I'm so lucky that I documented every version of me and where I was in the time my illness was going on. There are so many lessons here about visualizing your health, about finding gratitude in the worst situations, about trying to find a finish line that will actually never appear. About understanding the significance of the real-life values of family and friends and support. That the universe will always show up. That business is just part of being an artist. And being an artist is just part of life. Just creating the pathway of where we think we're going, that stillness is an activity. That we need stillness and isolation to recalibrate, to understand who we are. That bad habits of busyness can cause stress to the body and to the mind – that causes great illness. That the universe is really planning everything for you, and of your need to trust it. I went down to Mexico to chase a fear. That made me conclude this journal. As I've tried to re-enter normal life, I may have become a burden to myself, therefore becoming a burden to those around me. I was given the ability to be so vulnerable. During the process of my illness. And I have to learn how to reduce my vulnerability or my internal sharings with those around me so I don't remain a burden to them. In this past year, I've taken away so much. The hospital room became something so familiar. Something so comfortable. I found it so difficult to leave it.

And I experienced real PTSD and trauma, and still continue to. I've had great certainty with my life and where I should go and the work I need to do. And I've lost all of that as well. I can't remember what those things are anymore, but I'm sure I'll find them again. I'll find that purpose. I was inspired to take self-portraits and to journal because of what the late Ezra Caldwell did through his cancer battle that he lost. As well as through Mallory Smith's cystic fibrosis battle that she lost. If one person reads this or many people and it makes an impact, I think it will all be worth it. I think that's what our responsibility as artists anyway is – to just share what we are going through. To find relatability to others so that they can go through it as well and know that everything will be OK. Or that it's normal to go through a hard time. I really want to thank everyone for helping me get through this time. Grateful to have a new dog because of it. To have such deeper friendships and relationships with people. To have a different understanding of my health. To have such deep fear of life, but know I'll conquer that fear. I have a great debt to both Jill and Emma for helping me through this time. For living with me, staying in the hospital, switching off, and being such a strong support system in business and in my life. Thank you to Emma for being there and helping me create the work. And thank you to you, my love, with all the challenges this year has brought you and for supporting me. As lost as I've become, I know that you've become lost too. I know how fatigued you are from lifting so much weight of my stress and pain. I can never repay you for all the time you've given me and supported me for. I thank you for writing all these journal entries, and I know it's become too much for you, which is why this will be the last one. Thank you for writing. And I love you. Thanks for listening.

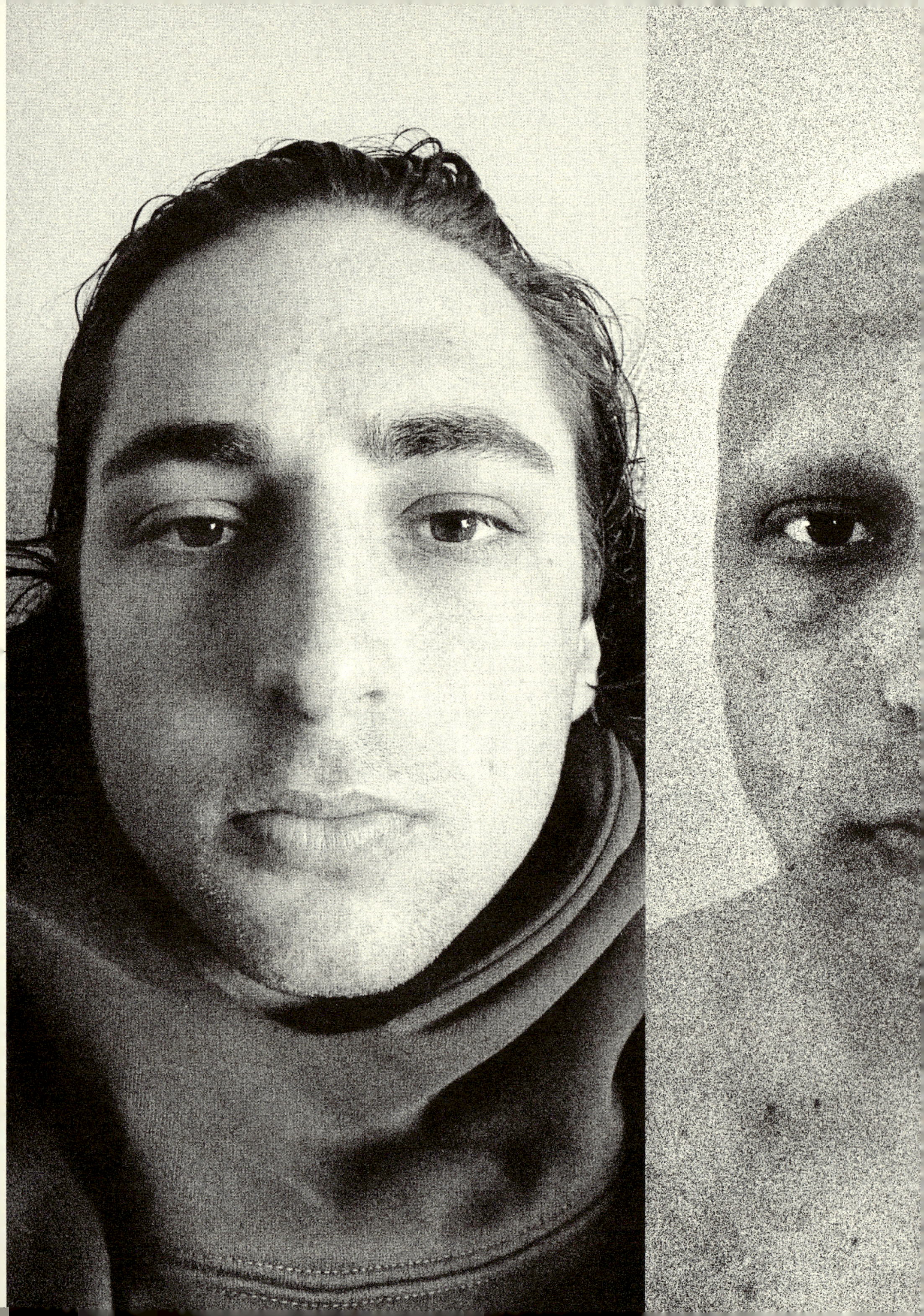

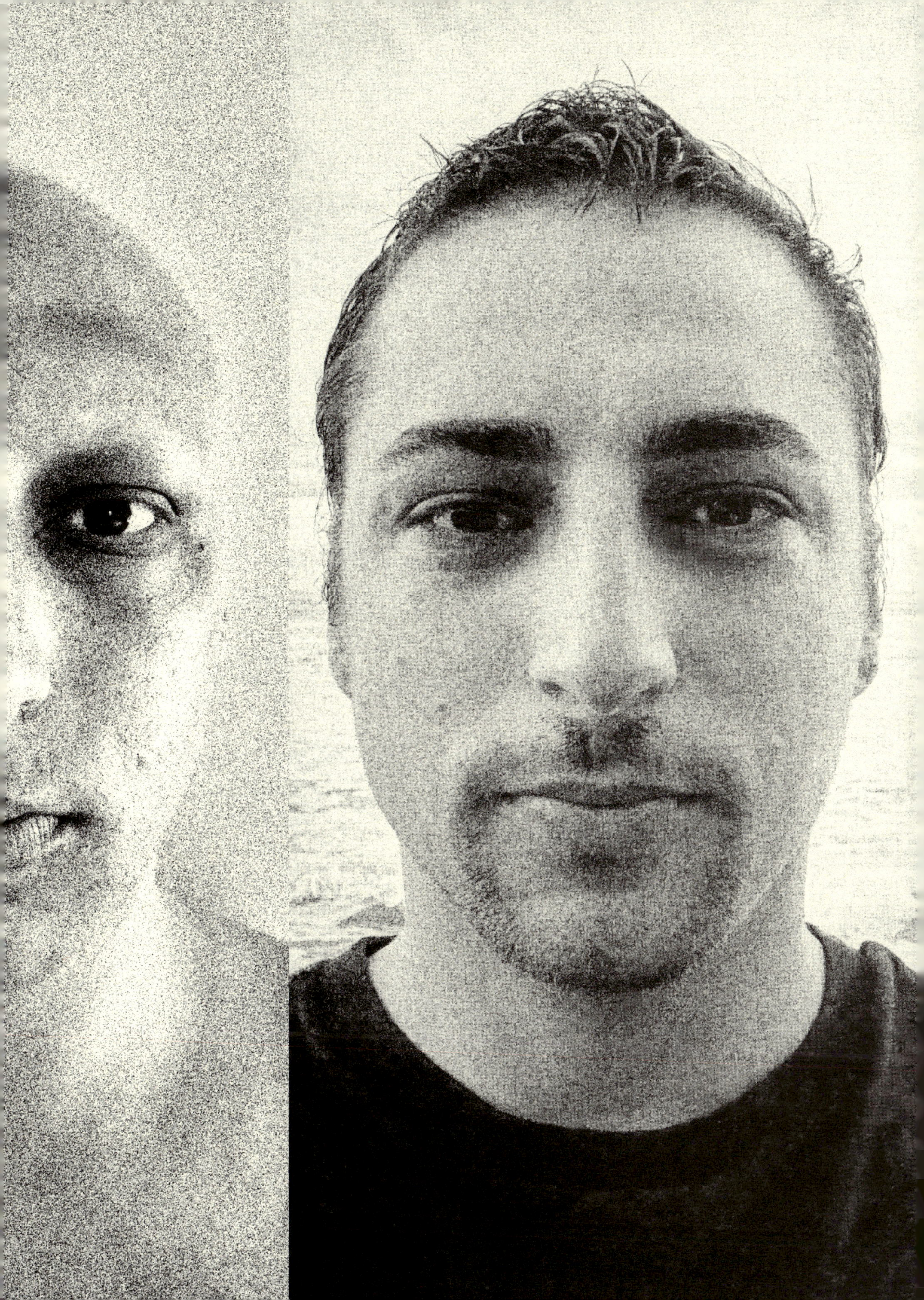

The Guest House.

This being human is a guest house.
Every morning a new arrival.

A joy, a depression, a meanness,
some momentary awareness comes
as an unexpected visitor.

Welcome and entertain them all!
Even if they are a crowd of sorrows,
who violently sweep your house
empty of its furniture,
still, treat each guest honorably.
He may be clearing you out
for some new delight.

The dark through, the shame, the malice.
meet them at the door laughing,
and invite them in.

Be grateful for whoever comes,
because each has been sent
as a guide from beyond.

Rumi

CLOSING

We all are born and die many times. It's most powerful when we are aware of it. Sometimes we die and are rebirthed in the same lifetime or in the same body. And others in new eras or forms.

July 25, 2024

The start of a meditation. Tapping in, quieting, listening. I appear in the hospital. Surgical light. Surgery room. But I'm on the table this time. The doctor's hovering over me. I thought maybe it was a past life, but no, it's this one. Heart surgery. My body exposed. Cut open. They are peering in, trying to solve the problem. It's not looking good. I cut in and out of this scene like a movie, and when I settle back in it's happening. My death. I'm dying. But it's OK. I reassure myself. Closing in. That's it. My body is moved to another table, but I don't see them place it there. I see it there, but I'm not there. That version is gone. My new spirit is here. All these people are here now, together. We are meant to be here.

I have to emerge and find this new version. It's his story, but it's also mine. We have always been in it together. So many hearts and lives connected along the way. We are all meant to live, experience, hold, let go, and be. We are connected. And we are separate. A balance. We are both at a new start now.

I'm grateful I could witness and experience us both moving on from past versions of ourselves and into a rebirth. It was my honor to document your story and be with you every step of the way. I'm so grateful you are on the other side. Cancer free. Healthy. A new outlook on life. A deeper connection to people around you and to your art. A focus on healing. A reminder of what is truly important in this precious life we are given.

Thank you for sharing your story, my love.

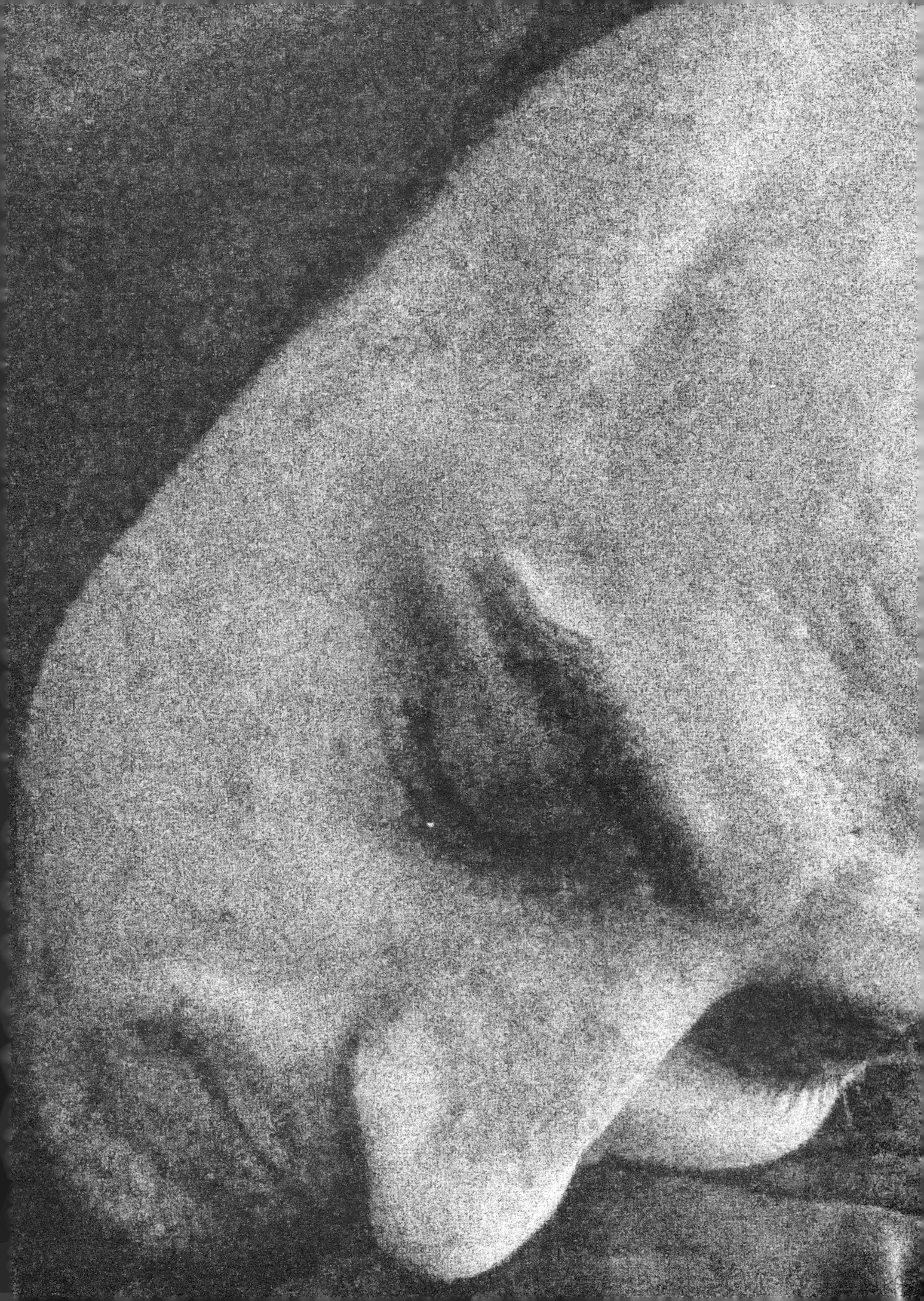

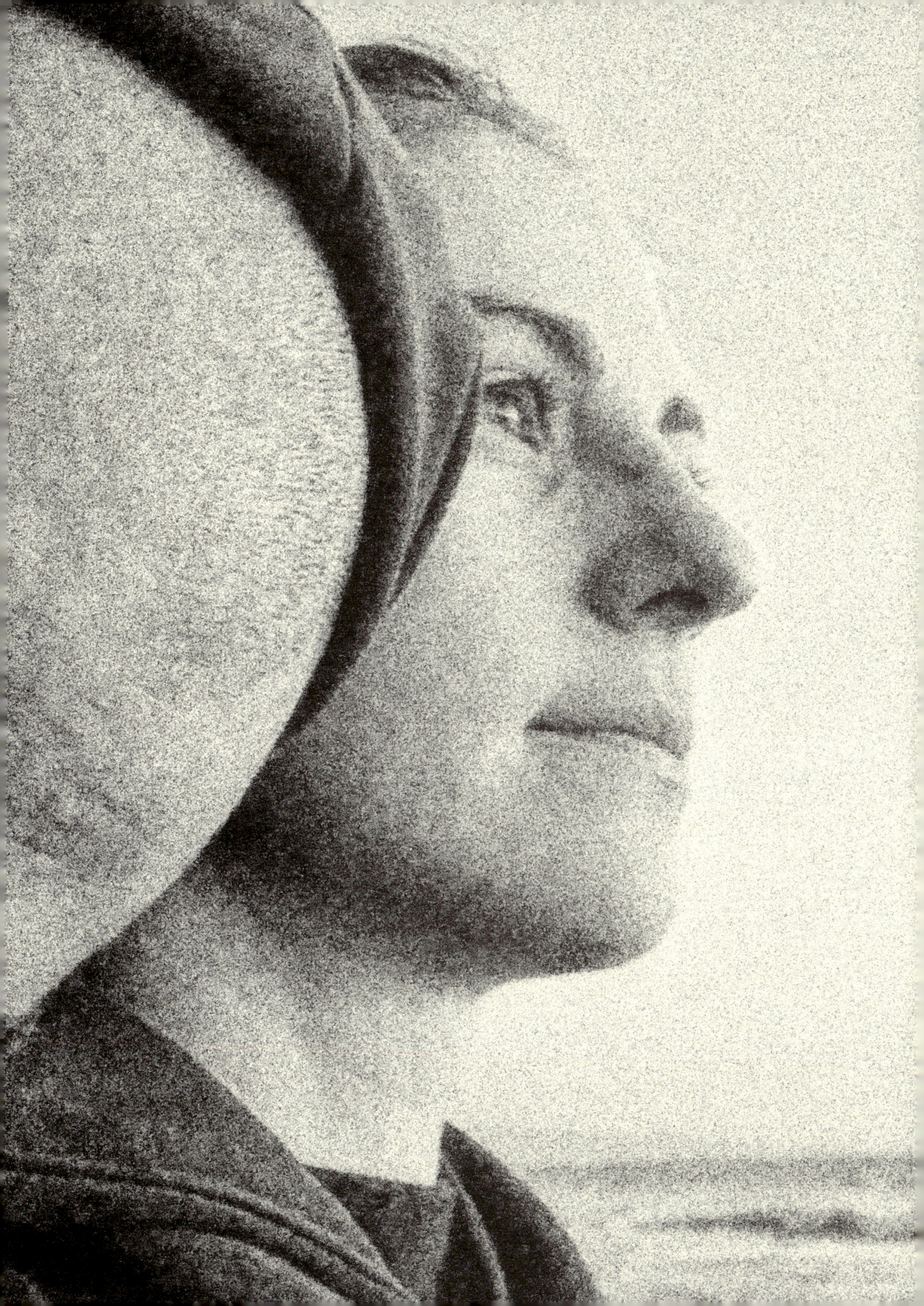

I want to give an acknowledgement to my mother, father, Danielle, Ronnie, Frank, Jonathan, Liza, Noah, Liam, Arlene, Ryan and Laura, Katelyn, Suzy and Stephen, Beth and Jason, Ron, Jodi, Shari, Jayne, Rob and Tara, Ryan, Robbie, Haley and Indy, Helene and Rich, Maria Mancuso, Ivan Cash, Robert Schulman, Ken Robin, Sequoyah, Daniel and Arabella Ezralow, Alex Bartlett, Nathan Birnbaum, Robert Bernstein, Donald Byrd, Kanye West, Glen Hansard, Will Adashek, David Tytler, Jessica Young, Nova, Steve Hackman, Renee Stewart, Tal Barnston, Anibal and Pilar Sandoval, Mila and Lucas, Lamonte Goode, Nic Walton, Antonio Sánchez, Yseult, Imogen Heap, Jordyn Gatti, Tessa Matthias, Simony Monteiro, Michele Denegri, Tanu Muino, Nikita Kuzmenko, Lewis Segal, Heather Gerlach, Brigitte and Gianna D'Annibale, Joshua Geyer, Marshall Birnbaum, Danny Errico, Jack Goodwin, Diane Shader Smith, Ronit Stone, Chelsey D'adesky, McCall Bronson, Ashley Navid, Daphna Nazarian, Natasha Mossanen Rahban, Rauf Yasit, Francisco Cruz, Peter Walker, Emily Kikta, Sean Apel, Mike Tyus, Joy Brown, Joanne Wiles, Danny Robinson, Marissa Lepor, Amy and Harold Masor, Dr. Shirley Impellizzeri, Dr. Gregory Flaxman, Eugene Cash, my extraordinary company of dancers, collaborators and board, extended family and close friends who have gotten me through, and the unbelievable doctors, nurses and caretakers at UCLA Health.

To Dr Caspian Oliai, Dr Mary Kwaan, and Dr Jenny Sauk for saving my life.

To my friends along the journey, Jade Christianne, Raffaella Dobles and Madlen Mossanen who we have lost to cancer. And my grandfather Gil Jacobson.

And a very special acknowledgment to Jill, Emma, and Sam for being directly by my side the entire time.

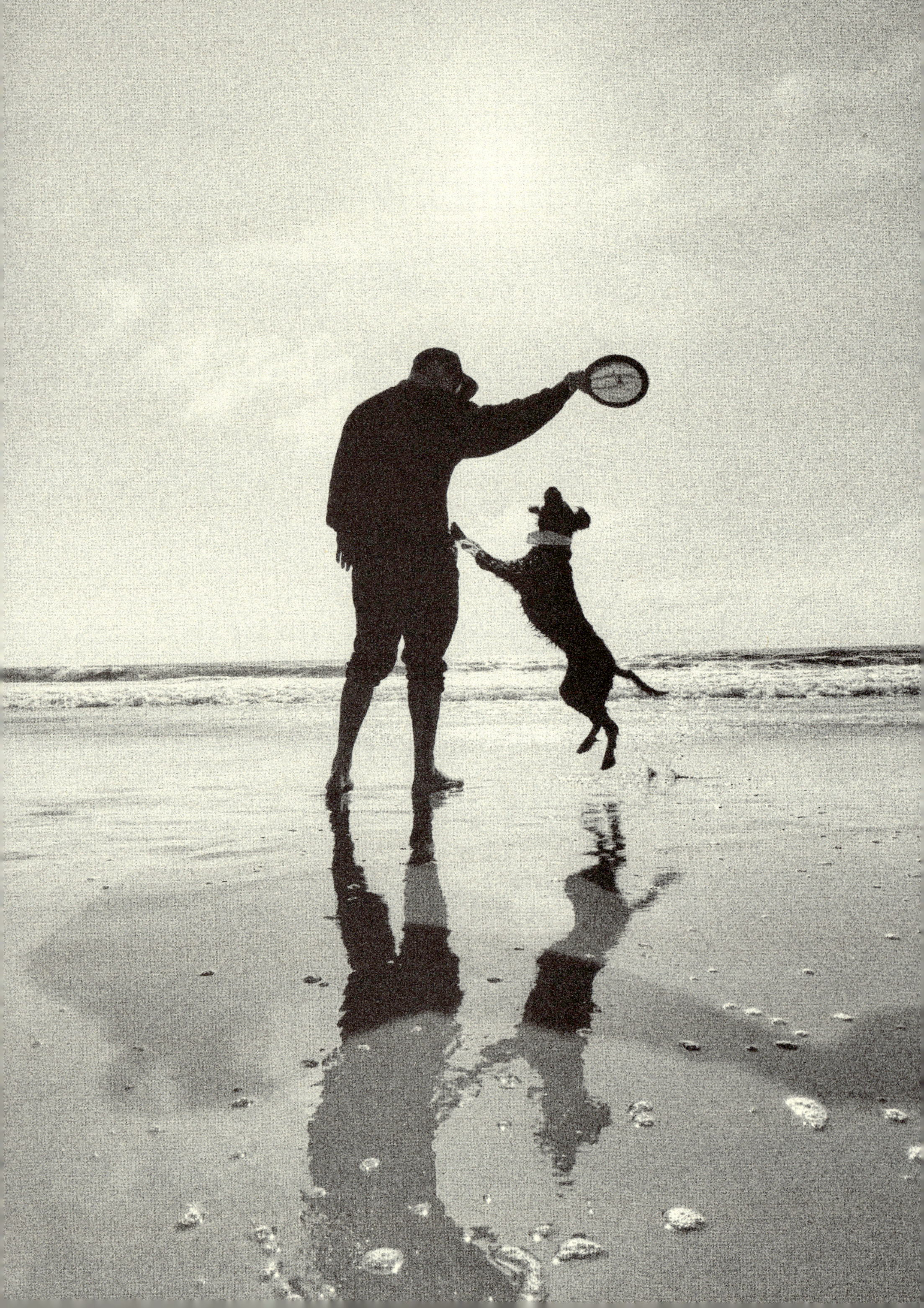

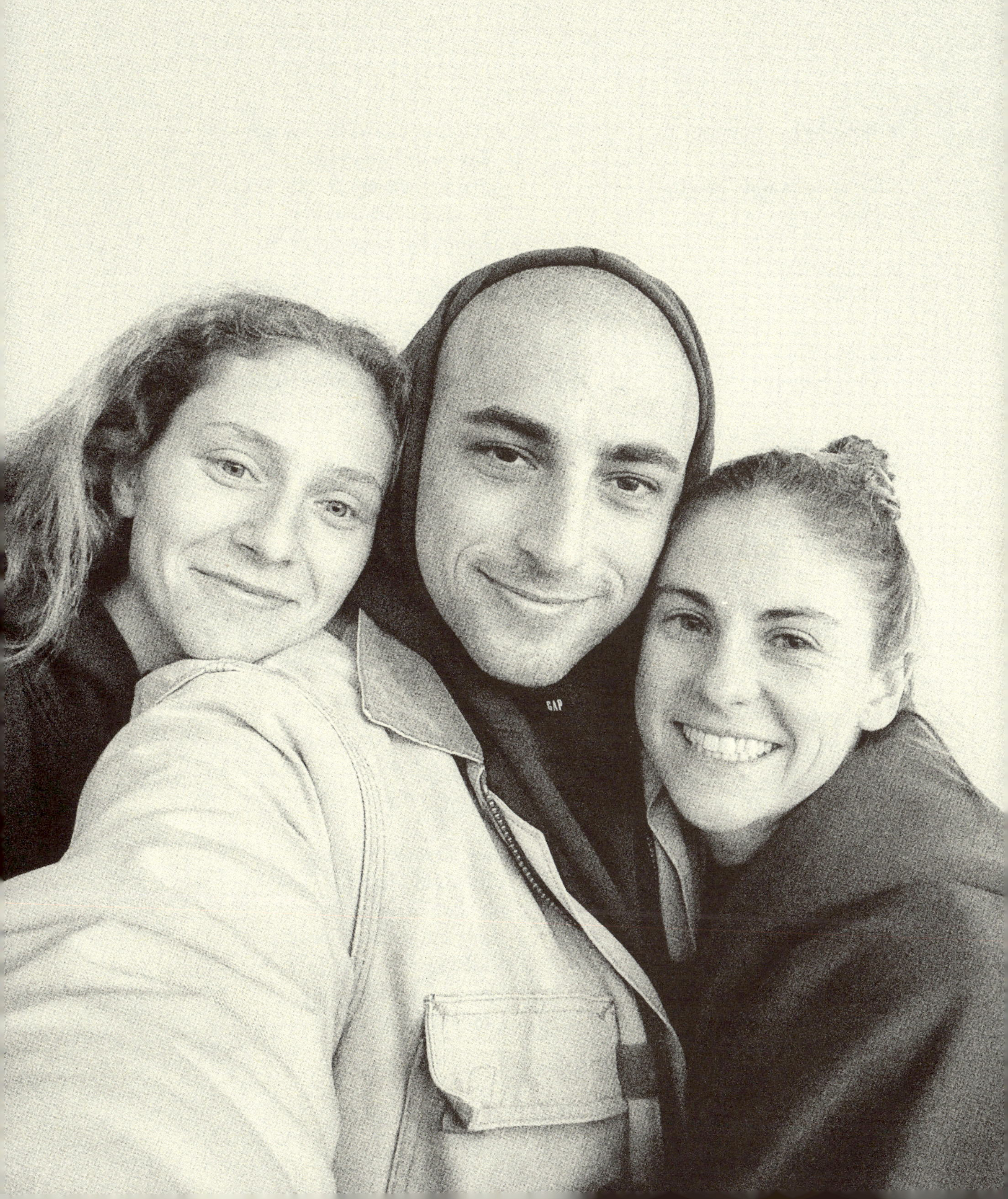
GAP

CEMENTED BEAUTY
A Cancer Story

A book by Jacob Jonas

Photographs and Texts by
Jacob Jonas

As dictated to
Jill Wilson

Foreword by
Glen Hansard

Creative Direction &
Additional Photography
Emma Rosenzweig-Bock

Design Director Erika Udvardi
Production Designer Emma Singleton
Photo Editor Ron Mey
Copy-Editor and Proofreader
Rich Cutler, Helius

This book was typeset in
EB Garamond

Co-Published by
Jacob Jonas The Company
jacobjonas.org

SpineSun, LLC,
spinesun.com

Atelier Éditions
atelier-editions.com

For Jacob Jonas The Company
Director: Jacob Jonas
Executive Producer: Jill Wilson
Producer/Art Director:
Emma Rosenzweig-Bock

For Atelier Éditions
Publisher: Pascale Georgiev
Editorial Assistant: Agnes Perotto-Wills

First Edition of 1,000
Printed in Mexico
on 100% ecological paper
from sustainable forests
ISBN 978-1-954957-13-8
Special Edition of 200
ISBN 978-1-954957-14-5